ANNALS OF
THE NEW YORK ACADEMY
OF SCIENCES

Volume 842

EDITORIAL STAFF

Executive Editor
BILL BOLAND

Managing Editor
JUSTINE CULLINAN

Associate Editor
STEVEN E. BOHALL

New York Academy of Sciences
2 East 63rd Street
New York, New York 10021

NEW YORK ACADEMY OF SCIENCES
(Founded in 1817)
BOARD OF GOVERNORS, October 1997–September 1998

RICHARD A. RIFKIND, *Chairman of the Board*
ELEANOR BAUM, *Vice Chairman of the Board*
RODNEY W. NICHOLS, *President and CEO* [ex officio]

Honorary Life Governors
WILLIAM T. GOLDEN   JOSHUA LEDERBERG

JOHN T. MORGAN, *Treasurer*

Governors

D. ALLAN BROMLEY	LAWRENCE B. BUTTENWIESER	PRAVEEN CHAUDHARI
RONALD L. GRAHAM	BILL GREEN	HENRY M. GREENBERG
JACQUELINE LEO	WILLIAM J. McDONOUGH	KATHLEEN P. MULLINIX
SANDRA PANEM	CHARLES RAMOND	SARA LEE SCHUPF
JAMES H. SIMONS	WILLIAM C. STEERE, JR.	TORSTEN WIESEL

MARTIN L. LEIBOWITZ, *Past Chairman of the Board*
HELENE L. KAPLAN, *Counsel* [ex officio]   CRAIG PURINTON, *Secretary* [ex officio]

SALIVARY GLAND BIOGENESIS AND FUNCTION

ANNALS OF THE NEW YORK ACADEMY OF SCIENCES

Volume 842

SALIVARY GLAND BIOGENESIS AND FUNCTION

Edited by Maria A. Kukuruzinska and Lawrence A. Tabak

New York Academy of Sciences
New York, New York
1998

Copyright © 1998 by the New York Academy of Sciences. All rights reserved. Under the provisions of the United States Copyright Act of 1976, individual readers of the Annals are permitted to make fair use of the material in them for teaching and research. Permission is granted to quote from the Annals provided that the customary acknowledgment is made of the source. Material in the Annals may be republished only by permission of the Academy. Address inquiries to the Executive Editor at the New York Academy of Sciences.

Copying fees: For each copy of an article made beyond the free copying permitted under Section 107 or 108 of the 1976 Copyright Act, a fee should be paid through the Copyright Clearance Center, Inc., 222 Rosewood Drive, Danvers, MA 01923. The fee for copying an article is $3.00 for nonacademic use; for use in the classroom it is $0.07 per page.

∞ The paper used in this publication meets the minimum requirements of American National Standard for Information Sciences—Permanence of Paper for Printed Library Materials. ANSI Z39.48-1984.

Softcover art: Confocal image (1 micron-thick optical section) of a 5-day-old hamster submandibular gland double stained for F-actin (red), using rhodamine-phalloidin, and beta 1 integrin (green), with a monoclonal mouse anti-hamster primary antibody and a fluorescein-conjugated anti-mouse secondary antibody. Beta 1 integrin is found primarily in the basal lamina, whereas F-actin is prominent in the apical regions of the ducts. Courtesy of Kelley Lennon, Douglas Cotanche, Sue Menko, and Maria A. Kukuruzinska.

Library of Congress Cataloging-in-Publication Data

Salivary gland biogenesis and function / edited by Marie A. Kukuruzinska and Lawrence A. Tabak.
    p. cm. — (Annals of the New York Academy of Sciences : v. 842)
    Includes bibliographical references and index.
    ISBN 1-57331-135-9 (cloth : alk. paper). — ISBN 1-57331-136-7 (pbk. : alk. paper)
    1. Salivary glands—Physiology—Congresses. 2. Salivary glands--Growth—Congresses. I. Kukuruzinska, Maria A. II. Tabak. Lawrence A., 1951- . III. Series.
    Q11.N5 vol. 842
    [QP191]
    500 s—dc21
    [573.3'5379]
                                                                  98-15976
                                                                                CIP

ComCom/RRD
Printed in the United States of America
ISBN 1-57331-135-9 (cloth)
ISBN 1-57331-136-7 (paper)
ISSN 0077-8923

ANNALS OF THE NEW YORK ACADEMY OF SCIENCES
Volume 842
April 15, 1998

SALIVARY GLAND BIOGENESIS AND FUNCTION[a]

Editors and Conference Organizers
MARIA A. KUKURUZINSKA AND LAWRENCE A. TABAK

CONTENTS

Preface. *By* Maria A. Kukuruzinska and Lawrence A. Tabak	ix
Preparing for the Twenty-first Century. *By* Harold Slavkin	xi
Glandular Structure and Gene Expression: Lessons from the Mammary Gland. *By* Mina J. Bissell	1

Part I. Development

Multifunctional Lens Crystallins and Corneal Enzymes: More than Meets the Eye. *By* JORAM PIATIGORSKY	7
The Roles of Stably Committed and Uncommitted Cells in Establishing Tissues of the Somite. *By* MINDY GEORGE-WEINSTEIN, JACQUELYN GERHART, MICHELE MATTIACCI-PAESSLER, EILEEN SIMAK, JENNIFER BLITZ, REBECCA REED, AND KAREN KNUDSEN	16
Regulation of the *Sex Combs Reduced* Gene in *Drosophila*. *By* JAMES A. KENNISON, MARTHA VÁZQUEZ, AND BRENDA J. BRIZUELA	28
Integrins and Development: How Might These Receptors Regulate Differentiation of the Lens. *By* SUE MENKO, NANCY PHILP, BOB VENEZIALE, AND JANICE WALKER	36
Integrins and Matrix Molecules in Salivary Gland Cell Adhesion, Signaling, and Gene Expression. *By* ROBERT M. LAFRENIE AND KENNETH M. YAMADA	42
Expression of *Rhizobium* Chitin Oligosaccharide Fucosyltransferase in Zebrafish Embryos Disrupts Normal Development. *By* CARLOS E. SEMINO, MIGUEL L. ALLENDE, JEROEN BAKKERS, HERMAN P. SPAINK, AND PHILLIPS P. ROBBINS	49

[a]This volume is the result of a conference, entitled **Salivary Gland Biogenesis and Function,** held in Arlie, Virginia on November 7–10, 1996.

Regulation and Formation of the *Drosophila* Salivary Glands. *By* DEBORAH J. ANDREW 55

Salivary Gland Nucleotide Receptors: Changes in Expression and Activity Related to Development and Tissue Damage. *By* JOHN T. TURNER, MINJUNG PARK, JEAN M. CAMDEN, AND GARY A. WEISMAN 70

Part II. Homeostasis

The Role of the Insulin-like Growth Factor I Receptor in Transformation and Apoptosis. *By* MARIANA RESNICOFF AND RENATO BASERGA 76

Apoptosis: A Modulator of Cellular Homeostasis and Disease States. *By* MARY J. DELONG 82

Nucleotide Sugars, Nucleotide Sulfate, and ATP Transporters of the Endoplasmic Reticulum and Golgi Apparatus. *By* PATRICIA BERNINSONE AND CARLOS B. HIRSCHBERG 91

Development of Salivary Gland Cell Lines for Studies of Signaling and Physiology. *By* STEPHEN P. SOLTOFF, SHELLEY A. GRUBMAN, AND DOUGLAS M. JEFFERSON 100

Transcriptional Regulation of Salivary Proline-rich Protein Gene Expression. *By* DAVID K. ANN AND H. HELEN LIN 108

Protein Secretion by Rat Parotid Acinar Cells: Pathways and Regulation. *By* J. DAVID CASTLE 115

Part III. Dysfunction

Salivary Abnormalities in Prader-Willi Syndrome. *By* P. SUZANNE HART 125

Acquired Salivary Dysfunction: Drugs and Radiation. *By* PHILIP C. FOX 132

Antigen Processing and Autoimmunity: Evaluation of mRNA Abundance and Function of HLA-linked Genes. *By* YINENG FU, GANG YAN, LIJIA SHI, AND DENISE FAUSTMAN 138

Clinical Implications of the Dry Mouth: Oral Mucosal Diseases. *By* J. L. JENSEN AND P. BARKVOLL 156

Part IV. The Future: Key Issues

Combination Gene Therapy for Salivary Gland Cancer. *By* BERT W. O'MALLEY JR. AND DAQING LI 163

Somatic Gene Transfer to Salivary Glands. *By* BRIAN C. O'CONNELL, C. DAVID LILLIBRIDGE, INDU AMBUDKAR, AND DAVID KRUSE 171

Studying Development of Disease Through Temporally Controlled Gene Expression in the Salivary Gland. *By* PRISCILLA A. FURTH, MINGLIN LI, AND LOTHAR HENNIGHAUSEN 181

In Vitro and *In Vivo* Models for the Reconstruction of Intercellular Signaling. *By* KAMAL H. BOUHADIR AND DAVID J. MOONEY 188

Part V. Poster Papers

Molecular Dissection of the Genetic Targets of ALG7 in the Serpentine Receptor-mediated Signal Transduction Pathway in Yeast. *By* KELLEY LENNON, ALBERTO BIRD, AND MARIA A. KUKURUZINSKA 195

Cholecystokinin as Neurotransmitter and Neuromodulator in Parasympathetic Secretion in the Rat Submandibular Gland. *By* NORIYASU TAKAI, TORU SHIDA, KENJI UCHIHASHI, YUTAKA UEDA, AND YO YOSHIDA 199

Transfection of COS Cells with Human Cystatin cDNA and Its Effect on HSV-1 Replication. *By* TARA R. WEAVER-HILTKE AND LIBUSE A. BOBEK 204

Salivary Acidic Proline-rich Proteins in Rheumatoid Arthritis. *By* J. L. JENSEN 209

Confocal Imaging of Gene Expression during Hamster Submandibular Gland Biogenesis. *By* RUI FERNANDES, MATTHEW FOX, DOUGLAS COTANCHE, KELLEY LENNON, AND MARIA A. KUKURUZINSKA 212

Lacrimal Gland Functions Are Differentially Controlled by Protein Kinase C Isoforms. *By* DRISS ZOUKHRI, ROBIN R. HODGES, CHRISTIAN SERGHERAERT, AND DARLENE A. DARTT 217

Autoantibodies in Salivary Hypofunction in the NOD Mouse. *By* THOMAS R. ESCH AND MARTIN A. TAUBMAN 221

* * *

Epilogue. *By* MARIA A. KUKURUZINSKA AND LAWRENCE A. TABAK 229

Index of Contributors 231

Financial assistance was received from:
- NATIONAL INSTITUTE OF DENTAL RESEARCH, NIH
- COLGATE-PALMOLIVE COMPANY
- BLOCK DRUG COMPANY, INC.
- MGI PHARMA, INC.
- SJÖGREN'S SYNDROME FOUNDATION
- NATIONAL SJÖGREN'S SYNDROME ASSOCIATION

The New York Academy of Sciences believes it has a responsibility to provide an open forum for discussion of scientific questions. The positions taken by the participants in the reported conferences are their own and not necessarily those of the Academy. The Academy has no intent to influence legislation by providing such forums.

Preface

MARIA A. KUKURUZINSKA[a] AND LAWRENCE A. TABAK[b]

[a]Division of Oral Biology, Boston University, School of Dental Medicine,
Boston, Massachusetts 02118, USA
[b]Department of Dental Research, University of Rochester,
Rochester, New York 14642, USA

Science-based approaches have been increasingly used for the prevention and treatment of numerous acquired and inherited disorders. Although salivary gland–derived health problems pose a significant disease burden, relatively few preventive and corrective therapeutics for these disorders exist. With population longevity increasing, the incidence of oral dysfunctions will only escalate in the future. The slow progress in this area of oral medicine stems from the paucity of molecular and cellular details regarding salivary gland biogenesis and function.

Much of our current knowledge of development and homeostasis derives from such biological model systems as muscle, lens, *Drosophila, Caenorhabditis elegans,* and yeast. Using these systems, a combination of genetic and molecular approaches has yielded revelations, not only about the genetic programs for growth, differentiation, and apoptosis, but also about their remarkable evolutionary conservation.

The current climate of rapid advances in the biomedical sciences has provided the impetus for organizing the salivary research conference. The goal was to bring to the forefront the latest science from diverse areas of development and tissue homeostasis. We felt that the most effective strategies for studies of salivary cell lineage, differentiation, death, and renewal would be defined through cross-fertilization of ideas from existing knowledge. The new information would then facilitate the design of rational therapeutics for salivary gland–related dysfunctions.

The picturesque and informal setting of the Airlie Center proved conducive and stimulating to discussion and exchanges of ideas. The meeting's success stemmed from the scientific accomplishments of, and the interactions among, the participants. This publication reflects the substance of the conference, the outcomes of which not only met our initial objectives, but surpassed our expectations.

We acknowledge the financial support for the conference from the National Institute of Dental Research (NIDR) and from corporate sponsors. In particular, we thank Dr. Eleni Kousvelari, Director for Extramural Research at the NIDR, for providing guidance throughout the planning and preparation phases. Without her vision of the future of biomedical research, this meeting would not have been possible. We would like also to express our gratitude to Dr. Dan Nathanson, Boston University School of Dental Medicine, for his help in the recruitment of corporate sponsorships.

Preparing for the Twenty-first Century

HAROLD SLAVKIN

National Institute of Dental Research, National Institutes of Health, Bethesda, Maryland 20892, USA

What will clinical dentistry be like in the twenty-first century? During the twentieth century, in no small measure because of the heroic efforts of the 1926 Gies Report and World War II, American dental education evolved from a secondary position in freestanding and often proprietary schools to become an integral part of research-intensive university professional education. This evolution provided dentistry with a formidable scientific basis for diagnosis, therapeutics, and disease prevention. The development of clinical skills coupled with advanced dental materials and therapeutics has truly been remarkable.

Now we approach the twenty-first century as a nation of changing demographics. Consider the "social math" of America. By 2010 nearly 40 million Americans will be 65 years of age or older. Expectations for "quality of life" now punctuate American values. Whereas in 1900 the human life span was 45 years, today it approaches 80 years. Whereas in 1900 the primary causes of mortality and morbidity were acute infectious diseases, today our challenges include complex viral infections as well as neoplastic diseases and chronic disabling diseases (e.g., chronic facial pain, skeletal-muscular degeneration, osteoarthritis, and cerebrovascular and coronary diseases and disorders). In fact, one American dies every hour of oral cancer. The practice of clinical dentistry in the twenty-first century will change by continuing (1) to integrate dental practice into comprehensive health care, (2) to increasingly advocate for health promotion, (3) to increase our knowledge of diagnostics and therapeutics, and (4) to use novel strategies for oral health care.

SALIVARY GLAND BIOGENESIS AND FUNCTION

Glandular Structure and Gene Expression

Lessons from the Mammary Gland[a]

MINA J. BISSELL[b]

Life Sciences Division, Lawrence Berkeley National Laboratory, One Cyclotron Road, MS 83-101, Berkeley, California 94720, USA

In the last decade, we have established "designer microenvironments" in culture[1] to maintain tissue-specific gene expression, and we have destabilized homeostasis in transgenic mice to study how tissue-specific gene expression is regulated in the mammary gland. We initially postulated,[2] and later provided evidence, that the extracellular matrix (ECM), in general, and the basement membrane (BM), in particular, regulate functional differentiation at multiple levels (FIG. 1; see Roskelley *et al.*[3] and references cited). The ECM also regulates growth factor expression as well as the expression of transcription factors involved in growth.[4,5] In collaboration with Zena Werb's laboratory (University of California, San Francisco) using transgenic mice, we have shown that the BM is essential for both morphogenesis and functional differentiation *in vivo* and that its loss leads also to apoptosis *in vivo* and in culture.[6-8] The ratio of ECM-degrading proteinases and their inhibitors are crucial, and a disturbance in this ratio leads to formation and dissemination of breast tumors in transgenic animals.[9,10] We thus propose that the ECM and their receptor integrins are central regulators of growth, differentiation, apoptosis, and cancer (FIG. 2).

More recently, we have shown that these studies have direct relevance to human breast cancer. In collaboration with Ole W. Petersen's laboratory (Copenhagen, Denmark), we developed a three-dimensional assay for distinguishing normal and malignant breast cells from primary tissues and cell lines.[11] In a basement membrane assay, non-malignant cells formed organized structures and regained morphological differentiation analogous to acini *in vivo*. Tumor cells, by contrast, formed masses of disorganized structures and continued to grow. We concluded that cultivation in three dimensions with access to a malleable basement membrane serves to rapidly distinguish normal and malignant cells. We further hypothesized that the ability to sense the BM correctly, and to form organotypic structure, was a function of a class of suppressor genes lost, as cells became disorganized and finally malignant.[11] In collaboration with Pat Steeg's laboratory (National Cancer Institute), we showed that a putative "metastasis suppressor gene," NM23, exhibited a growth-suppressive phenotype once transfected into metastatic and aggressive breast cells grown in three dimensions.[12] An examination of these cultures indicated that transfected cells could form a continuous BM.

We now have begun a comprehensive study of a human breast "progression series" developed in the Petersen and Briand laboratories.[13] The cells were derived from reduction mammaplasty and were passaged in minimal and defined medium for more than 200 generations. They eventually became malignant when epidermal growth factor was removed in midpassage.[14] As such, these cells constitute the only known "spon-

---

[a] This work was supported by the Office of Health and Environmental Research of the U.S. Department of Energy under contract DE-AC03-76-SF00098 and the National Institutes of Health (CA64786 and CA57621).

[b] Tel: (510) 486-4365; fax: (510) 486-5586; e-mail: mjbissell@lbl.gov

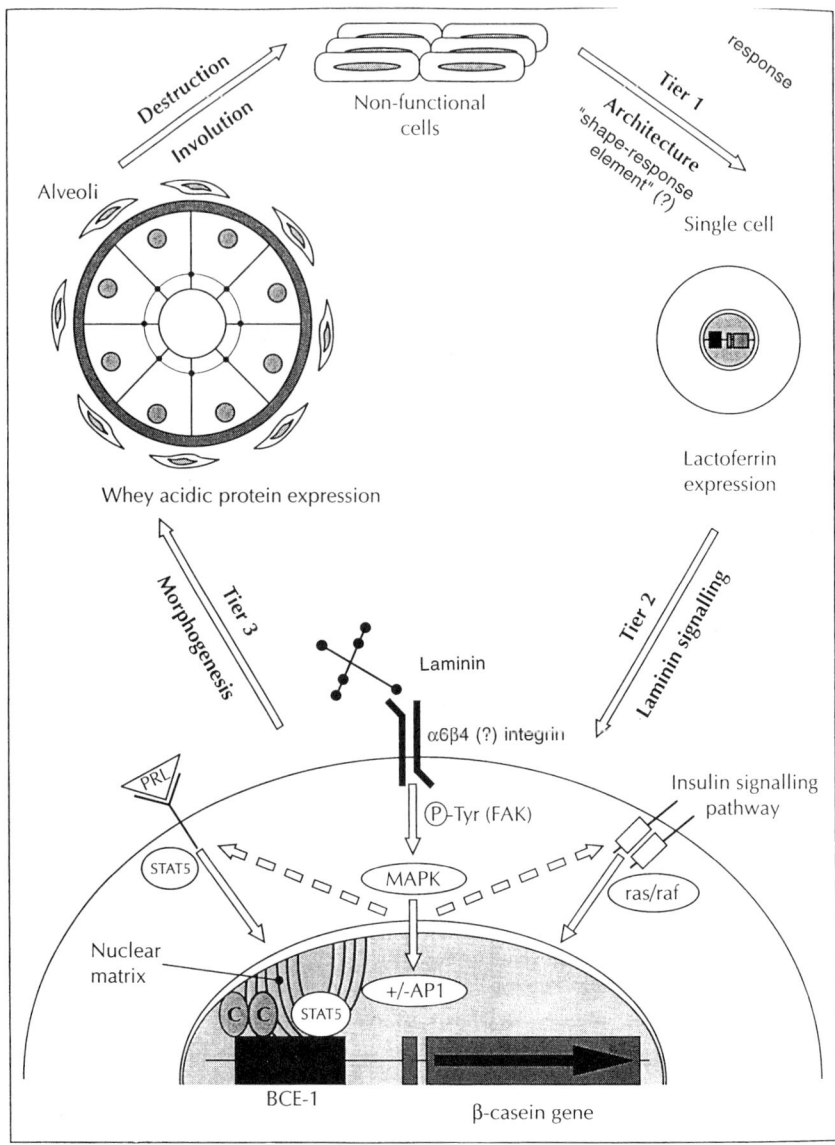

FIGURE 1. A hierarchy of ECM-dependent signals regulates mammary gland development. The first tier of the hierarchy is mediated by architectural changes in cell shape that result in lactoferrin expression. This can be brought about by a basement membrane matrix, by laminin, or by an inert substrata, such as polyhema. The second tier of the hierarchy is mediated by laminin-specific biochemical signals that activate an ECM-response element (BCE-1) and induce endogenous β-casein expression. The third tier in the hierarchy is by "tissue morphogenesis" brought about by a malleable BM leading to the formation of alveoli in tissue culture models and serves to allow whey acidic protein (WAP) expression. Destruction of the hierarchy is mediated by matrix metalloproteases and results in involution. C = CCAATT/enhancer binding protein; FAK = focal adhesion kinase; MAPK = mitogen-activated protein kinase; PRL = prolactin.[3]

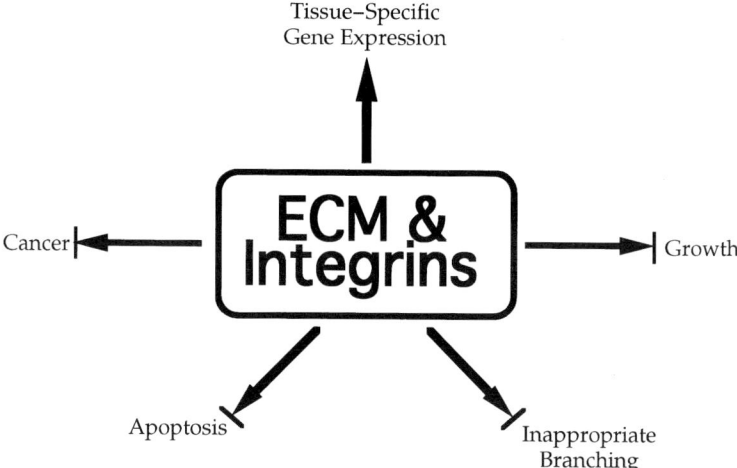

FIGURE 2. ECM-mediated signals inhibit inappropriate branching, apoptosis, growth, and the development of cancer but positively influence tissue-specific gene expression in the mammary gland.

taneously" transformed human breast epithelial culture model. These cells do not exhibit different morphologies or growth rates on tissue culture plastic. When grown in our assay, however, they sort into "normal" and "malignant" phenotypes, as described above. Even after cells gain a mutation in P53 and develop other deletions and amplifications in many of their chromosomes, as shown by comparative genomic hybridization (CGH; unpublished data in collaboration with J. Gray and D. Pinkel laboratories, UCSF/LBNL), they still form organized acini and cease growth. Only a very late subpopulation, grown in a defined medium in the absence of growth factors, forms colonies that resemble the malignant phenotype, but that are not tumorigenic (unpublished). Thus, we can distinguish a "premalignant" phenotype in our three-dimensional assay. The tumorigenic cells were derived from this population after injection in the nude mice.

These findings allowed us to postulate that the structure of the acini may be a dominant organizing force in maintaining breast function. We therefore asked how an early passage that formed normal structure differed from its malignant counterpart. We defined the behavior of a phenotypically normal population at passage 50 (referred to as S1-50), and its eventual malignant counterpart T4, in terms of growth, cytoskeletal structure, and integrin composition.[15] T4 cells had profound changes in organization of adhesion molecules, cytoskeleton, growth, and all other functions studied. Surprisingly, however, once treated with a function-blocking β_1 integrin antibody to "normalize" the level of β_1 integrin at the cell surface, these cells reverted to a near normal phenotype. All parameters measured had normalized. This included DNA synthesis, the number of cells in the acini, P21 and cyclin D-1 levels, interaction of E-cadherin with catenins, formation of BM, and organization of actin (FIG. 3; for details, please refer to the original paper of Weaver *et al.*[15]). This reversion was not due to selection and was reversible once the antibody was removed.

We conclude that the organization of the tissue (breast acini) is dominant over the cellular genome. Thus, form and function are intimately related in epithelia, and unless

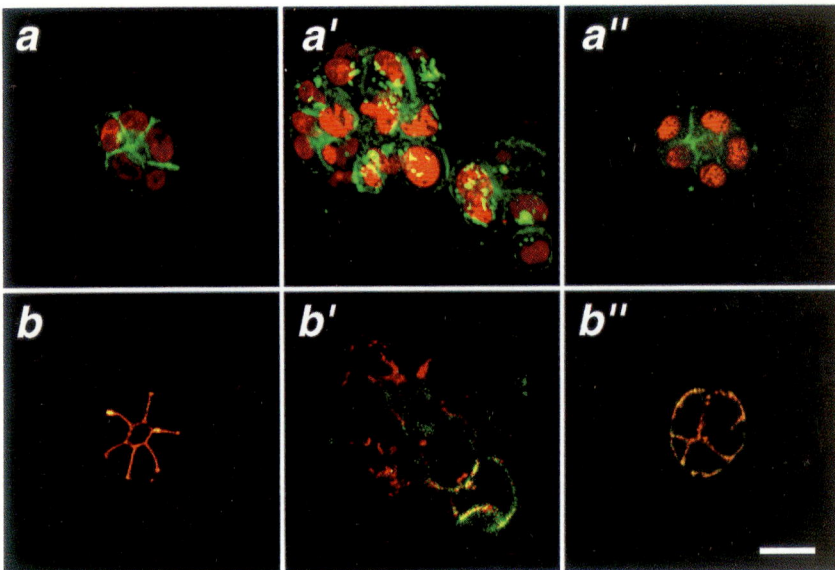

FIGURE 3. Reversion of human breast cancer cells to a normal phenotype by β_1-integrin function-blocking antibodies in a three-dimensional basement membrane assay. It shows confocal double fluorescence microscopic images of nonmalignant, phenotypically normal acini (left); tumorigenic, disorganized colonies (middle); and reverted, phenotypically normal acini (right). All colonies were double-stained for F-actin (green) and nuclei (propidium iodide, red) (top), or E-cadherin (green) and β-catenin (Texas red) (bottom). (Top panels) Both the nonmalignant and β_1-integrin function-blocking antibody-treated reverted tumor acini showed basally localized nuclei and organized filamentous F-actin, whereas tumorigenic colonies had disorganized, hatched bundles of actin and pleiomorphic nuclei. (Bottom panels) In the nonmalignant and β_1-integrin function-blocking antibody-treated reverted tumor acini, E-cadherin and β-catenin were colocalized and superimposed at the cell–cell junctions, whereas in the tumor colonies, these proteins were randomly dispersed throughout the cells. All cultures were cryosectioned (5 µ) after 10–12 d of cutting inside a reconstituted basement membrane. (Cover image of *The Journal of Cell Biology,* Volume 137, Number 1, April 7, 1997.)

we understand this relationship at the subcellular, cellular, and tissue levels, we will not understand breast or other epithelial cancers.

REFERENCES

1. STOKER, A.W., C.H. STREULI, M. MARTINS-GREEN & M.J. BISSELL. 1990. Designer microenvironments for the analysis of cell and tissue function. Curr. Opin. in Cell Biol. **2:**864–874.
2. BISSELL, M.J., H.G. HALL & G. PARRY. 1982. How does the extracellular matrix direct gene expression? J. Theor. Biol. **99:**31–68.
3. ROSKELLEY, C.D., A. SREBROW & M.J. BISSELL. 1995. A hierarchy of ECM-mediated signalling regulates tissue-specific gene expression. Curr. Opin. Cell Biol. **7:**736–747.
4. STREULI, C.H., C. SCHMIDHAUSER, M. KOBRIN, M.J. BISSELL & R. DERYNCK. 1993. Extracellular matrix regulates expression of the TGF-β gene. J. Cell Biol. **120:**253–260.

5. DESPREZ, P.Y., E. HARA, M.J. BISSELL & J. CAMPISI. 1995. Suppression of mammary epithelial cell differentiation by the helix-loop-helix protein, Id-1. Mol. Cell Biol. **15:**3398–3404.
6. SYMPSON, C.J., R.S. TALHOUK, C.M. ALEXANDER, J.R. CHIN, M.J. BISSELL & Z. WERB. 1994. Targeted expression of stromelysin to the mouse mammary gland provides evidence for a role of proteinases in branching morphogenesis and the requirement for an intact basement membrane for tissue-specific gene expression. J. Cell. Biol. **125:** 681–693.
7. BOUDREAU, N., C.J. SYMPSON, Z. WERB & M.J. BISSELL. 1995. Suppression of ICE and apoptosis in mammary epithelial cells by extracellular matrix. Science **267:**891–893.
8. BOUDREAU, N., Z. WERB & M.J. BISSELL. 1996. Suppression of apoptosis by basement membrane requires three-dimensional tissue organization and withdrawal from the cell cycle. Proc. Natl. Acad. Sci. USA **93:**3509–3513.
9. SYMPSON, C.J., M.J. BISSELL & Z. WERB. 1995. Mammary gland tumor formation in transgenic mice overexpressing stromelysin-1. Semin. Cancer Biol. **6:**159–163.
10. WERB *et al.* In preparation.
11. PETERSEN, O.W., L. RØNNOV-JESSEN, A.R. HOWLETT & M.J. BISSELL. 1992. Interaction with basement membrane serves to rapidly distinguish growth and differentiation pattern of normal and malignant human breast epithelial cells. Proc. Natl. Acad. Sci. USA **89:**9064–9068.
12. HOWLETT, A.R., O.W. PETERSEN, P.S. STEEG & M.J. BISSELL. 1994. A novel function for the nm23-H1 gene: Overexpression in human breast carcinoma cells leads to the formation of basement membrane and growth arrest. J. Natl. Cancer Inst. **86:**1838–1844.
13. BRIAND, P., O.W. PETERSEN & B. VAN DEURS. 1987. A new diploid nontumorigenic human breast epithelial cell line isolated and propagated in chemically defined medium. *In Vitro* Cell. Dev. Biol. **23:**181–188.
14. BRIAND, P., K.V. NIELSEN, M.W. MADSEN & O.W. PETERSEN. 1996. Trisomy 7p and malignant transformation of human breast epithelial cells following epidermal growth factor withdrawal. Cancer Res. **56:**2039–2044.
15. WEAVER, V.M., O.W. PETERSEN, F. WANG, C.A. LARABELL, P. BRIAND, C. DAMSKY & M.J. BISSELL. 1997. Reversion of the malignant phenotype of human breast cells in three-dimensional culture and *in vivo* using integrin blocking antibodies. J. Cell Biol. **137:**231–246.

OTHER RELEVANT REFERENCES FROM OUR LABORATORY (SINCE 1995)

ALEXANDER, C.M., E.W. HOWARD, C.J. SYMPSON, M.J. BISSELL & Z. WERB. 1996. Rescue of stromelysin-1-induced mammary epithelial cell apoptosis and entactin degradation by a TIMP-1 transgene. J. Cell Biol. **135:**6, 1669–1677.
ASHKENAS, J., J. MUSCHLER & M.J. BISSELL. 1997. The extracellular matrix in epithelial biology: Shared molecules and common themes in distant phyla. Dev. Biol. **180:**433–444.
BISSELL, M.J. 1997. The central role of basement membrane in functional differentiation, apoptosis and cancer: A personal account. Cell Death Reprod. Physiol. In press.
BOUDREAU, N., C. MYERS & M.J. BISSELL. 1995. From laminin to lamin: Regulation of tissue-specific gene expression by the ECM. Trends Cell Biol. **5:**1–4.
BOUDREAU, N., S.T. REDDY, A.W. STOKER, C. FAIRMAN & M.J. BISSELL. 1996. The embryonic environment and the extracellular matrix suppress oncogenic transformation by Rous sarcoma virus in the chick embryo. Mol. Cell. Differ. **3:**261–274.
HIRAI, Y., A. LOCHTER, S. GALOSY, S. KOSHIDA & M.J. BISSELL. 1998. Epimorphin, not hepatocyte growth factor or epidermal growth factor, functions as a morphoregulatory molecule for mammary epithelial cells. J. Cell Biol. **140:**159–169.
HOWLETT, A.R., N. BAILEY, C. DAMSKY, O.W. PETERSEN & M.J. BISSELL. 1995. Cellular growth and survival are mediated by β-1 integrins in normal human breast epithelium but not in breast carcinoma. J. Cell Sci. **108:**1945–1957.
JONES, P.L., N. BOUDREAU, C.A. MEYERS, H.P. ERICKSON & M.J. BISSELL. 1995. A novel function for tenascin: Transcriptional regulation of beta-casein gene expression. J. Cell Sci. **108:**519–527.
LELIEVRE, S., V.M. WEAVER & M.J. BISSELL. 1996. Extracellular matrix signalling from the cellu-

lar membrane skeleton to the nuclear skeleton: A model of gene regulation. Recent Prog. Horm. Res. **52:**417–432.

LELIEVRE, S., V.M. WEAVER, C.A. LARABELL & M.J. BISSELL. 1997. Extracellular matrix and nuclear matrix interactions may regulate apoptosis and tissue-specific gene expression: A concept whose time has come. *In* Advances in Molecular and Cell Biology. R.H. Getzenberg, Ed.: **24:**1–55. JAI Press Inc., Greenwich, CT.

LIN, C.Q., P. DEMPSEY, C. COFFEY & M.J. BISSELL. 1995. Extracellular matrix regulates whey acidic protein gene expression by suppression of TGF-α in mouse mammary epithelial cells: Studies in culture and in transgenic mice. J. Cell Biol. **129:**1115–1126.

LOCHTER, A., S. GALOSY, J. MUSCHLER, N. FREEDMAN, Z. WERB & M.J. BISSELL. 1997. A molecular program that leads to loss of differentiated phenotype of mammary epithelial cells is triggered by the matrix metalloproteinase stromelysin-1. J. Cell Biol. **139:**1861–1872.

LOCHTER, A., C.J. SYMPSON, N. TERRACIO, Z. WERB & M.J. BISSELL. 1997. Stromelysin-1 dependent invasion of basement membrane-like matrices and altered matrix-dependent regulation of stromelysin-1 gene expression by mouse mammary tumor cells. J. Biol. Chem. **272:**5007–5015.

LUND, L., J. ROMER, N. THOMASSET, H. SOLBERG, C. PYKE, M.J. BISSELL, K. DANO & Z. WERB. 1996. Two distinct phases of apoptosis in mammary gland involution: Proteinase-independent and -dependent pathways. Development **122:**181–193.

MARTINS-GREEN, M. & M.J. BISSELL. 1995. Cell-ECM interactions in development. Sem. Dev. Biol. **6:**149–159.

MYERS, C.A., C. SCHMIDHAUSER, J. MELLENTIN-MICHELOTTI, G. FRAGOSO, C.D. ROSKELLEY, G. CASPERSON, R. MOSSI, P. PUJUGUET, G. HAGER & M.J. BISSELL. 1998. Characterization of BCE-1: A transcriptional enhancer regulated by prolactin and extracellular matrix and modulated by the state of histone acetylation. Mol. Cell. Biol. In press.

PETERSEN, O.W., L. RONNOV-JESSEN & M.J. BISSELL. 1995. The microenvironment of the breast: The overall roles of the stroma and the extracellular matrix in function and dysfunction. Breast J. **1:**22–35.

PETERSEN, O.W., L. RONNOV-JESSEN, V.M. WEAVER & M.J. BISSELL. 1997. Differentiation and cancer in the mammary gland. Adv. Cancer Res. In press.

PUJUGUET, P. & M.J. BISSELL. 1997. Extracellular matrix signaling in differentiation, apoptosis and cancer. Helix **6:**16–25.

RØNNOV-JESSEN, L., O.W. PETERSEN, V. KOTELIANSKI & M.J. BISSELL. 1995. The origin of the myofibroblasts in breast: Recapitulation of tumor environment in culture unravels heterogeneity and implicates fibroblasts and vascular smooth muscle cells but not pericytes in conversion. J. Clin. Invest. **95:**859–873.

RØNNOV-JESSEN, L., O.W. PETERSEN & M.J. BISSELL. 1996. Cellular changes involved in conversion of normal to malignant breast: The importance of the stromal reaction. Physiol. Rev. **76:**69–125.

STREULI, C.H., C. SCHMIDHAUSER, N. BAILEY, P. YURCHENCO, A. SKUBITZ & M.J. BISSELL. 1995. A domain within laminin that mediates tissue-specific gene expression in mammary epithelia. J. Cell Biol. **120:**253–260.

WERB, Z., C.J. SYMPSON, C.M. ALEXANDER, N. THOMASSET, L. LUND, A. MACAULEY, J. ASHKENAS & M.J. BISSELL. 1996. Extracellular matrix remodeling and the regulation of epithelial-stromal interactions during differentiation and involution. Kidney Int. **49:**S68–S74.

Multifunctional Lens Crystallins and Corneal Enzymes

More than Meets the Eye

JORAM PIATIGORSKY[a]

Laboratory of Molecular and Developmental Biology, National Eye Intitute, National Institutes of Health, Building 6/Room 201, Bethesda, Maryland 20892-2730, USA

ABSTRACT: The abundant water-soluble proteins, called crystallins, of the transparent, refractive eye lens have been recruited from metabolic enzymes and stress-protective proteins by a process called "gene sharing." Many crystallins are also present at lower concentration in nonocular tissues where they have nonrefractive roles. The complex expression pattern of the mouse αB-crystallin/small heat shock protein gene is developmentally controlled at the transcriptional level by a combinatorial use of shared and lens-specific regulatory elements. A number of crystallin genes, including that for αB-crystallin, are activated by Pax-6, a conserved transcription factor for eye evolution. Aldehyde dehydrogenase class 3 and transketolase are metabolic enzymes comprising extremely high proportions of the water-soluble proteins of the cornea and may have structural as well as enzymatic roles, reminiscent of lens enzyme-crystallins. Inductive processes appear to be important for the corneal-preferred expression of these enzymes. The use of the same protein for entirely different functions by a gene-sharing mechanism may be a general strategy based on evolutionary tinkering at the level of gene regulation.

INTRODUCTION

A primary function of the eye lens and cornea of vertebrates is to refract light and form an image on the retina. The eye lens of vertebrates is a transparent, avasular, noninnervated, encapsulated tissue comprising an anterior layer of cuboidal epithelial cells and a posterior array of elongated fiber cells[1] (FIG. 1). The central fiber cells lose their organelles, including their cell nuclei and are filled with a high concentration (80–90%) of water-soluble proteins called crystallins. Lens cells cannot be renewed because they are entrapped by a capsule surrounding the lens, and the lens fiber cell proteins cannot turnover inasmuch as the fibers lack a cell nucleus. Consequently, the crystallins must be stable proteins that can survive throughout the life of the organism. In the case of humans and some other vertebrates, this can be a very long time indeed. The cornea of the vertebrate eye is transparent and avascular, like the lens, but there are also a number of differences. The bulk of the cornea is an extracellular matrix (stroma, see below). The cornea also has anterior epithelial cells that are nucleated and constantly being renewed. Consequently, corneal epithelial cell proteins do not need to be stable for life like the lens crystallins. Moreover, the cornea is situated on the surface of the eye, making it the primary line of defense against environmental insults.

Many invertebrates, including cephalopods (squid, octopus, cuttlefish) and cnidarians (jellyfish), among other species, also have complex eyes with transparent cellular lenses and surface corneas. The lenses of invertebrates may have refractive properties that are similar to that of vertebrates (especially the cephalopod lenses) and accumu-

---

[a] Tel: (301) 496-9467; fax: (301) 402-0781; e-mail: joram@helix.nih.gov

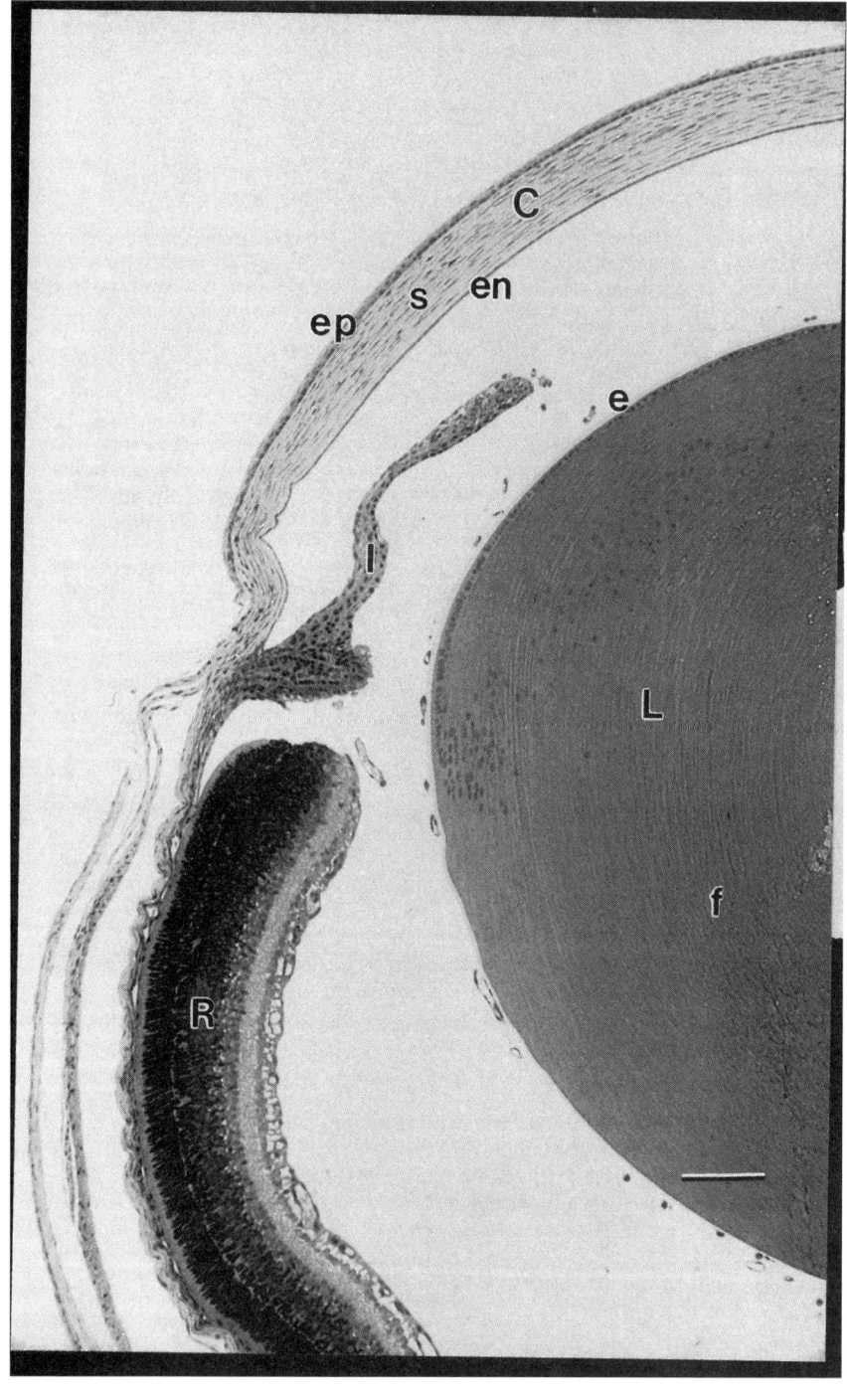

late high concentrations of crystallins. Hardly anything is known about the biology and proteins of the corneas of invertebrates.

LENS CRYSTALLINS

The crystallins are responsible for the transparent and refractive properties of the lens and have thus always been considered as highly specialized proteins. Comparative studies have revealed, as indicated in TABLE 1, that the lens crystallins of vertebrates and invertebrates are surprisingly diverse.[2-4] Some crystallins are present in all vertebrates (α- and $\beta\gamma$-crystallins), whereas a growing list of others are found only in selected species (the taxon-specific crystallins). An unexpected finding that emerged from the crystallin sequences is that many of these proteins, previously believed to be lens specific, are either closely related or identical to enzymes or stress proteins used in many tissues for nonrefractive purposes. The first clear indication that crystallins are borrowed proteins was the homolgy of the α-crystallins to the small heat shock proteins of *Drosophila*.[5,6] Later, it was established that the αB-crystallin gene is stress inducible, constitutively expressed in many different tissues and overexpressed in a variety of diseases, including neurodegenerative and cellular growth disorders.[7] By contrast, the α-A-crystallin gene, which is an evolutionary sibling of the αB gene, is (almost) lens specific, is not inducible by physiological stress, and, except for the cataract in the αA-crystallin knockout mouse,[8] has not been associated with any diseases.

In contrast to the numerous investigations that have been performed on the vertebrate crystallins, very few studies have been conducted on invertebrate lenses.[4] We have investigated the crystallins of cephalopods,[9] jellyfish,[10] and, very recently, scallops (Piatigorsky and Horwitz, unpublished). These studies have established that the general principle of recruiting crystallins from enzymes with stress-related functions is operative throughout the animal kingdom; one of these (aldehyde dehydrogenase, used in cephalopods and scallops) is also used as a crystallin in vertebrates (elephant shrew). In addition, several novel proteins that probably serve nonrefractive functions, as judged by their expression outside of the lens, have been identified from jellyfish. The analysis of the major cephalopod crystallins (S-crystallins/glutathione S-transferase) has led to an evolutionary model for crystallin recruitment that differs in part from that used by vertebrates; multiple duplications, sequence changes, and an insertion of a new exon have given rise to an extensive set of modified, lens-specific S-crystallins, which, except for one family member (SL11), lack enzymatic activity. In this model the ancestral glutathione S-transferase gene never became highly expressed in the lens, and complete separation of function occurred within the family.

GENE SHARING

A very important fact is that individual stress-crystallins (*e.g.*, αB-crystallin/small heat shock protein) and enzyme-crystallins (*e.g.*, τ-crystallin/α-enolase or δ2-crystallin/argininosuccinate lyase) that are expressed preferentially in the lens are often en-

---

FIGURE 1. Portion of eye from a three-day postnatal mouse showing the cornea (C) with its epithelium (ep), stroma (s), and endothelium (en) indicated; the lens (L) with its epithelium (e) and fibers (f) indicated; and the iris (I) and retina (R). The mouse eye opens approximately 14 days after birth, at which time the corneal epithelial cells become multilayered. Hematoxylin/eosin stain. $\times$ 110, bar=100 µm. (Micrograph courtesy of Dr. W. Gerald Robison Jr.).

TABLE 1.

Lens Crystallins

Vertebrates
    α (small heat shock proteins/chaperones; all vertebrates)
    βγ (members of microbial stress protein superfamily; all vertebrates)
    ε (lactate dehydrogenase B; ducks, crocodiles)
    δ (argininosuccinate lyase; birds, reptiles)
    τ (α-enolase; turtles, ducks, other selected vertebrates)
    ζ (novel quinone oxidoreductase; guinea pig, camel, degu, llama, rock cavy)
    μ (relative of bacterial ornithine cyclodeaminase; australian marsupials)
    η (retinaldehyde dehydrogenase; elephant shrews)
    ρ (relative of aldo-keto reductase; frogs)
    λ (relative of hydroxyl CoA dehydrogenase; rabbits, hares)
    π (glyceraldehyde-3-phosphate dehydrogenase; geckos)

Invertebrates
    S (glutathione S-transferase and its relatives; cephalopods)
    Ω/L (relative of aldehyde dehydrogenase; cephalopods, especially octopus; scallops; squid light organ)
    J (novel proteins; jellyfish)
    Drosocrystallin (novel protein; *Drosophila*)

Abundant Corneal Enzymes

aldehyde dehyrogenase class 3 (mammals)
aldehyde dehydrogenase class 1/2 (some fish)
transketolase (mammals)
α-enolase (mammals, chickens)
peptidyl-prolyl *cis-trans* isomerase (also known as cyclophilin; chicken)
δ1-crystallin (chicken)

coded in the same genes as the ubiquitous proteins that are expressed to a much lesser extent in other tissues.[11–13] We have called this dual role for crystallins "gene sharing."[11,14] Gene sharing is defined as having a protein with two or more entirely different functions encoded in, or sharing, the same gene. It implies that the innovation of a new function (refraction for a crystallin) from a ubiquitous protein (heat shock protein or metabolic enzyme) may be associated strictly with changes in the regulation of its gene.[15–17]

LENS CRYSTALLINS ARE MULTIFUNCTIONAL PROTEINS

In principle the multifunctional properties of the crystallins would allow them to play more than one role in the lens. Although it remains unresolved whether the lens depends upon the inherent enzymatic abilities of the taxon-specific crystallins when they accumulate to high concentrations as refractive proteins, it is likely that the lens does exploit the heat shock protein-related ability of the α-crystallins to protect against protein aggregation during aging.[18] This chaperone effect of the α-crystallins represents a beautiful fusion of two abilities—refraction to provide normal function, and protection against protein aggregation to guard against cataract—in one tissue as a consequence of gene sharing. This has alerted us to the possibility that the crystallins may have even additional functions that are used in the lens or in other tissues. One discovery we have made recently that has kindled our interest is the *in vitro* ability of the αA- and αB-crystallins to undergo autophosphorylations on specific serines.[19] In addition to characterizing these reactions, we are exploring the possibility that autophosphorylation reflects a signal transduction or other metabolic role involving the crystallins. This would be very important in itself and would change our thinking of the α-crystallins as being solely structural proteins to being proteins with metabolic functions as well, similar to the enzyme-crystallins.

DOES THE CORNEA HAVE MULTIFUNCTIONAL "CRYSTALLINS"?

Although different structurally from the lens, the cornea is also transparent and a major contributor to the refractive power of the eye. The cornea contains a 5–6 cell layer anterior epithelium, a thick stroma filled with a collagenous matrix harboring keratocytes, and a posterior layer of endothelial cells responsible for keeping the organ dehydrated. Like the lens, the cornea is derived embryologically from the surface ectoderm. Interestingly, it has been shown already some time ago that BCP 54, a major corneal protein, comprises 20–40% of the water-soluble protein of the bovine cornea.[20,21] BCP 54 is present in all mammalian corneas examined and is aldehyde dehydrogenase class 3 (ALDH3),[22,23] a tumor-inducible detoxification enzyme.[24] ALDH3 is located principally in the corneal epithelial cells. The unexpectedly high concentration of ALDH3 in the cornea is reminiscent of the enzyme-crystallins in the lens.

It has now been shown that the corneal epithelial cells of vertebrates, including humans, accumulate different enzymes in a taxon-specific manner at crystallin concentrations,[25] as does the lens (see TABLE 1). Another enzyme that amounts to 10% of the total corneal protein of the mouse and is found at much lower concentrations in other tissues is transketolase (TKT).[26,27] Because the concentrations of individual enzymes of the cornea range from 10% to 40% of the total water-soluble protein in this tissue, it seems very likely that they are serving structural as well as enzymatic roles in the cells. Although it is almost certain that ALDH3 and TKT protect the cornea from oxidative stresses imposed by light,[24,26] ALDH3 also appears to be responsible for absorption of UV light.[22] Indeed, the fact that ALDH3 and a few other proteins constitute the bulk of the water-soluble proteins of the bovine cornea has led them to be called absorbins.[28] Thus, the few major water-soluble proteins of the cornea are enzymes with stress-protective functions, and it is likely that these, as the enzyme-crystallins of the lens, have structural as well as enzymatic roles.

THE αA- AND αB-CRYSTALLIN/SMALL HEAT SHOCK PROTEIN GENES

We have identified positive *cis* elements that are used for the regulation of the mouse and chicken αA-crystallin promoter.[8,29] It is interesting to note that there are a number of differences in the arrangement and use of the *cis* elements and *trans* factors that regulate the orthologous αA-crystallin gene of mice and chickens, despite the fact that the αA-crystallin promoter of both species is lens specific when introduced as a transgene in transgenic mice. Negative control is also involved in the regulation of the αA-crystallin genes. For example, a composite element in the chicken promoter uses cAMP-responsive element-binding protein (CREB) or cAMP-responsive element-modulatory protein (CREM) in the lens for activation and AP-1 (Fra2 and JunD) in fibroblasts for repression.

In marked contrast to the high degree of lens specialization of the αA-crystallin gene, the mouse αB-crystallin/small heat shock protein gene has a very complex pattern of expression (heart, skeletal muscle, lung, kidney, brain, eye, among other tissues) that is transcriptionally regulated.[30–32] An additional complicating feature of αB-crystallin gene expression is that it uses at least two transcription start sites, a major one at +1 and a minor one at –474.[33] The upstream start site is used predominantly in the lung and brain. Nothing is known yet about the control mechanisms responsible for directing the utilization of the +1 or –474 transcription start sites. Interestingly, the developing heart is the first tissue to express the αB-crystallin gene. An extensive series of site-specific mutagenesis experiments have revealed at least five control elements within a muscle-preferred enhaner element located at position –427/–259 of the gene.[34,35] Three of these elements (αBE1, 2, and 3) are shared by many tissues, whereas one (αBE4) appears to be used only in the heart and another (MRF) primarily, but not exclusively, in skeletal muscle and heart. Deletion experiments indicate that αBE1, in particular, is critical for both muscle and lens expression. Gel-shift tests using specific antisera have indicated that αBE4 uses serum response factor (SRF) or a related protein for heart expression, and MRF uses one or more MyoD/myogenin family members in skeletal muscle and USF in the heart. The factors using the shared αBE1, 2, and 3 control elements have not been identified yet and remain as an important area of future investigation.

Finally, transgenic mice and transfection experiments have identified two lens-specific control elements (LSR1 and LSR2) proximal to the αB-crystallin enhancer.[36] These both bind the paired domain of Pax-6 and can be activated by Pax-6 in cotransfection experiments using fibroblasts.[37] In addition to Pax-6, LSR1 and LSR2 bind to and can be activated by retinoic acid receptors (RARβ and RXRβ heterodimers) (Gopal-Srivastava and Piatigorsky, unpublished). Pax-6 and RARβ/RXRβ are additive in their stimulating effect of the αB-crystallin promoter. Quantitative considerations of transgenic mouse and transfection experiments indicate that the enhancer, LSR1 and LSR2, must interact for maximizing lens expression of the αB-crystallin gene. Whereas much work remains to construct a comprehensive view of the constitutive expression of the αB-crystallin/small heat shock protein gene, our results show that a special combination of shared and tissue-specific control elements has evolved to recruit this multifunctional protein to become a refractive crystallin of the lens while keeping its other function(s) in other tissues.

THE IMPORTANCE OF PAX-6

Pax-6 is a paired-domain, homeodomain transcription factor that has been associated with numerous eye defects. Pax-6 from *Drosophila,* mouse, or squid can stimulate the production of ectopic eyes when overexpressed in the fly wing, antenna, or leg.[38,39] Pax-6 appears to be the first of a cascade of transcription factors that form a conserved regulatory network for eye development throughout evolution. In addition to activating the mouse αB-crystallin promoter, Pax-6 can also activate the chicken and mouse αA-, chicken δ1-, and guinea pig ζ-crystallin promoters.[29]

We have found recently that Pax-6 can also repress crystallin promoter activity (Duncan, Cvekl, Haynes II, and Piatigorsky, in preparation). The chicken βB1-crystallin gene contains a powerful, lens-specific promoter that functions only in the lens fiber cells.[40] Current experiments indicate that the βB1-crystallin promoter can be activated by another homeodomain-containing transcription factor called Prox 1 (Duncan, Tomarev, and Piatigorsky, unpublished). *In situ* hybridization and immunocytochemical experiments have indicated that Pax-6 is present predominantly in the epithelium of embryonic chicken lenses, where βB1-crystallin is not expressed, and Prox 1 accumulates in the cortical regions of the embryonic lens fibers, where βB1-crystallin gene expression commences.[41] These spatial localizations support the possibility that the differential effects of Prox 1 and Pax-6 on crystallin genes have *in vivo* significance.

It is not known whether or not Pax proteins influence crystallin transcription in invertebrates. The squid Pax-6 gene has been cloned,[39] as has a fragment of a Pax homologue from jellyfish (Piatigorsky and Norman, unpublished). Further experiments are required to test whether the squid or jellyfish crystallin genes are either activated or repressed by these Pax transcription factors.

Finally, it is not known whether Pax-6 affects the transcription of ALDH3 or TKT in the cornea. Pax-6 is expressed in the developing chicken[42] and postnatal mouse[42] (Kays and Piatigorsky, unpublished) cornea. Although it is likely that constitutive, tissue-specific expression contributes to the high expression of the abundant corneal enzymes, it is likely that inductive effects are also very important for their high expression in the cornea. ALDH3[43] and TKT[26] do not accumulate in the corneal epithelial cells until eye opening in mice, when the cornea is exposed to light. Moreover, there are multiple, stress-responsive sequence motifs in the 5′ flanking region of the ALDH3[44,45] and TKT[46] genes.

FINAL COMMENTS

The contrast between having stress induction contributing to corneal expression of putative enzyme-crystallins and developmental control at the transcriptional level governing lens expression of crystallins has clinical and basic science implications. From a medical viewpoint, inductive versus developmental control would clearly affect gene therapy. From an evolutionary viewpoint, this difference is consistent with the possibility that the biology and mechanisms of gene expression in the corneal epithelial cells reflect those that were operative in the ancestral lens before it became internalized within the eye. It would seem, therefore, that study of these two distinct eye tissues, cornea and lens, should fuse to produce a more complete portrait of the evolution of crystallin gene expression, with the abundant water-soluble enzymes of the cornea representing the early stages of crystallin recruitment, and the lens crystallins comprising abundant enzymes and stress proteins representing the modern evolutionary adaptations.

ACKNOWLEDGMENTS

I thank Drs. Stanislav I. Tomarev and Christina M. Sax for useful comments after critically reading this manuscript, and Dr. W. Gerald Robison Jr. for providing FIGURE 1.

REFERENCES

1. PIATIGORSKY, J. 1981. Lens differentiation in vertebrates. A review of cellular and molecular features. Differentiation **19:** 134–153.
2. WISTOW, G. & J. PIATIGORSKY. 1988. Lens crystallins: The evolution and expression of proteins for a highly specialized tissue. Annu. Rev. Biochem. **57:** 479–504.
3. BLOEMENDAL, H. & W.W. DE JONG. 1991. Lens proteins and their genes. Prog. Nucleic Acid Res. Mol. Biol. **41:** 259–281.
4. TOMAREV, S.I. & J. PIATIGORSKY. 1996. Lens crystallins of invertebrates. Diversity and recruitment from detoxification enzymes and novel proteins. Eur. J. Biochem. **235:** 449–465.
5. INGOLIA, T.D. & E.A. CRAIG. 1982. Four small Drosophila heat shock proteins are related to each other and to mammalian α-crystallin. Proc. Natl. Acad. Sci. USA **79:** 2360–2364.
6. DE JONG, W.W. *et al.* 1993. Evolution of the α-crystallin/small heat shock family. Mol. Biol. Evol. **10:** 103–126.
7. SAX, C.M. & J. PIATIGORSKY. 1994. Expression of the α-crystallin/small heat shock protein/molecular chaperone genes in the lens and other tissues. Adv. Enzymol. Relat. Areas Mol. Biol. **69:** 155–201.

8. BRADY, J.P. *et al.* 1997. Targeted disruption of the mouse αA-crystallin gene induces cataract and cytoplasmic inclusion bodies containing the small heat shock protein αB-crystallin. Proc. Natl. Acad. Sci. USA **94:** 884–889.
9. TOMAREV, S.I. *et al.* 1995. Glutathione S-transferase and S-crystallins of cephalopods: Evolution from active enzyme to lens refractive protein. J. Mol. Evol. **41:** 1048–1056.
10. PIATIGORSKY, J. *et al.* 1993. J1-crystallins of the cubomedusan jellyfish lens constitute a novel family encoded in at least three intronless genes. J. Biol. Chem. **268:** 11894–11901.
11. PIATIGORSKY, J. *et al.* 1988. Gene sharing by δ-crystallin and argininosuccinate lyase. Proc. Natl. Acad. Sci. USA **85:** 3479–3483.
12. HENDRIKS, W. *et al.* 1988. Duck lens ε-crystallin and lactate dehydrogenase B are identical: A single-copy gene product with two distinct functions. Proc. Natl. Acad. Sci. USA **85:** 7114–7118.
13. WISTOW, G.J. *et al.* 1989. τ-Crystallin/α-enolase: One gene encodes both an enzyme and a lens structural protein. J. Cell Biol. **107:** 2729–2736.
14. PIATIGORSKY, J. & G. WISTOW. 1989. Enzyme/crystallins: Gene sharing as an evolutionary strategy. Cell **57:** 197–199.
15. PIATIGORSKY, J. & G. WISTOW. 1991. The recruitment of crystallins: New functions precede gene duplication. Science **252:** 1078–1079.
16. PIATIGORSKY, J. 1992. Lens crystallins. Innovation associated with changes in gene regulation. J. Biol. Chem. **267:** 4277–4280.
17. WISTOW, G.J. 1993. Lens crystallins: Gene recruitment and evolutionary dynamism. Trends Biochem. Sci. **18:** 301–306.
18. HORWITZ, J. 1992. α-Crystallin can function as a molecular chaperone. Proc. Natl. Acad. Sci. USA **89:** 10449–10453.
19. KANTOROW, M. & J. PIATIGORSKY. 1994. α-Crystallin/small heat shock protein has autokinase activity. Proc. Natl. Acad. Sci. USA **91:** 3112–3116.
20. HOLT, W.S. & J.H. KINOSHITA. 1973. The soluble proteins of the bovine cornea. Invest. Ophthalmol. **12:** 114–126.
21. ALEXANDER, R.J. *et al.* 1981. Isolation and characterization of BCP 54, the major soluble protein of bovine cornea. Exp. Eye Res. **32:** 205–216.
22. ABEDINIA, M. *et al.* 1990. Bovine corneal aldehyde dehydrogenase: The major soluble protein with a possible dual protective role for the eye. Exp. Eye Res. **51:** 419–426.
23. COOPER, D.L. *et al.* 1990. Bovine corneal protein 54K (BCP54) is a homologue of the tumor-associated (class 3) rat aldehyde dehydrogenase (RATALD). Gene **98:** 201–207.
24. LINDAHL, R. 1992. Aldehyde dehydrogenases and their role in carcinogenesis. Crit. Rev. Biochem. Mol. Biol. **27:** 283–335.
25. CUTHBERTSON, R.A. *et al.* 1992. Taxon-specific recruitment of enzymes as major soluble proteins in the corneal epithelium of three mammals, chicken, and squid. Proc. Natl. Acad. Sci. USA **89:** 4004–4008.
26. SAX, C.M. *et al.* 1996. Transketolase is a major protein in the mouse cornea. J. Biol. Chem. **272:** 33568–33574.
27. GUO, J. *et al.* 1997. Heterogenous expression of transketolase in ocular tissues. Curr. Eye Res. **16:** 467-474.
28. MITCHELL, J. & R.J. CENEDELLA. 1995. Quantitation of ultraviolet light-absorbing fractions of the cornea. Cornea **14:** 266–272.
29. CVEKL, A. & J. PIATIGORSKY. 1996. Lens development and crystallin gene expression: Many roles for Pax-6. BioEssays **18:** 621–630.
30. DUBIN, R.A. *et al.* 1991. Expression of the murine αB-crystallin gene in lens and skeletal muscle: Identification of a muscle-preferred enhancer. Mol. Cell. Biol. **11:** 4330–4349.
31. HAYNES, J.I. *et al.* 1996. Spatial and temporal activity of the αB-crystallin/small heat shock protein gene promoter in transgenic mice. Dev. Dyn. **207:** 75–88.
32. BENJAMIN, I.J. *et al.* 1997. Temporospatial expression of the small HSP/αB-crystallin in cardiac and skeletal muscle during mouse development. Dev. Dyn. **208:** 75–84.
33. FREDERIKSE, P.H. *et al.* 1994. Structure and alternate tissue-preferred transcription initiation of the mouse αB-crystallin/small heat shock protein gene. Nucleic Acids Res. **22:** 5686–5694.
34. GOPAL-SRIVASTAVA, R. & J. PIATIGORSKY. 1993. The murine αB-crystallin/small heat shock

protein enhancer: Identification of αBE-1, αBE-2, αBE-3, and MRF control elements. Mol. Cell. Biol. **13:** 7144–7152.
35. GOPAL-SRIVASTAVA, R. *et al.* 1995. Regulation of the murine αB-crystallin/small heat shock protein gene in cardiac muscle. Mol. Cell. Biol. **15:** 7081–7090.
36. GOPAL-SRIVASTAVA, R. & J. PIATIGORSKY. 1994. Identification of a lens-specific regulatory region (LSR) of the murine αB-crystallin gene. Nucleic Acids Res. **22:** 1281–1286.
37. GOPAL-SRIVASTAVA, R. *et al.* 1996. Pax-6 and αB-crystallin/small heat shock protein gene regulation in the murine lens. Interaction with the lens-specific regions, LSR1 and LSR2. J. Biol. Chem. **271:** 23029–23036.
38. HALDER, G. *et al.* 1995. Induction of ectopic eyes by targeted expression of the eyeless gene in *Drosophila*. Science **267:** 1788–1792.
39. TOMAREV, S.I. *et al.* 1997. Squid Pax-6 and eye development. Proc. Natl. Acad. Sci. USA **94:** 2421–2426.
40. DUNCAN, M.K. *et al.* 1996. Developmental regulation of the chicken βB1 crystallin promoter in transgenic mice. Mech. Dev. **57:** 79–89.
41. TOMAREV, S.I. *et al.* 1996. Chicken homeobox gene Prox 1 related to *Drosophila prospero* is expressed in the developing lens and retina. Dev. Dyn. **206:** 354–367.
42. KOROMA, B.M. *et al.* 1997. The Pax-6 homeobox gene is expressed throughout the corneal and conjunctival epithelia. Invest. Ophthalmol. Vis. Sci. **38:** 108–120.
43. DOWNES, J. & R. HOLMES. 1992. Development of aldehyde dehydrogenase and alcohol dehydrogenase in mouse eye: Evidence for light-induced changes. Biol. Neonate **61:** 118–123.
44. ASMAN, D.C. *et al.* 1993. Organization and characterization of the rat class 3 aldehyde dehydrogenase gene. J. Biol. Chem. **268:** 12530–12536.
45. HSU, L.C. *et al.* 1996. The human aldehyde dehydrogenase 3 gene (ALDH3): Identification of a new exon and diverse mRNA isoforms, and functional analysis of the promoter. Gene Expression **6:** 87–99.
46. SALAMON, C., M. CHERVENAK, J. PIATIGORSKY & C.M. SAX. 1998. The mouse transketolase (TKT) gene: Cloning, characterization, and functional promoter analysis. Genomics. In press.

The Roles of Stably Committed and Uncommitted Cells in Establishing Tissues of the Somite

MINDY GEORGE-WEINSTEIN,[b] JACQUELYN GERHART, MICHELE MATTIACCI-PAESSLER, EILEEN SIMAK, JENNIFER BLITZ, REBECCA REED, AND KAREN KNUDSEN[a]

Department of Anatomy, Philadelphia College of Osteopathic Medicine, 4170 City Avenue, Philadelphia, Pennsylvania 19131, USA
[a]Lankenau Medical Research Center, Wynnewood, Pennsylvania, USA

> ABSTRACT: Somites are blocks of embryonic mesoderm tissue that give rise to skeletal muscle, cartilage, and other connective tissues. The development of different tissues within the somite is influenced by adjacent structures, in particular, the neural tube and notochord. Results of experiments performed *in vivo* and *in vitro* suggest that somites contain populations of cells stably programmed to undergo either skeletal myogenesis or chondrogenesis and a population uncommitted to either pathway. The fate of the uncommitted cells would depend on a transfer of information from the committed cells. Communication between committed and uncommitted cells is regulated by cell and tissue interactions that either activate or inhibit this process.

Skeletal muscle formation occurs during the embryonic and fetal periods of development and in response to injury of adult muscle.[1,2] The process begins when replicating muscle precursor cells withdraw from the cell cycle, initiate the synthesis of contractile proteins, align, and fuse to form multinucleated myofibers.[3] This is followed by innervation and attachment to tendons. Practically all skeletal muscle precursor cells originate from embryonic structures called somites.[4] Somites are blocks of mesoderm tissue that lie along either side of the developing spinal cord or neural tube and the notochord (FIGURES 1A and B). They form by pinching off from the rostral end of the segmental plate mesoderm.

Initially somites consist of a compact mass of cells that within a few hours form a circular epithelium. Several hours later they become partitioned into three tissues, the myotome, dermatome, and sclerotome (FIG. 1B). The myotome forms the skeletal muscles of the trunk. The dermatome gives rise to the connective tissue of the back and also contains skeletal muscle precursors that migrate into the limb bud. The sclerotome differentiates into the cartilages of vertebrae and ribs.[4]

Tissues lying in close proximity to the somite influence the pathway of differentiation of its cells.[5-32] The development of the chondrogenic sclerotome is promoted by the notochord, most likely through the secretion of Sonic hedgehog.[19,29-32] Wnts 1, 3, and 4 are secreted by the dorsal neural tube, and in combination with Sonic hedgehog, promote myogenesis within the myotome.[18,32]

The mechanisms whereby molecules secreted by the neural tube and notochord regulate differentiation within the somite are unknown. If somite cells have the potential

---

[b] Tel: (215) 871-6541; fax: (215) 871-6540; e-mail: mindyw@pcom.edu

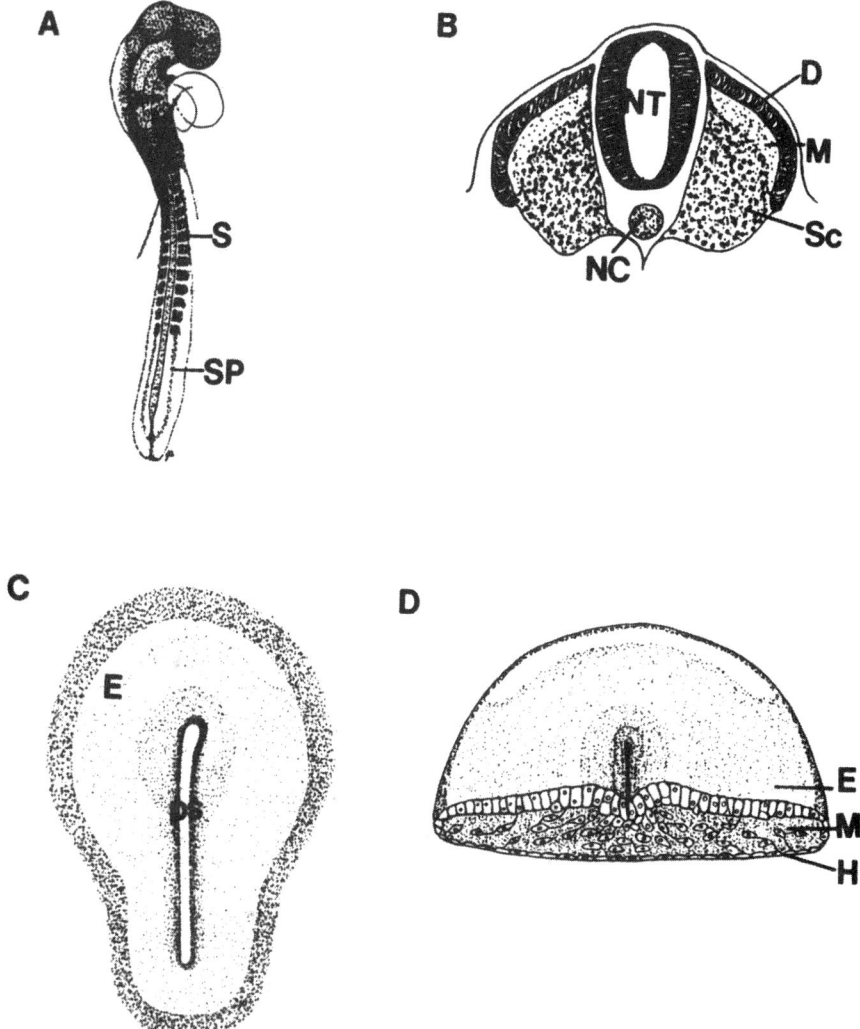

FIGURE 1. Stage 4 and 14 chick embryos. **A:** The stage-14 embryo contains somites (S) that form from the rostral end of the segmental plate mesoderm (SP). **B:** A transverse section through the stage 14 embryo showing the neural tube (NT), notochord (NC), and tissues that develop from the somite: the dermatome (D), myotome (M), and sclerotome (Sc). **C:** A view of the dorsal surface of the stage 4 embryo showing the epiblast (E) and primitive streak (ps). **D:** A transverse section through the stage 4 embryo. Cells of the epiblast layer (E) ingress through the primitive streak to form the mesoderm (M). The hypoblast (H) is eventually replaced by ingressing epiblast cells that form the endoderm.

to differentiate along multiple pathways, then extrinsic factors such as Wnts and Sonic hedgehog would be required to instruct them to follow a specific pathway of development. Alternatively, if somite cells are irreversibly committed to develop along a single pathway, signaling molecules may permit them to differentiate. Support for the notion that cells of the newly formed somite are multipotential comes from experiments in which the position of the somite was changed relative to its surrounding tissues. These manipulations alter the cells' normal pathway of differentiation from myogenesis to chondrogenesis, and vice versa.[11,12,20,23,27,28,33] Additional support for the existence of multipotentiality comes from the observation that single cells labeled within the segmental plate mesoderm give rise to progeny found in both myogenic and chondrogenic regions of the somite.[34] Together, these results suggest that the segmental plate mesoderm and newly formed somites contain cells whose fate is directed by the environment.

By contrast, transplantation and cell culture experiments support a model in which at least some segmental plate cells are inherently programmed to follow separate pathways of differentiation. Segmental plate tissue implanted into the limb bud forms both skeletal muscle and cartilage.[35] Cell culture analyses have revealed that somite and segmental plate cells can differentiate in the absence of the neural tube or notochord. When these tissues are isolated, dissociated to produce a single cell suspension, and cultured at relatively high density, they form skeletal muscle and chondroblasts (FIGURES 2A–D).[36,37] Some cells differentiate in the absence of cell division, suggesting that myogenic or chondrogenic potential is an inherent property of subpopulations of segmental plate cells. The presence of myogenic cells *in vivo* also is supported by the finding that mRNA for the skeletal muscle specific, basic helix-loop-helix transcription factor MyoD[38] is detected in segmental plate tissue by reverse transcription-polymerase chain reaction (RT-PCR).[39]

Evidence suggesting that the segmental plate contains subpopulations of cells stably committed to differentiate into either muscle or chondroblasts can be reconciled with the ability of somite cells to switch from a myogenic to chondrogenic fate after changing their environment by proposing that these tissues contain both committed and uncommitted cells. We propose that cells stably committed to the myogenic or chondrogenic lineage are randomly distributed throughout the segmental plate and somites and that they regulate the pathway of differentiation of their uncommitted neighbors. Evidence for the presence of randomly distributed, stably committed cells in the somite comes from transplantation studies. Both the myogenic dorsal region and chondrogenic ventral region of the somite give rise to muscle and cartilage when they are implanted separately into the limb bud.[35] Furthermore, after excision of the neural tube, MyoD mRNA can be detected in cells of the sclerotome region of the somite.[40]

The presence of randomly distributed, stably committed myogenic and chondrogenic cells also would explain the apparent change in cell fate that occurs when the position of the newly formed somite is altered relative to its surrounding tissues.[11,12,20,23,27,28,30,34] A committed muscle precursor cell present in the presclerotomal region would be activated after a rotation that placed it in proximity to the myogenesis-promoting dorsal neural tube. The activated muscle precursor would then recruit its uncommitted neighbors to form a myogenic myotome. When the dermamyotome is rotated and positioned closer to the notochord, a stably committed chondrogenic cell present in this region would become activated to recruit surrounding cells to form the sclerotome.

In summary, we propose that the segmental plate mesoderm and newly formed somites contain populations of cells stably programmed to undergo either skeletal myogenesis or chondrogenesis and a population uncommitted to either pathway. The

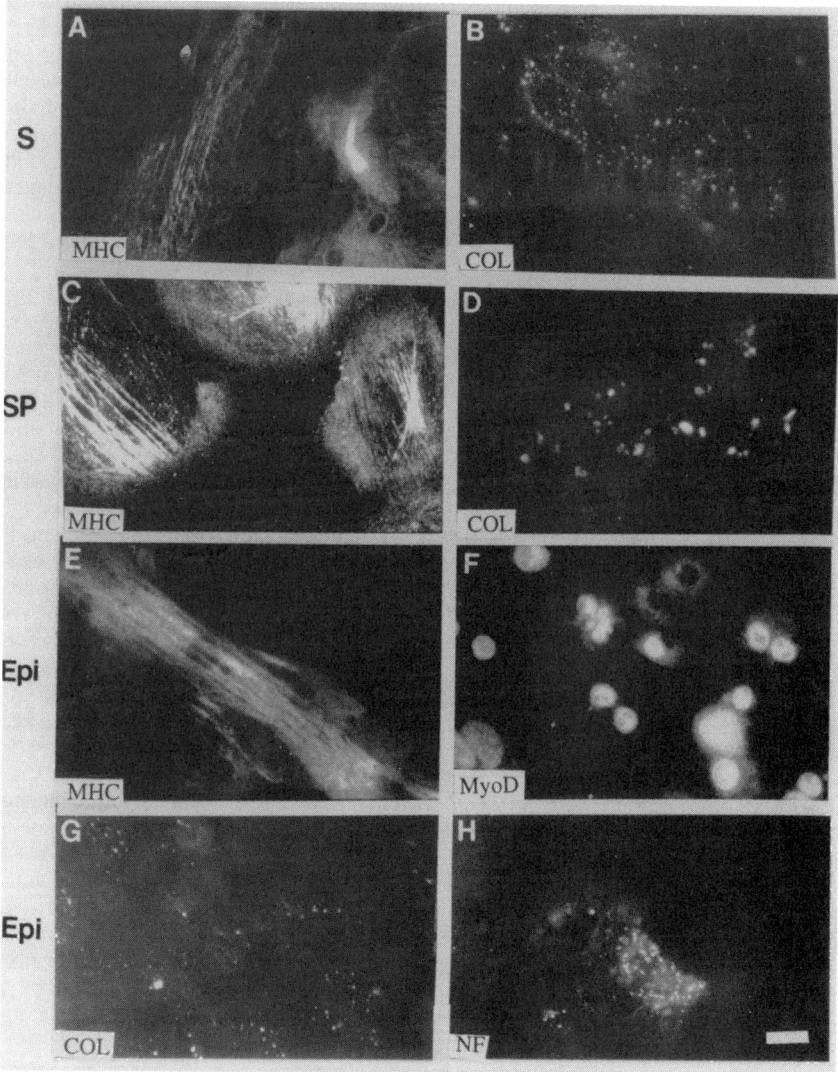

FIGURE 2. Differentiation of somite, segmental plate, and epiblast cells *in vitro*. Cultures were prepared from the 8 most caudal pairs of somites or segmental plates from stage 13 and 14 embryos. Epiblasts (Epi) were obtained from stage 4, primitive streak stage embryos. Cells were cultured for 48 hours, fixed, and labeled with antibodies to sarcomeric myosin heavy chain (MHC),[96] type II collagen (COL),[99] MyoD,[104] or neurofilament protein (NF). Somite and segmental plate cells differentiated into skeletal muscle and chondroblasts. Epiblast cells differentiated into skeletal muscle, neurons, and cells synthesizing type II collagen. Bar = 12 μm in A, C, D, and H; and 17 μm in B, E, F, and G.

fate of the uncommitted cells would depend on the transfer of information from the stably committed cells. In turn, the transfer of information from the committed cells is regulated by cell-cell and tissue interactions that either activate or inhibit this process.

These premises raise several questions regarding the mechanisms of induction of differentiation in the somite. First, what is the nature of the population of uncommitted cells? Cell culture[36,39,41] and transplantation studies[35] suggest that although these cells are not stably committed, they do have a propensity for differentiating into skeletal muscle. When somite and segmental plate cells are isolated from surrounding tissues and cultured in serum-free medium, most undergo skeletal myogenesis (TABLE 1).[37] Furthermore, the paired box genes Pax-3 and -7 initially are expressed throughout the segmental plate and later become restricted to myogenic regions of the somite.[11,25,28,42] The recruitment of uncommitted cells to the chondrogenic lineage correlates with the downregulation of Pax-3 and -7 and upregulation of Pax-1 and -9[23-26,29-31,43-48] and the basic helix-loop-helix protein scleraxis.[49] The apparent dominance of the myogenic pathway may reflect a more potent or preexisting influence of the stably committed myogenic cells over the uncommitted population.

The second question arising from our model focuses on the timing, location, and mechanism of emergence of the stably committed myogenic and chondrogenic precursor cells in the embryo. Cells with the potential to differentiate into skeletal muscle are present in the chick embryo prior to the formation of the first pairs of somites.[50-55] In an effort to determine when and how cells develop the potential to form skeletal muscle, we turned our attention to the tissue that gives rise to the segmental plate mesoderm: the epiblast. During gastrulation, some epiblast cells ingress through the primitive streak and then migrate laterally to form the mesoderm and endoderm layers (FIGURES 1C and D). Other epiblast cells remain in the dorsal layer and develop into ectoderm and neurectoderm.

Epiblasts were separated from the mesoderm, hypoblast, and primitive streak, enzymatically dissociated, plated at high density, and grown in protein- and hormone-free medium.[41] Although *in vivo* the epiblast gives rise to all tissues of the embryo,[56-59] the dominant pathway of differentiation *in vitro* is skeletal myogenesis (TABLE 2, FIG. 2E).[41] MyoD mRNA is present in the epiblast *in vivo,* and its expression is rapidly upregulated *in vitro* such that within two hours of plating 99% of the cells contain MyoD protein in the nucleus (FIG. 2F).[41] Within five days after plating, greater than 80% of epiblast cells contain myosin, the skeletal muscle–specific troponin T (TABLE 2) and 12101 antigen, titin, and α-actinin.[41] Some cells were capable of contracting. By contrast, only 1% of epiblast cells obtained from embryos prior to primitive streak formation differentiate into skeletal muscle *in vitro* (TABLE 2).[37,39,41] Thus a fundamental change occurs

TABLE 1. Myogenesis in Somite and Segmental Plate Cultures[a]

	Percent Myosin Positive: 48 hours
Somite Cells	73 ± 10 (20)
Segmental Plate Cells	68 ± 6 (17)

[a]The 8 most caudal pairs of somites and segmental plates were isolated from stage 13 and 14 chick embryos,[95] as described previously.[36] Tissues were dissociated and 2×10^4 cells in 10 μL of medium, containing sera and embryo extract, were plated onto tissue culture dishes coated with gelatin and fibronectin. One hour after plating, dishes were flooded with protein and hormone-free DMEM/F12 medium. Cells were fixed and labeled with the MF20 monoclonal antibody to sarcomeric myosin heavy chain[96] after 48 hours in culture. Results are the mean ± standard deviation. Number of cultures scored is indicated in parenthesis. Greater than 200 cells were scored per culture. Percent myosin positive equals number of fluorescent cells divided by total cells × 100.

TABLE 2. Differentiation of Epiblast Cells *in Vitro*[a]

	Prestreak Epiblast Cells		Primitive Streak Stage Epiblast Cells	
	Percent Positive 48 hours	Percent Positive 120 hours	Percent Positive 48 hours	Percent Positive 120 hours
Myosin	0 (11)	1 ± 1 (10)	33 ± 3 (5)	83 ± 4 (4)
Skeletal troponin T		1 ± 1 (4)	10 ± 6 (3)	81 ± 2 (4)
Neurofilament protein	0 (9)	.4 ± .3 (4)	1 ± 2 (3)	.2 ± .3 (6)
Type II collagen	0 (5)	1 ± 1 (4)	2 ± 1 (3)	.4 ± 1 (5)
Notochord antigen	0 (3)	1 ± 1 (5)	1 ± 1 (3)	1 ± 1 (5)

[a]Epiblast cells from preprimitive streak stage embryos (Eyal-Giladi and Kochav's stages X and XI;[97] Hamburger and Hamilton's stage 1[95]) and primitive streak stage embryos (Hamburger and Hamilton's stages 3 and 4) were plated as described in TABLE 1. Dishes were flooded with serum-free medium. After 48 and 120 hours in culture, cells were fixed and labeled with antibodies to sarcomeric myosin heavy chain (MF20),[96] skeletal muscle–specific troponin T,[98] neurofilament protein (2H3), type II collagen (CIICI),[99] or notochord antigen (NOT-1).[100] Values are the mean ± standard deviation. Number of cultures scored is indicated in parenthesis. Percent positive equals number of fluorescent cells divided by total cells × 100.

within the epiblast during primitive streak formation that results in a dramatic increase in the number of cells that can form muscle *in vitro*.

Nonmuscle cell types, including neurons, notochord cells, and cells synthesizing type II collagen, also are present in cultures of epiblast cells from primitive streak and preprimitive streak stage embryos (TABLE 2).[39,41] These cells emerge even when greater than 90% of the surrounding cells in primitive streak stage cultures form muscle. This suggests that the epiblast of the freshly laid, pregastrulating chick embryo contains small numbers of cells stably programmed to follow different pathways of development. Holtzer et al.[50] proposed that these cells were founder cells for different lineages. In invertebrate embryos, founder cells have been defined as those that are autonomously specified to follow a particular pathway of development and are responsible for establishing tissues by a direct transfer of information to neighboring cells.[60-65]

Finally, if founder cells for the myogenic and chondrogenic lineages are responsible for recruiting uncommitted cells to follow the same pathway of development, how is this accomplished? We hypothesize that the spread of information from the committed cells to their uncommitted neighbors occurs, in part, by neutralizing inhibitory signals generated by cell and tissue interactions. For example, the lateral plate mesoderm maintains those myogenic somite cells that migrate into the limb in the precursor state.[12] In addition, the differentiation of epiblast cells is repressed when they are cultured in the presence of the underlying mesoderm.[41] This inhibitory effect is specific for the mesoderm because myogenesis occurs normally when epiblast cells are co-cultured with the extraembryonic area opaca, primitive streak, or neural tube.[41]

A role for cell-cell interactions in the inhibition of differentiation is suggested by comparing cell culture studies in which segmental plates and newly formed somites are plated as intact tissues versus a single cell suspension. When cultured as intact tissues, differentiation does not occur unless the neural tube and/or notochord are present.[13-18] By contrast, if the tissues are dissociated to produce a single cell suspension and then plated, these mesoderm cells readily undergo myogenesis and chondrogenesis.[36] Similarly, myogenesis is delayed when epiblasts are plated as an intact epithelium instead of a single cell suspension.[41]

One candidate for an inhibitor of differentiation within the segmental plate and newly formed somites is the cell surface protein Notch. Notch is present in the segmental plate mesoderm of the mouse[66–69] and chicken embryos.[70] Forced expression of Notch inhibits myogenesis in the *Xenopus* embryo and in cultured mouse cells by interfering with the activity of MyoD.[70–73] It is possible that Notch inhibits communication between founder cells and uncommitted cells in the somite as occurs in various tissues of invertebrate embryos.[74] Release of somite cells from the inhibitory Notch influence may be mediated by Wnts produced by the neural tube, inasmuch as Wnts have been shown to block the Notch pathway in *Drosophila* embryos.[75] In addition, two nuclear helix-loop-helix proteins, Id and Twist, are present in the somites and can inhibit the activity of MyoD.[76–79] Thus, multiple mechanisms may be operating to prevent premature differentiation.

Release from inhibition alone is not sufficient for the onset of muscle differentiation. Myogenesis is promoted by close contact between cells. Formation of skeletal muscle in epiblast cultures occurs to a much greater extent when they are plated at high density rather than low density.[39] This phenomenon, called the community effect,[80] also is important for myogenesis of cells from the *Xenopus laevis* embryo[80–82] and from mouse somite cells.[83] This effect appears to be mediated by a class of cell-cell adhesion molecules called cadherins. Cadherins are a family of transmembrane proteins that bind homotypically to cadherins on adjacent cells.[84,85] The cytoplasmic domain binds the catenins that link the cadherin to the cytoskeleton.[86–89] As epiblast cells enter the primitive streak to form the mesoderm, there is a switch in expression from E- to N-cadherin.[90,91] A similar change in cadherin expression occurs when epiblast cells are placed in culture.[37] Antibodies that specifically block cell-cell adhesion mediated by N-cadherin inhibit myogenesis of chick embryo epiblast, segmental plate, and somite cells *in vitro* (TABLE 3).[37] Furthermore, injection of dominant negative N-cadherin mRNA into 2–4 cell *Xenopus* embryos suppresses the expression of MyoD.[92]

It is probable that other cadherins besides N-cadherin can promote myogenesis in the somite. The N-cadherin-null transgenic mouse dies by embryonic day 10 but forms recognizable, albeit abnormal, somites.[93] Cells isolated from the somites of these mice can differentiate into skeletal muscle *in vitro*. Although these somite cells are missing

TABLE 3. Effect of Antibodies to N-Cadherin on Myogenesis[a]

	Epiblast Percent Myosin[+]	Segmental Plate Percent Myosin[+]	Somite Percent Myosin[+]
No antibodies	14 ± 6 (7)	69 ± 5 (8)	71 ± 6 (11)
N-Cadherin IgG	2 ± 1 (8)		
N-Cadherin Fab	5 ± 3 (4)		
N-Cadherin NCD2 mAb	0 (6)	11 ± 5 (4)	20 ± 9 (7)
N-Cadherin 7.2.3 MAb	24 ± 9 (5)	71 ± 4 (4)	73 ± 2 (4)

[a]Stage 3 and 4 epiblast cells and stage 13 and 14 segmental plate and somite cells were incubated in the presence or absence of antibodies for the first 24 hours in culture, and then fixed and labeled with the MF20 monoclonal antibody (MAb) to sarcomeric myosin heavy chain.[96] N-cadherin IgGs and Fabs[101,102] were used at a concentration of 200 μg/mL. The NCD2[103] and 7.2.3[37] monoclonal antibodies were used at 100 μg/mL. Results are the mean ± standard deviation. Number of cultures scored is indicated in parenthesis. Greater than 200 cells were scored per culture. Percent myosin[+] equals number of fluorescent cells divided by total cells × 100. Only function-perturbing antibodies to N-cadherin (N-cadherin IgG and Fab, and NCD2 MAb) inhibited the differentiation of epiblast cells. NCD2 MAb also inhibited muscle differentiation in somite and segmental plate cultures. The nonfunction perturbing 7.2.3 MAb to N-cadherin did not affect the differentiation of epiblast, segmental plate, or somite cells.

N-cadherin, they do express another cadherin(s). This is not surprising, considering that developing skeletal muscle cells express multiple cadherins.[94]

In conclusion, we postulate that stably committed founder cells for multiple lineages, including skeletal muscle and chondroblasts, are present in the chick embryo prior to gastrulation. These founder cells are responsible for recruiting their uncommitted neighbors within the somite to form the myogenic myotome or chondrogenic sclerotome. The recruitment process is regulated by cell and tissue interactions that either activate or inhibit the transfer of information from founder cells to uncommitted cells. This model suggests that both instructive and permissive interactions are important for the regulation of cell fate. Surrounding tissues send signals that permit the stably programmed founder cells to instruct their uncommitted neighbors to differentiate along the same pathway as themselves. This mechanism of cell fate determination would provide the early embryo with the ability to regulate the initial size of tissues through the proliferation of uncommitted cells and their recruitment to different lineages. Some degree of plasticity would be built into the embryo by positioning the stably committed cells randomly within a given tissue. Disruption of development in a limited area could be compensated for by surviving stably committed cells and uncommitted cells present in adjacent areas.

REFERENCES

1. KELLY, A.M. & S.I. ZACHS. 1969. The histogenesis of rat intercostal muscle. J. Cell Biol. **42:** 135–153.
2. BISCHOFF, R. 1994. The satellite cell and muscle regeneration. *In* Myology. A.G. Engel & C. Franzini-Armstrong, Eds.: 97–118. McGraw Hill. New York, New York.
3. OKAZAKI, K. & H. HOLTZER. 1966. Myogenesis: Fusion, myosin synthesis and the mitotic cycle. Proc. Natl. Acad. Sci. USA **56:** 1484–1486.
4. CHRIST, B. & C.P. ORDAHL. 1995. Early stages of chick somite development. Anat. Embryol. **191:** 381–396.
5. STERN, H.M. & S.D. HAUSCHKA. 1995. Neural tube and notochord promote *in vitro* myogenesis in single somite explants. Dev. Biol. **167:** 87–103.
6. MUCHMORE, W.B. 1951. Differentiation of the trunk mesoderm in *Amblystoma maculatum*. J. Exp. Zool. **118:** 137–185.
7. STRUDEL, G. 1955. L'action morphogene du tube nerveux et de la corde sur la differenciation des vertebres et des muscles vertebraux chez l'embryon de poulet. Arch. Anat. Micros. Morphol. Exp. **44:** 209–235.
8. TEILLET, M.A. & N.M. LE DOUARIN. 1983. Consequences of neural tube and notochord excision on the development of the peripheral nervous system in the chick embryo. Dev. Biol. **98:** 192–211.
9. RONG, P.M., M. TEILLET, C. ZILLER & N.M. LE DOUARIN. 1992. The neural tube/notochord complex is necessary for vertebral but not limb and body wall striated muscle differentiation. Development **115:** 657–672.
10. CHRIST, B., B. BRAND-SABERI, M. GRIM & J. WILTING. 1992. Local signalling in dermomyotomal cell type specification. Anat. Embryol. **186:** 505–510.
11. BOBER, E., B. BRAND-SABERI, C. EBENSPERGER, J. WILTING, R. BALLING, B. PATERSON, H.H. ARNOLD & B. CHRIST. 1994. Initial steps of myogenesis in somites are independent of influence from axial structures. Development **120:** 3073–3082.
12. POURQUIE, O., M. COLTEY, C. BREANT & N. LE DOUARIN. 1995. Control of somite patterning by signals from the lateral plate. Proc. Natl. Acad. Sci. USA **92:** 3219–3223.
13. AVERY, G., M. CHOW & H. HOLTZER. 1956. An experimental analysis of the development of the spinal column. V. Reactivity of chick somites. J. Exp. Zool. **132:** 409–425.
14. VIVARELLI, E. & G. COSSU. 1986. Neural control of early myogenic differentiation in cultures of mouse somites. Dev. Biol. **117:** 319–325.
15. KENNY-MOBBS, T. & P. THOROGOOD. 1987. Autonomy of differentiation in avian brachial somites and the influence of adjacent tissues. Development **100:** 449–462.

16. BUFFINGER, N. & F.E. STOCKDALE. 1994. Myogenic specification somites: Induction by axial structures. Development **120:** 1443–1452.
17. MUNSTERBERG, A.E. & A.B. LASSAR. 1995. Combinatorial signals from the neural tube, floor plate and notochord induce myogenic bHLH gene expression in the somite. Development **121:** 651–660.
18. STERN, H.M., A.M.C. BROWN & S.D. HAUSCHKA. 1995. Myogenesis in paraxial mesoderm: Preferential induction by dorsal neural tube and by cells expressing Wnt-1. Development **121:** 3675–3786.
19. HOLTZER, H. & S.R. DETWILER. 1953. An experimental analysis of the development of the spinal column. III. Induction of skeletogenous cells. J. Exp. Zool. **123:** 335–370.
20. WATTERSON, R., I. FOWLER & B.J. FOWLER. 1954. The role of the neural tube and notochord in development of the axial skeleton of the chick. Am. J. Anat. **95:** 337–400.
21. GROBSTEIN, C. & H. HOLTZER. 1955. In vitro studies of cartilage induction in mouse somite mesoderm. J. Exp. Zool. **128:** 333–356.
22. LASH, J., S. HOLTZER & H. HOLTZER. 1957. An experimental analysis of the development of the spinal column. VI. Aspects of cartilage induction. Exp. Cell Res. **13:** 292–303.
23. BRAND-SABERI, B., C. EBENSPERGER, J. WILTING, R. BALLING & B. CHRIST. 1993. The ventralizing effect of the notochord on somite differentiation in chick embryos. Anat. Embryol. **188:** 238–245.
24. DIETRICH, S., F.R. SCHUBERT & P. GRUSS. 1993. Altered Pax gene expression in murine notochord mutants: The notochord is required to initiate and maintain ventral identity in the somite. Mech. Dev. **44:** 189–207.
25. GOULDING, M.D., A. LUMSDEN & P. GRUSS. 1993. Signals from the notochord and floor plate regulates the region-specific expression of two Pax genes in the developing spinal cord. Development **117:** 1001–1016.
26. KOSEKI, H., H. WALLIN, J. WILTING, Y. MIZUTANI, A. KISPERT, C. EBENSPERGER, B. HERRMANN, B. CHRIST & R. BALLING. 1993. A role for Pax-1 as a mediator of notochordal signals during the dorsoventral specification of vertebrae. Development **119:** 649–660.
27. POURQUIE, O., M. COLTEY, M. TEILLET, C. ORDAHL & N. M. LE DOUARIN. 1993. Control of dorsoventral patterning of somitic derivatives by notochord and floor plate. Proc. Natl. Acad. Sci. USA **90:** 5242–5246.
28. GOUDLING, M., A.L. LUMSDEN & A.J. PAQUETTE. 1994. Regulation of Pax-3 expression in the dermomyotome and its role in muscle development. Development **120:** 957–971.
29. FAN, C.-M. & M. TESSIER-LAVIGNE. 1994. Patterning of mammalian somites by surface ectoderm and notochord: Evidence for sclerotome induction by a hedgehog homolog. Cell **79:** 1175–1186.
30. JOHNSON, R.L., E. LAUFER, R.D. RIDDLE & C. TABIN. 1994. Ectopic expression of Sonic hedgehog alters dorsal-ventral patterning of somites. Cell **79:** 1165–1173.
31. FAN, C.-M., J.A. PORTER, C. CHIANG, D.T. CHANG, P.A. BEACHY & M. TESSIER-LAVIGNE. 1995. Long-range sclerotome induction by sonic hedgehog: Direct role of the amino-terminal cleavage product and modulation by the cyclic AMP signaling pathway. Cell **81:** 457–465.
32. MUNSTERBERG, A.E., J. KITAJEWSKI, D.A. BUMCROT, A.P. MCMAHON & A.B. LASSAR. 1995. Combinatorial signaling by Sonic hedgehog and Wnt family members induces myogenic bHLH gene expression in the somite. Genes & Dev. **9:** 2911–2922.
33. AOYAMA, H. & K. ASAMOTO. 1988. Determination of somite cells: Independence of cell differentiation and morphogenesis. Development **104:** 15–28.
34. STERN, C.D., S.E. FRASER, R.J. KEYNES & D.R.N. PRIMMETT. 1988. A cell lineage analysis of segmentation in the chick embryo. Development **104** (Suppl.): 231–244.
35. WACHTLER, F., B. CHRIST & M. JACOB. 1982. Grafting experiments on determination and migratory behavior of presomitic, somitic and somatopleural cells in avian embryos. Anat. Embryol. **164:** 369–378.
36. GEORGE-WEINSTEIN, M., J. GERHART, G. FOTI & J.W. LASH. 1994. Maturation of myogenic and chondrogenic cells in the presomitic mesoderm of the chick embryo. Exp. Cell Res. **211:** 263–274.
37. GEORGE-WEINSTEIN, M., J. GERHART, J. BLITZ, E. SIMAK & K. KNUDSEN. 1997. N-cadherin

promotes the commitment and differentiation of skeletal muscle precursor cells. Dev. Biol. **185:** 14–24.
38. DAVIS, R.L., H. WEINTRAUB & A.B. LASSAR. 1987. Expression of a single transfected cDNA converts fibroblasts to myoblasts. Cell **5:** 987–1000.
39. GEORGE-WEINSTEIN, M., J. GERHART, R. REED, A. STEINBERG, M. MATTIACCI, H. WEINTRAUB & K. KNUDSEN. 1996. Intrinsic and extrinsic regulation of the development of myogenic precursors in the chick embryo. Basic Appl. Myology **6:** 417–430.
40. BOBER, E., B. BRAND-SABERI, C. EBENSPERGER, J. WILTING, R. BALLING, B. PATERSON, H.-H. ARNOLD & B. CHRIST. 1994. Initial steps of myogenesis in somites are independent of influence from axial structures. Development **120:** 3073–3082.
41. GEORGE-WEINSTEIN, M., J. GERHART, R. REED, J. FLYNN, B. CALLIHAN, M. MATTIACCI, C. MIEHLE, G. FOTI, J.W. LASH & H. WEINTRAUB. 1996. Skeletal myogenesis: The preferred pathway of chick embryo epiblast cells *in vitro*. Dev. Biol. **173:** 279–291.
42. WILLIAMS, B.A. & C.P. ORDAHL. 1994. Pax-3 expression in segmental mesoderm marks early stages in myogenic cell specification. Development **120:** 785–796.
43. LOVE, J. & R. TUAN. 1993. Pair-rule gene expression in the somitic stage chick embryo: Association with somite segmentation and border formation. Differentiation **54:** 73–83.
44. DEUTSCHE, U., G.R. DRESSLER & P. GRUSS. 1988. Pax-1, a member of a paired box homologous murine gene family, is expressed in segmental structures during development. Cell **53:** 617–625.
45. WALLIN, J., J. WILTING, H. KOSEKI, R. FRITSCH, B. CHRIST & R. BALLING. 1994. The role of Pax-1 in axial skeleton development. Development **120:** 1109–1121.
46. EBENSPERGER, C., J. WILTING, B. BRAND-SABERI, Y. MIZUTANI, B. CHRIST, R. BALLING & H. KOSEKI. 1995. Pax-1, a regulator of sclerotome development is induced by notochord and floor plate signals in avian embryos. Anat. Embryol. **191:** 279–310.
47. DIETRICH, S. & P. GRUSS. 1995. Undulated phenotypes suggest a role for PAX-1 for the development of vertebral and extravertebral structures. Dev. Biol. **167:** 529–548.
48. SMITH, C.A. & R.S. TUAN. 1995. Functional involvement of Pax-1 in somite development: Somite dysmorphogenesis in chick embryos treated with Pax-1 paired-box antisense oligodeoxynucleotide. Teratology **52:** 333–345.
49. CSERJESI, P., D. BROWN, K.L. KOGON, G.E. LYONS, N.G. COPELAND, D.J. GILBERT, N.A. JENKINS & E.N. OLSON. 1995. Scleraxis: A basic helix-loop-helix protein that prefigures skeletal formation during mouse embryogenesis. Development **121:** 1099–1110.
50. HOLTZER, H., J. BIEHL, R. PAYETTE, J. SASSE, M. PACIFICI & S. HOLTZER. 1983. Cell diversification: Differing roles of cell lineages and cell-cell interactions. *In* Limb Development and Regeneration, Part B. P.F. Goetinck & J.A. MacCabe, Eds.: 271–280. A.R. Liss Publishers. New York, New York.
51. KRENN, V., P. GORKA, F. WACHTLER, B. CHRIST & J.H. JACOB. 1988. On the origin of cells determined to form skeletal muscle in avian embryos. Anat. Embryol. **179:** 49–54.
52. CHOI, J., T. SCHULTHEISS, M. LU, F. WACHTLER, N. KURUC, W.W. FRANKE, D. BADER, D.A. FISCHMAN & H. HOLTZER. 1989. Founder cells for the cardiac and skeletal myogenic lineages. *In* Cellular and Molecular Biology of Muscle Development. L.H. Kedes & F.E. Stockdale, Eds.: 27–36. A.R. Liss, Inc. New York, New York.
53. HOLTZER, H., T. SCHULTHEISS, C. DILULLO, J. CHOI, M. COSTA, M. LU & S. HOLTZER. 1990. Autonomous expression of the differentiation programs of cells in the cardiac and skeletal myogenic lineages. Ann. N. Y. Acad. Sci. **599:** 158–169.
54. CHEN, Y.P. & M. SOLURSH. 1991. The determination of myogenic and cartilage cells in the early chick embryo and the modifying effect of retinoic acid. Roux's Arch. Dev. Biol. **200:** 162–171.
55. VON KIRSCHLOFER, K., M. GRIM, B. CHRIST & F. WACHTLER. 1994. Emergence of myogenic and endothelial cell lineages in avian embryos. Dev. Biol. **163:** 270–278.
56. ROSENQUIST, G.C. 1966. A radioautographic study of labeled grafts in the chick blastoderm. Development from primitive streak stages to stage 12. Contrib. Embryol. Carnegie Inst. **38:** 71–110.
57. FONTAINE, J. & N. LE DOUARIN. 1977. Analyses of endoderm formation into avian blastoderm by the use of quail-chick chimeras. The problem of the neural ectodermal origin of the cells of the APUD series. J. Embryol. Exp. Morph. **74:** 1–14.

59. STERN, C. & D.R. CANNING. 1990. Origin of cells giving rise to mesoderm and endoderm in chick embryo. Nature **343:** 273–275.
60. PREISS, J.R. & J.N. THOMSTON. 1987. Cellular interactions in early *C. elegans* embryos. Cell **48:** 241–250.
61. STERNBERG, P.W. 1991. Control of cell lineage and cell fate during nematode development. Curr. Top. Dev. Biol. **25:** 177–225.
62. HORVITZ, H.R. & I. HERSKOWITZ. 1992. Mechanisms of asymmetric cell division: Two Bs or not two Bs that is the question. Cell **68:** 237–255.
63. GURDON, J.B. 1992. The generation of diversity and pattern in animal development. Cell **68:** 185–199.
64. GREENWALD, I. & G.M. RUBIN. 1992. Making a difference: The role of cell-cell interactions in establishing separate identities for equivalent cells. Cell **68:** 271–281.
65. SCHNABEL, R. 1995. Duels without obvious sense: Counteracting inductions involved in body wall muscle development in the *Caenorhabditis elegans* embryo. Development **121:** 2219–2232.
66. FRANCO DEL AMO, F., D.E. SMITH, P.J. SWIATEK, M. GENDRON-MEGUIRE, R.J. GREENSPAN, A.P. MCMAHON & T. GRIDLEY. 1992. Expression of Motch, a mouse homolog of *Drosophila notch,* suggests an important role in early postimplantation mouse development. Development **115:** 737–744.
67. REAUME, A.G., R.A. CONLON, R. ZIRNGIBL, T.P. YAMAGUCHI & J. ROSSANT. 1992. Expression analysis of a Notch homologue in the mouse embryo. Dev. Biol. **154:** 377–387.
68. KOPAN, R. & H. WEINTRAUB. 1993. Mouse Notch: Expression in hair follicles correlates with cell fate determination. J. Cell Biol. **121:** 631–641.
69. KOPAN, R., J.S. NYE & H. WEINTRAUB. 1994. The intracellular domain of mouse Notch: A constitutively activated repressor of myogenesis directed at the basic helix-loop-helix region of MyoD. Development **120:** 2385–2396.
70. MYAT, A., D. HENRIQUE, D. ISH-HOROWICZ & J. LEWIS. 1996. A chick homologue of serrate and its relationship with notch and delta homologues during central neurogenesis. Dev. Biol. **174:** 233–247.
71. SASAI, Y., R. KAGEYAMA, Y. TAGAWA, R. SHIGEMOTO, S. NAKANISHI. 1992. Two mammalian helix-loop-helix factors structurally related to Drosophila hairy and Enhancer of split. Genes & Dev. **6:** 2620–2634.
72. JENNINGS, B., J. DE CELIS, C. DELIDAKIS, A. PREISS & S. BRAY. 1995. Role of Notch and achaete-scute complex in the expression of Enhancer of split bHLH proteins. Development **121:** 3745–3752.
73. JARRIAULT, S., C. BROU, F. LOGEAT, E.H. SCHROETER, R. KOPAN & A. ISRAEL. 1995. Signalling downstream of activated mammalian Notch. Nature **377:** 356–358.
74. ARTAVANIS-TSAKONAS, S., K. MATSUNO & M.E. FORTINI. 1995. Notch signaling. Science **268:** 225–232.
75. AXELROD, J.D., K. MATSUNO, S. ARTAVANIS-TSAKONAS & N. PERRIMON. 1996. Interaction between Wingless and Notch signaling pathways mediated by Dishevelled. Science **271:** 1826–1832.
76. WANG, Y., R. BENEZRA & D.A. SASSOON. 1992. Id expression during mouse development: A role in morphogenesis. Dev. Dyn. **194:** 222–230.
77. BENEZRA, R., R.L. DAVIS, D. LOCKSHON, D.L. TURNER & H. WEINTRAUB. 1990. The protein Id: A negative regulator of helix-loop-helix DNA binding proteins. Cell **61:** 49–59.
78. JEN, Y., H. WEINTRAUB & R. BENEZRA. 1992. Overexpression of Id protein inhibits the muscle differentiation program: *In vivo* association of Id with E2A proteins. Genes & Dev. **6:** 1466–1479.
79. SPICER, D.B., J. RHEE, W.L. CHEUNG & A.B. LASSAR. 1996. Inhibition of myogenic bHLH and MEF2 transcription factors by the bHLH protein twist. Science **272:** 1476–1480.
80. GURDON, J.B. 1988. A community effect in animal development. Nature **336:** 772–774.
81. SARGENT, T.D., M. JAMRICH & I.B. DAWID. 1986. Cell interactions and the control of gene activity during early development of *Xenopus laevis.* Dev. Biol. **114:** 238–246.
82. GURDON, J.B., K. KATO & N.D. HOPWOOD. 1992. Muscle gene activation in *Xenopus* requires intercellular communication during gastrula as well as blastula stages. Development (Suppl.) **137:** 137–142.

83. Cossu, G., R. Kelly, S. Di Donna, E. Vivarelli & M. Buckingham. 1995. Myoblast differentiation during mammalian somitogenesis is dependent upon a community effect. Dev. Biol. **92:** 2254–2258.
84. Takeichi, M. 1988. The cadherins: Cell-cell adhesion molecules controlling animal morphogenesis. Development **102:** 639–655.
85. Takeichi, M. 1991. Cadherin cell adhesion receptors as a morphogenetic regulator. Science **251:** 1451–1455.
86. Aberle, H., S. Blutz, J. Stappert, H. Weissing, R. Kemler & H. Hosschuetzky. 1994. Assembly of the cadherin-catenin complex *in vitro* with recombinant proteins. J. Cell Sci. **107:** 3655–3663.
87. Jou, T.-S., D.B. Stewart, J. Stappert, W.J. Nelson & J.A. Marrs. 1995. Genetic and biochemical dissection of protein linkages in the cadherin-catenin complex. Proc. Natl. Acad. Sci. USA **92:** 5067–5071.
88. Knudsen, K. A., A. Peralta Soler, K.R. Johnson & M.J. Wheelock. 1995. Interaction of α-actinin with the cadherin/catenin cell-cell adhesion complex via a-catenin. J. Cell Biol. **130:** 1–11.
89. Rimm, D. L., E.R. Koslov, P. Kebriaei, C.D. Cianci & J.S. Morrow. 1995. α1(E)-catenin is an actin-binding and -bundling protein mediating the attachment of F-actin to the membrane adhesion complex. Proc. Natl. Acad. Sci. USA **92:** 8813–8817.
90. Edelman, G.M., W.J. Gallin, A. Delouvee, B.A. Cunningham & J.-P. Thiery. 1989. Early epochal maps of two different cell adhesion molecules. Proc. Natl. Acad. Sci. USA **80:** 4384–4388.
91. Hatta, K. & M. Takeichi. 1986. Expression of N-cadherin adhesion molecules associated with early morphogenetic events in chick development. Nature **320:** 447–449.
92. Holt, C.E., P. Lemaire & J.B. Gurdon. 1994. Cadherin-mediated cell interactions are necessary for the activation of MyoD in *Xenopus mesoderm*. Proc. Natl. Acad. Sci. USA **91:** 10844–10848.
93. Radice, G.L., H. Rayburn, H. Matsunami, K.A. Knudsen, M. Takeichi & R. Hynes. 1997. Developmental defects in mouse embryos lacking N-cadherin. Dev. Biol. **181:** 64–78.
94. McDonald, K.A., A.F. Horwitz & K.A. Knudsen. 1995. Adhesion molecules and skeletal myogenesis. Semin. Dev. Biol. **6:** 105–116.
95. Hamburger, V. & H.L. Hamilton. 1951. A series of normal stages in development of the chick embryo. J. Morphol. **88:** 49–92.
96. Bader, D., T. Masaki & D.A. Fischman. 1982. Immunochemical analysis of myosin heavy chain during avian myogenesis *in vivo* and *in vitro*. J. Cell Biol. **95:** 763–770.
97. Eyal-Giladi, H. & S. Kochav. 1976. From cleavage to primitive streak formation: A complementary normal table and a new look at the first stages of the development of the chick. Dev. Biol. **49:** 321–337.
98. Shimizu, N. & Y. Shimada. 1985. Immunochemical analysis of troponin T isoforms in embryonic, adult, regenerating, and denervated chicken fast skeletal muscle. Dev. Biol. **111:** 324–334.
99. Holmdahl, R., K. Rubin, L. Klareskog, E. Larsson & H. Wigzell. 1986. Characterization of the antibody response in mice with type II collagen-induced arthritis, using monoclonal anti-type II collagen antibodies. Arthritis Rheum. **29:** 400–410.
100. Yamada, T., M. Placzek, H. Tanaka, J. Dodd & T.M. Jessel. 1991. Control of the cell pattern in the developing nervous system: Polarizing activity of the floor plate notochord. Cell **64:** 635–647.
101. Peralta Soler, A. & K. Knudsen. 1994. N-cadherin involvement in cardiac involvement in cardiac myocyte interaction and myofibrillogenesis. Dev. Biol. **162:** 9–17.
102. Wheelock, M. J. & K.A. Knudsen. 1991. N-cadherin-associated proteins in chicken muscle. Differentiation **46:** 35–42.
103. Hatta, K. & M. Takeichi. 1986. Expression of N-cadherin adhesion molecules associated with early morphogenetic events in chick development. Nature **320:** 447–449.
104. Yablonka-Reuveni, Z. & A.J. Rivera. 1994. Temporal expression of regulatory and structural muscle proteins during myogenesis of satellite cells on isolated adult rat fibers. Dev. Biol. **164:** 588–603.

Regulation of the *Sex Combs Reduced* Gene in *Drosophila*

JAMES A. KENNISON,[a,d] MARTHA VÁZQUEZ,[b] AND BRENDA J. BRIZUELA[c]

[a]*Laboratory of Molecular Genetics, National Institute of Child Health and Human Development, National Institutes of Health, Bethesda, Maryland 20892-2785, USA*
[b]*Departamento de Genética y Fisiología Molecular, Instituto de Biotecnología, UNAM, Cuernavaca, Morelos 62250, México*
[c]*Howard Hughes Medical Institute, Department of Biological Chemistry, University of California, Los Angeles, Los Angeles, California 90024-1737, USA*

> ABSTRACT: The *Sex combs reduced* gene of the Antennapedia complex specifies the identities of the anterior thoracic and posterior head segments, including the primordium of the larval salivary gland. The *Sex combs reduced* transcription unit spans over 30 kb of genomic DNA, with another 40 kb of upstream *cis*-regulatory sequences. The pattern of *Sex combs reduced* transcription is set in the early embryo by the segmentation genes and is then maintained by two competing sets of proteins, the Polycomb group and the trithorax group. One of the trithorax group genes required for activation, the *brahma* gene, encodes an evolutionarily conserved DNA-stimulated ATPase that is part of a large protein complex. This complex facilitates the action of sequence-specific, DNA-binding proteins in regulating target genes, possibly by altering chromatin structure.

INTRODUCTION

The larval salivary gland of *Drosophila* forms during embryogenesis in a region of the fly called parasegment 2. The identity of parasegment 2 is specified by the homeotic *Sex combs reduced (Scr)* gene of the Antennapedia complex. That the formation of the salivary gland is determined by *Scr* was shown by altering *Scr* expression.[1,2] Mutants that lack *Scr* function failed to develop salivary glands in the normal location. By contrast, ectopic expression of *Scr* proteins in the wrong part of the embryo caused the appearance of ectopic salivary glands. Thus, *Scr* specifies the formation of salivary glands. Although *Scr* proteins are expressed both dorsally and ventrally in a two-parasegment region of the embryo, salivary glands develop only in the ventral part of the first of the two parasegments. In another paper in this series, Deborah Andrew will discuss the factors that restrict the development of salivary glands to only this subset of the *Scr*-expressing cells of the embryo. We will focus here on the *cis*-regulatory elements and the *trans*-acting factors that are responsible for defining and maintaining the patterns of *Scr* expression. The *trans*-acting factors are encoded by four groups of genes, shown in FIGURE 1. The first group of genes, the segmentation genes, not only divide the embryo into segments, but also set the initial domains of expression of *Scr* and the other homeotic genes. The second group of genes that limit *Scr* expression are the other HOM genes, the homeotic genes of the Antennapedia and bithorax complexes. Finally, the last two groups of genes, the Polycomb and trithorax group genes,

---

[d] Address for correspondence: James A. Kennison, Bldg. 6B, Room 3B-331, NIH, Bethesda, MD 20892-2785. Tel: (301) 496-8399; fax: (301) 496-0243; e-mail: jkl5o@nih.gov

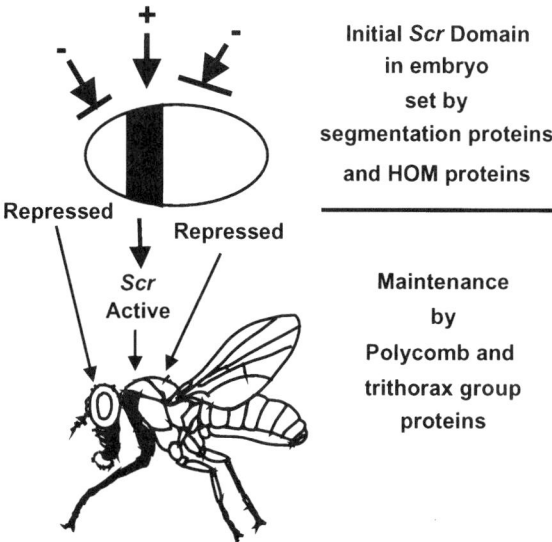

FIGURE 1. A hierarchy of genes regulates the expression and function of *Scr*. The initial domains of *Scr* expression are determined by the segmentation proteins and refined by cross-regulatory interactions among the other HOM genes. After early embryogenesis, both *Scr* repression and activation are maintained throughout embryogenesis and larval growth until differentiation of the adult structures during pupation. Repression is maintained by the Polycomb group proteins and activation by the trithorax group proteins.

help to maintain these patterns of homeotic gene expression through many cell divisions.

STRUCTURE OF THE *SCR* GENE AND ITS *CIS*-REGULATORY ELEMENTS

The *Scr* transcription unit spans about 30 kb of genomic DNA and encodes a homeodomain-containing protein.[3-7] *Scr* protein is thought to control pathways of development by binding directly to DNA sequences in target genes and activating or repressing transcription.[8,9] At least one mammalian homologue, the mouse *HOX-1.3* protein, functions in *Drosophila* to mimic some *Scr* functions.[10] In addition to the 30 kb transcription unit, the *Scr* gene includes an additional 40 kb of upstream *cis*-regulatory sequences.[7,11,12] The *Scr* transcription unit and its upstream regulatory region are shown in FIGURE 2. Many of the *cis*-regulatory elements appear to be redundant, but so far, only one enhancer element for driving *Scr* expression in the salivary gland has been identified. This element is within a 6 kb genomic DNA fragment from a region that is about 20 kb upstream of the *Scr* transcription unit.[11,12] Although the *fushi tarazu (ftz)* transcription unit is between this enhancer element and the *Scr* promoter, the enhancer element activates the *Scr* promoter while ignoring the *ftz* promoter.[11,13,14] The molecular mechanism for this promoter specificity remains to be determined.

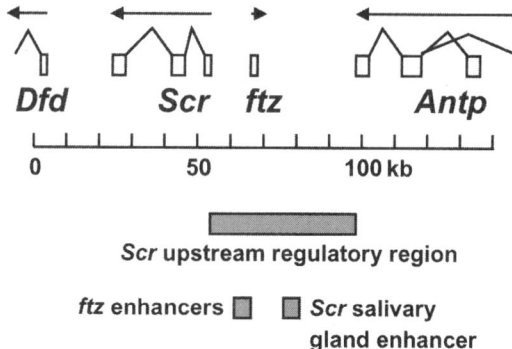

FIGURE 2. The *Scr* gene spans a region of about 70 kb of genomic DNA. The transcription units in the *Scr* region of the genome are shown at the top of the FIGURE by the arrows indicating the length and direction of each transcription unit. Only the 5' end of the *Deformed (Dfd)* and the 3' end of the Antennapedia *(Antp)* transcription units are shown. The open boxes directly below each transcription unit show the exons that are spliced to generate the transcripts for each gene. Several of the small introns in *Antp* and *ftz* are not shown. The horizontal line in the middle indicates the genomic DNA (in kb) spanning this region. The shaded boxes at the bottom of the FIGURE indicate some of the known *cis*-regulatory regions, including the 40 kb *Scr* upstream regulatory region, the *ftz* enhancers, and the *Scr* salivary gland enhancer.

TRANS-ACTING FACTORS THAT REGULATE *SCR* EXPRESSION

When the *Scr* gene is first transcribed in the early embryo, the initial domains of expression are set by the action of the segmentation genes,[4] the genes that also act to divide the embryo into segments. Cross-regulatory interactions among the HOM genes also help to define these initial domains. *Antennapedia,* which is expressed in a region of the embryo just posterior to *Scr,* represses *Scr* expression in the epidermis, but positively regulates *Scr* in the mesoderm.[4,15] Transcriptional silencing of *Scr* is maintained in the regions that are anterior and posterior to its initial domain throughout embryogenesis and larval growth by the action of at least a dozen transcriptional repressors called the Polycomb (PC) group genes.[16–18] The PC group genes were first identified because PC group mutations cause derepression of *Scr* in the cells that form the second and third legs of the adult. The ectopic *Scr* expression causes these cells to differentiate structures characteristic of the first leg in place of second- and third-leg structures.[19] There is a row of very distinctive bristles called the sex comb that is normally found on the first leg of adult males. PC group mutations cause the appearance of sex combs on all three legs of adult males and have names such as *Polycomb, extra sex combs,* and *Additional sex combs.*[16,18] PC group mutations not only derepress *Scr* in the cells that form the adult, but also derepress *Scr* in the embryo.[4,19–21]

Many of the PC group genes have been cloned[18,22,23] and appear to encode chromatin-associated proteins that are thought to silence homeotic genes either by forming chromatin structures that block binding of transcription factors, or by preventing proteins bound to upstream *cis*-regulatory elements from interacting with basal transcription factors bound at the promoter.[22,24–27] Regardless of the molecular mechanisms of PC group silencing, the extra sex combs phenotype caused by *Scr* derepression in the cells that form the adult cuticle provides a good assay for *Scr* function. We have used this phenotype to identify genes that are required for *Scr* expression or function during larval growth.[28,29] These genes are members of a group of positive regulators of the homeotic genes. This group is called the trithorax (TRX) group of genes, after one of its best-characterized members, *trithorax*.[18,30,31] The rationale that we have used to identify new TRX group genes is straightforward. For most genes in *Drosophila*, the amount of gene product is proportional to the number of copies of the gene. Flies with only a single copy of an autosomal gene have only half as much gene product as flies with two copies. Although such reductions in amount of gene product usually have no phenotypes in wild-type flies, they are often not sufficient under more limiting conditions. The *Scr* derepression phenotype in the adult legs provides a very sensitive assay for *Scr* function. Mutations that are lethal when homozygous can be isolated in heterozygotes by their suppression of the *Scr* derepression phenotype. We have isolated mutations in five known and thirteen new TRX group genes.[28] Because we believe that the new TRX group genes are required for determining cell fates, we have given them names that have connotations with fate in different languages. As examples, *brahma* is one of the Hindu gods of fate, *moira* is a Greek word for fate, and *kismet* is a Turkish word for fate. Although isolated because of their functions during larval growth, many of the TRX group genes are also required for *Scr* expression or function during embryogenesis.[32–38]

THE *BRAHMA* PROTEIN IS REQUIRED FOR *SCR* TRANSCRIPTION

Among the TRX group genes required for *Scr* transcription, we have characterized the *brahma* (*brm*) gene extensively.[32,39] Embryos that lack a functional *brm* gene die late in embryogenesis with few defects. These mutant embryos, however, have high levels of maternally encoded wild-type *brm* transcripts deposited in the unfertilized egg. When the levels of these maternally encoded transcripts are reduced, developmental defects are seen as early as the cellular blastoderm stage. Thus, the maternally encoded *brm* proteins are necessary for early embryogenesis. Both the maternal and zygotic *brm* transcripts appear to encode identical proteins of 1638 amino acids. The *brm* protein is very similar to a yeast transcriptional activator called *SWI2/SNF2*. Two mammalian *brm* homologues have also been identified, *HBRM* and *BRG1* in humans and *MBRM* and *BRG1* in the mouse.[40–43] The evolutionary relationships among these proteins is shown in FIGURE 3. Both *HBRM* and *BRG1* are about equally divergent from the *Drosophila brm* protein (about 50% identical across the entire protein). They are about 75% identical to each other but more than 90% identical to their homologues from mouse.

What is the function of the *brm*-related proteins in transcription? Both the *Drosophila* and yeast proteins are required for the transcriptional activation of multiple genes. In yeast, *SWI2/SNF2* is required for inducible, but not basal, transcription of target genes.[44] We are not sure what constitutes basal transcription in *Drosophila*, inasmuch as almost every gene appears to be developmentally regulated when examined carefully. The yeast, *Drosophila*, and mammalian *brm*-related proteins are all part of large protein complexes (called SWI/SNF complexes) of about two million Da in molecular mass.[45–50] The SWI/SNF complexes are not required for *in vitro* transcription from naked DNA but can facilitate transcription when chromatin templates are used.[50–52] This has lead to the suggestion that the SWI/SNF complexes remodel chromatin structure to facilitate the binding of proteins to their target sites.[53,54] This is shown in FIGURE 4. The SWI/SNF complexes may be part of the even larger RNA polymerase II holoenzyme.[55] Recently, we have been able to demonstrate genetic interactions between mutations in *brm* and *Taf110* (which encodes the 110 kDa subunit of the basal transcription factor TFIID) in *Drosophila*, again suggesting a direct interaction between the SWI/SNF complexes and the basal transcription factors bound at pro-

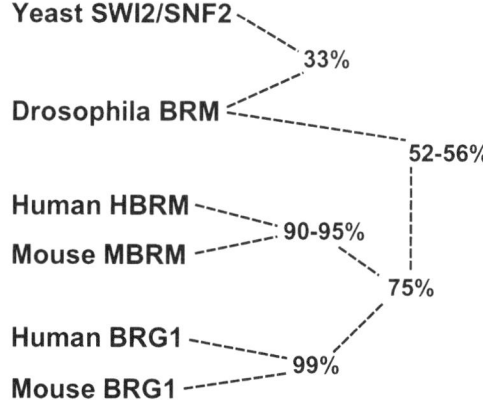

FIGURE 3. The brm-related proteins from yeast, *Drosophila,* and mammals are highly conserved. The percentages are the approximate amino acid sequence identities between various members of the family.

moters. In addition to multiple mammalian SWI/SNF complexes,[47,48] other chromatin remodeling complexes have been isolated.[56,57]

One of the conserved domains within the *brm*-related family of proteins is a region of about 700 amino acids that appears to be a DNA-stimulated ATPase domain.[33,58] This domain has been found in several other *Drosophila* proteins, including *ISWI*,[59] the *89B helicase*,[60] and *CHD1*.[61,62] *ISWI* is part of a chromatin remodeling complex called NURF (nucleosome remodeling factor),[57,63] and the *89B helicase* may be encoded by another of the TRX group genes, *moira*.[33] It will be very interesting to determine which of the other TRX group genes encode subunits of chromatin remodeling complexes. In addition, it is expected that other TRX group proteins will play different roles in regulating transcription or function of the *Scr* gene during development.

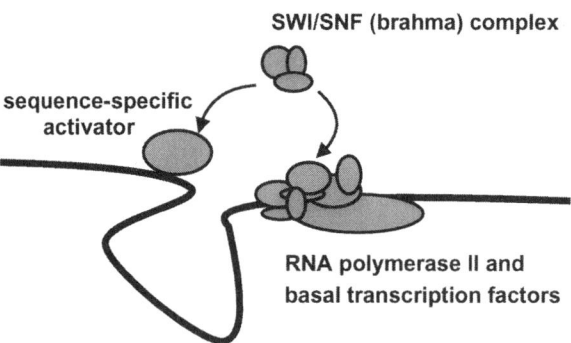

FIGURE 4. The SWI/SNF protein complexes may act to facilitate binding of either sequence-specific activator proteins, basal transcription factors, or both, to their respective target DNA sequences. Different SWI/SNF complexes may facilitate the binding of different sequence-specific activators.

REFERENCES

1. PANZER, S., D. WEIGEL & S.K. BECKENDORF. 1992. Organogenesis in *Drosophila melanogaster*: Embryonic salivary gland determination is controlled by homeotic and dorsoventral patterning genes. Development **114:** 49–57.
2. ANDREW, D.J., M.A. HORNER, M.G. PETITT, S.M. SMOLIK & M.P. SCOTT. 1994. Setting limits on homeotic gene function: Restraint of *Sex combs reduced* activity by *teashirt* and other homeotic genes. EMBO J. **13:** 1132–1144.
3. KUROIWA, A., U. KLOTER, P. BAUMGARTNER & W.J. GEHRING. 1985. Cloning of the homeotic *Sex combs reduced* gene in *Drosophila* and *in situ* localization of its transcripts. EMBO J. **4:** 3757–3764.
4. RILEY, P.D., S.B. CARROLL & M.P. SCOTT. 1987. The expression and regulation of *Sex combs reduced* protein in *Drosophila* embryos. Genes 4 Dev. **1:** 716–730.
5. MAHAFFEY, J.W. & T.C. KAUFMAN. 1987. Distribution of the *Sex combs reduced* gene products in *Drosophila melanogaster*. Genetics **117:** 51–60.
6. LEMOTTE, P.K., A. KUROIWA, L.I. FESSLER & W.J. GEHRING. 1989. The homeotic gene *Sex combs reduced* of Drosophila: Gene structure and embryonic expression. EMBO J. **8:** 219–227.
7. PATTATUCCI, A.M., D.C. OTTESON & T.C. KAUFMAN. 1991. A functional and structural analysis of the *Sex combs reduced* locus of *Drosophila melanogaster*. Genetics **129:** 423–441.
8. HAYASHI, S. & M.P. SCOTT. 1990. What determines the specificity of action of Drosophila homeodomain proteins. Cell **63:** 883–894.
9. AFFOLTER, M., A. SCHIER & W.J. GEHRING. 1990. Homeodomain proteins and the regulation of gene expression. Curr. Opin. Cell Biol. **2:** 485–495.
10. ZHAO, J.J., R.A. LAZZARINI & L. PICK. 1993. The mouse *Hox-1.3* gene is functionally equivalent to the *Drosophila Sex combs reduced* gene. Genes & Dev. **7:** 343–354.
11. GINDHART JR., J.G., A.N. KING & T.C. KAUFMAN. 1995. Characterization of the cis-regulatory region of the Drosophila homeotic gene *Sex combs reduced*. Genetics **139:** 781–795.
12. GORMAN, M.J. & T.C. KAUFMAN. 1995. Genetic analysis of embryonic cis-acting regulatory elements of the Drosophila homeotic gene *Sex combs reduced*. Genetics **140:** 557–572.
13. HAFEN, E., A. KUROIWA & W.J. GEHRING. 1984. Spatial distribution of transcripts from the segmentation gene *fushi tarazu* during Drosophila embryonic development. Cell **37:** 833–841.
14. HIROMI, Y., A. KUROIWA & W.J. GEHRING. 1985. Control elements of the Drosophila segmentation gene *fushi tarazu*. Cell **43:** 603–613.
15. REUTER, R. & M.P. SCOTT. 1990. Expression and function of the homoeotic genes *Antennapedia* and *Sex combs reduced* in the embryonic midgut of *Drosophila*. Development **109:** 289–303.
16. JÜRGENS, G. 1985. A group of genes controlling the spatial expression of the bithorax complex in *Drosophila*. Nature **316:** 153–155.
17. PARO, R. 1993. Mechanisms of heritable gene repression during development of Drosophila. Curr. Opin. Cell Biol. **5:** 999–1005.
18. KENNISON, J.A. 1995. The Polycomb and trithorax group proteins of *Drosophila*: Trans-regulators of homeotic gene function. Annu. Rev. Genet. **29:** 289–303.
19. PATTATUCCI, A.M. & T.C. KAUFMAN. 1991. The homeotic gene *Sex combs reduced* of *Drosophila melanogaster* is differentially regulated in the embryonic and imaginal stages of development. Genetics **129:** 443–461.
20. GLICKSMAN, M.A. & D.L. BROWER. 1990. Persistent ectopic expression of *Drosophila* homeotic genes resulting from maternal deficiency of the *extra sex combs* gene product. Dev. Biol. **142:** 422–431.
21. MCKEON, J. & H.W. BROCK. 1991. Interactions of the *Polycomb* group of genes with homeotic loci of *Drosophila*. Roux's Arch. Dev. Biol. **199:** 387–396.
22. PIRROTTA, V. & L. RASTELLI. 1994. *White* gene expression, repressive chromatin domains and homeotic gene regulation in *Drosophila*. Bioessays **16:** 549–556.

23. MOEHRLE, A. & R. PARO. 1994. Spreading the silence: Epigenetic transcriptional regulation during *Drosophila* development. Dev. Gene. **15:** 478–484.
24. ZINK, D. & R. PARO. 1995. *Drosophila* Polycomb-group regulated chromatin inhibits the accessibility of a *trans*-activator to its target DNA. EMBO J. **14:** 5660–5671.
25. SCHLOSSHERR, J., H. EGGERT, R. PARO, S. CREMER & R.S. JACK. 1994. Gene inactivation in *Drosophila* mediated by the *Polycomb* gene product or by position-effect variegation does not involve major changes in the accessibility of the chromatin fibre. Mol. Gen. Genet. **243:** 453–462.
26. BIENZ, M. & J. MÜLLER. 1995. Transcriptional silencing of homeotic genes in *Drosophila*. Bioessays **17:** 775–784.
27. CHAN, C.-S., L. RASTELLI & V. PIRROTTA. 1994. A *Polycomb* response element in the *Ubx* gene that determines an epigenetically inherited state of repression. EMBO J. **13:** 2553–2564.
28. KENNISON, J.A. & J.W. TAMKUN. 1988. Dosage-dependent modifiers of Polycomb and Antennapedia mutations in Drosophila. Proc. Natl. Acad. Sci. USA **85:** 8136–8140.
29. KENNISON, J.A. & J.W. TAMKUN. 1992. Trans-regulation of homeotic genes in *Drosophila*. New Biol. **4:** 91–96.
30. SHEARN, A. 1989. The *ash-1, ash-2* and *trithorax* genes of *Drosophila melanogaster* are functionally related. Genetics **121:** 517–525.
31. KENNISON, J.A. 1993. Transcriptional activation of *Drosophila* homeotic genes from distant regulatory elements. Trends Genet. **9:** 75–79.
32. BRIZUELA, B.J., L. ELFRING, J. BALLARD, J.W. TAMKUN & J.A. KENNISON. 1994. Genetic analysis of the *brahma* gene of *Drosophila melanogaster* and polytene chromosome subdivisions 72AB. Genetics **137:** 803–813.
33. BRIZUELA, B.J. & J.A. KENNISON. 1997. The *Drosophila* homeotic gene *moira* regulates expression of *engrailed* and HOM genes in imaginal tissues. Mech. Dev. **65:** 209–220.
34. HARDING, K.W., G. GELLON, N. MCGINNIS & W. MCGINNIS. 1995. A screen for modifiers of *Deformed* function in Drosophila. Genetics **140:** 1339–1352.
35. TRIPOULAS, N.A., E. HERSPERGER, D. LA JEUNESSE & A. SHEARN. 1994. Molecular genetic analysis of the *Drosophila melanogaster* gene *absent, small or homeotic discs1 (ash1)*. Genetics **137:** 1027–1038.
36. COHEN, B., E.A. WIMMER & S.M. COHEN. 1991. Early development of leg and wing primordia in the *Drosophila* embryo. Mech. Dev. **33:** 229–240.
37. INGHAM, P.W. & J.R.S. WHITTLE. 1980. *Trithorax*: A new homoeotic mutation of *Drosophila melanogaster* causing transformations of abdominal and thoracic imaginal segments. I. Putative role during embryogenesis. Mol. Gen. Genet. **179:** 607–614.
38. GAUSZ, J., G. BENCZE, H. GYURKOVICS, M. ASHBURNER, D. ISH-HOROWICZ & J.J. HOLDEN. 1979. Genetic characterization of the 87C region of the third chromosome of *Drosophila melanogaster*. Genetics **93:** 917–934.
39. TAMKUN, J.W., R. DEURING, M.P. SCOTT, M. KISSINGER, A.M. PATTATUCCI, T.C. KAUFMAN & J.A. KENNISON. 1992. *Brahma*: A regulator of Drosophila homeotic genes structurally related to the yeast transcriptional activator SNF2/SWI2. Cell **68:** 561–572.
40. KHAVARI, P.A., C.L. PETERSON, J.W. TAMKUN, D.B. MENDEL & G.R. CRABTREE. 1993. BRG1 contains a conserved domain of the *SWI2/SNF2* family necessary for normal mitotic growth and transcription. Nature **366:** 170–174.
41. RANDAZZO, F.M., P. KHAVARI, G. CRABTREE, J. TAMKUN & J. ROSSANT. 1994. *brg1:* A putative murine homologue of the *Drosophila brahma* gene, a homeotic gene regulator. Dev. Biol. **161:** 229–242.
42. CHIBA, H., M. MURAMATSU, A. NOMOTO & H. KATO. 1994. Two human homologues of *Saccharomyces cerevisiae SWI2/SNF2* and *Drosophila brahma* are transcriptional coactivators cooperating with the estrogen receptor and the retinoic acid receptor. Nucleic Acids Res. **22:** 1815–1820.
43. MUCHARDT, C. & M. YANIV. 1993. A human homologue of *Saccharomyces cerevisiae SNF2/SWI2* and *Drosophila brm* genes potentiates transcriptional activation by the glucocorticoid receptor. EMBO J. **12:** 4279–4290.
44. PETERSON, C.L. & I. HERSKOWITZ. 1992. Characterization of the yeast SWI1, SWI2, and SWI3 genes, which encode a global activator of transcription. Cell **68:** 573–583.

45. DINGWALL, A.K., S.J. BEEK, C.M. MCCALLUM, J.W. TAMKUN, G.V. KALPANA, S.P. GOFF & M.P. SCOTT. 1995. The *Drosophila* snr1 and brm proteins are related to yeast SWI/SNF proteins and are components of a large protein complex. Mol. Biol. Cell **6:** 777–791.
46. CAIRNS, B.R., Y.-J. KIM, M.H. SAYRE, B.C. LAURENT & R.D. KORNBERG. 1994. A multisubunit complex containing the *SWI1/ADR6, SWI2/SNF2, SWI3, SNF5,* and *SNF6* gene products isolated from yeast. Proc. Natl. Acad. Sci. USA **91:** 1950–1954.
47. WANG, W., J. COTE, Y. XUE, S. ZHOU, P.A. KHAVARI, S.R. BIGGAR, C. MUCHARDT, G.V. KALPANA *et al.* 1996. Purification and biochemical heterogeneity of the mammalian SWI-SNF complex. EMBO J. **15:** 5370–5382.
48. WANG, W., Y. XUE, S. ZHOU, A. KUO, B.R. CAIRNS & G.R. CRABTREE. 1996. Diversity and specialization of mammalian SWI/SNF complexes. Genes Dev. **10:** 2117–2130.
49. PETERSON, C.L., A. DINGWALL & M.P. SCOTT. 1994. Five *SWI/SNF* gene products are components of a large multisubunit complex required for transcriptional enhancement. Proc. Natl. Acad. Sci. USA **91:** 2905–2908.
50. KWON, H., A.N. IMBALZANO, P.A. KHAVARI, R.E. KINGSTON & M.R. GREEN. 1994. Nucleosome disruption and enhancement of activator binding by a human SW1/SNF complex. Nature **370:** 477–481.
51. IMBALZANO, A.N., H. KWON, M.R. GREEN & R.E. KINGSTON. 1994. Facilitated binding of TATA-binding protein to nucleosomal DNA. Nature **370:** 481–485.
52. COTÉ, J., J. QUINN, J.L. WORKMAN & C.L. PETERSON. 1994. Stimulation of GAL4 derivative binding to nucleosomal DNA by the yeast SWI/SNF complex. Science **265:** 53–60.
53. WINSON, F. & M. CARLSON. 1992. Yeast SNF/SWI transcriptional activators and the SPT/SIN chromatin connection. Trends Genet. **8:** 387–391.
54. PETERSON, C.L. 1996. Multiple SWItches to turn on chromatin? Curr. Opin. Genet. Dev. **6:** 171–175.
55. WILSON, C.J., D.M. CHAO, A.N. IMBALZANO, G.R. SCHNITZLER, R.E. KINGSTON & R.A. YOUNG. 1996. RNA polymerase II holoenzyme contains SWI/SNF regulators involved in chromatin remodeling. Cell **84:** 235–244.
56. CAIRNS, B.R., Y. LORCH, Y. LI, M.C. ZHANG, L. LACOMIS, H. ERDJUMENTBROMAGE, P. TEMPST, J. DU *et al.* 1996. RSC, an essential, abundant chromatin-remodeling complex. Cell **87:** 1249–1260.
57. TSUKIYAMA, T. & C. WU. 1995. Purification and properties of an ATP-dependent nucleosome remodeling factor. Cell **83:** 1011–1020.
58. LAURENT, B.C., I. TREICH & M. CARLSON. 1993. The yeast SNF2/SWI2 protein has DNA-stimulated ATPase activity required for transcriptional activation. Genes Dev. **7:** 583–591.
59. ELFRING, L.K., R. DEURING, C.M. MCCALLUM, C.L. PETERSON & J.W. TAMKUN. 1994. Identification and characterization of *Drosophila* relatives of the yeast transcriptional activator SNF2/SWI2. Mol. Cell. Biol. **14:** 2225–2234.
60. GOLDMAN-LEVI, R., C. MILLER, J. BOGOCH & N.B. ZAK. 1996. Expanding the Mot1 subfamily: 89B helicase encodes a new *Drosophila melanogaster* SNF2-related protein which binds to multiple sites on polytene chromosomes. Nucleic Acids Res. **24:** 3121–3128.
61. DELMAS, V., D.G. STOKES & R.P. PERRY. 1993. A mammalian DNA-binding protein that contains a chromodomain and an SNF2/SWI2-like helicase domain. Proc. Natl. Acad. Sci. USA **90:** 2414–2418.
62. STOKES, D.G. & R.P. PERRY. 1995. DNA-binding and chromatin localization properties of CHD1. Mol. Cell. Biol. **15:** 2745–2753.
63. TSUKIYAMA, T., C. DANIEL, J. TAMKUN & C. WU. 1995. *ISWI,* a member of the SWI2/SNF2 ATPase family, encodes the 140 kDa subunit of the nucleosome remodeling factor. Cell **83:** 1021–1026.

Integrins and Development: How Might These Receptors Regulate Differentiation of the Lens

SUE MENKO,[a] NANCY PHILP, BOB VENEZIALE, AND JANICE WALKER

Department of Pathology, Anatomy and Cell Biology, Thomas Jefferson University, 571 Jefferson Alumni Hall, 1020 Locust Street, Philadelphia, Pennsylvania 19107, USA

> ABSTRACT: Integrins transduce both internal signals and signals from the matrix. These interactions between integrins, their extracellular matrix ligands, and their cytoskeletal partners play an important role in the regulation of cellular differentiation. We have shown them to be important in lens cell differentiation. In the lens capsule there is a compartmentalization of matrix components with fibronectin, primarily localized to the anterior capsule, and tenascin in the posterior capsule. Integrins are developmentally regulated in the lens. $\alpha 5\beta 1$ integrin, like fibronectin, is primarily associated with the lens epithelial cells, where together they are likely to be important in regulation of adhesion and proliferation. $\alpha 6A\beta 1$, the integrin laminin receptor, is expressed at its highest levels in the equatorial epithelium and the peripheral fiber cells, both migratory populations. Because laminin is uniformly distributed in the lens capsule, such changes in $\alpha 6A$ integrin expression are likely critical to the cell's ability to regulate its response to laminin in the matrix. The organization of cytoskeletal molecules associated with the integrin cytoplasmic face also changes with development. In the epithelial regions of the lens, where the initiation of lens cell differentiation occurs, expression of the cytoskeletal proteins involved in cell-substrate interactions, talin, α-actinin, and the signaling proteins, are high. In the fiber cell region of the lens, where the cells establish stable cell-cell contacts, vinculin predominates and becomes highly associated with the cytoskeletal fraction. The role of integrins in lens development is not only regulated by changes in the expression of different integrin receptors but is also closely correlated with the expression and organization of the molecules with which they associate.

Regulation of cellular differentiation is, in part, dependent upon the interplay among the integrins, their extracellular matrix ligands, and their cytoskeletal partners. As transmembrane receptors, the integrins serve as a link in both outside-in and inside-out signaling events critical to many aspects of differentiation and development.[1] In transmitting information from their matrix environment, the integrin cytoplasmic domains initiate a signaling cascade, through the MAP kinase pathway, which leads to alterations in gene expression.[2] Therefore, changes in expression or organization of the matrix environment can regulate the initiation or maintenance of the differentiated state of a cell, outside-in signaling. Integrins also respond to signals from within the cell, undergoing either changes in expression or changes in conformation, both of which result in altering the way a cell interacts with its environment, inside-out signaling. Changes in integrin conformation have been shown to alter its affinity for its ligand.[3] This most likely results in a change in the association of the cytoskeleton with the cytoplasmic domain of the receptor. Therefore, the organization of cytoskeletal proteins into focal adhesion complexes is likely to serve as a regulator of cell differentiation.

Changes in the expression of extracellular matrix components have long been known to effect differentiation and development.[4-7] Recently, it has been demonstrated that ini-

---

[a] Tel: (215) 503-7845; fax: (215) 923-3808.

tiation of the differentiation of kidney, lung, and salivary gland epithelia can be correlated with the expression of a specific form of the basal lamina component laminin, known as laminin-1.[8–10] Many different integrins have been demonstrated to play specific roles in differentiation and development. Expression of the integrin laminin receptor, α6β1, is specifically correlated with the differentiation of kidney and salivary gland epithelia.[8,11] Changes in the affinity state of α5β1, a fibronectin receptor, play an important role in both keratinocyte and skeletal muscle differentiation.[12,13] The ability of myoblasts to initiate their differentiation and become postmitotic myocytes requires a reduction in affinity of α5β1 for fibronectin, but not a downregulation in α5β1 itself.[13] In keratinocyte differentiation α5β1 loses its affinity for fibronectin, allowing the cells to move away from the substratum, and only later becomes downregulated.[12] Because of the ability to change its affinity state, it is clear that the level of integrin expression does not regulate integrin function. Fibronectin-α5β1 integrin interactions are important in regulating cell motility[13,14] and in intracellular signaling through focal adhesion kinase (FAK).[15,16] In addition, α5 integrin has been shown to be required for cell proliferation, linked to a cell's fibroblast growth factor (FGF) responsiveness.[17]

We have examined the role of extracellular matrix expression, integrin expression, and cytoskeletal organization in the unique differentiation events that lead to the morphogenesis of a lens. Few systems lend themselves as beautifully to deciphering the interplay between integrins, their extracellular matrix ligands, and cytoplasmic-associated cytoskeletal and signaling molecules in differentiation as the lens. This is because a 10-day chick embryo lens exhibits a continuum of differentiation from the anterior epithelial cells to the mature fiber cells. Four distinct zones of differentiation are easily identified in the lens: (1) The anterior epithelium, a monolayer of undifferentiated but committed lens epithelial cells, serves as a progenitor population. (2) The equatorial epithelium, where initiation of lens fiber cell differentiation begins, is found along the equator of the lens and is separated from the anterior epithelium by a proliferative zone. The fiber cell region of the lens can be dissected into two zones. (3) The peripheral fiber cells, which contain cells undergoing fiber cell maturation, continue to differentiate as they migrate towards the central zone of the lens. Their differentiation involves cell elongation, cell migration, and loss of nuclei and organelles. (4) The central or core fiber cells of the lens are terminally differentiated.

The developing lens, from the time it pinches off from head ectoderm as the lens vesicle, is surrounded by a matrix known as the lens capsule. It has been shown by us and others that basement membrane proteins laminin and type IV collagen[18] are distributed in all regions of the capsule in the developing lens. The uniformity in distribution of the basal lamina proteins in the lens capsule was surprising because lens cells at all stages of differentiation associate with the capsule. If the matrix components of the capsule are instructive in events leading to lens differentiation, then one would expect a regulation of matrix components with lens epithelial cell differentiation. Upon further examination of other matrix molecules, we have found that to be the case. Fibronectin and tenascin are compartmentalized within the embryonic lens capsule. In a 10-day chick embryo lens, fibronectin is found limited to the anterior capsule, in association with the anterior epithelium. Fibronectin extends into the capsule in contact with the most anterior regions of the equatorial epithelium. By contrast, tenascin is expressed in the posterior capsule, in association with fiber cells, and extends through the capsule in the equatorial region, stopping at the interface of the equatorial epithelium with the anterior epithelium. The association of the lens epithelial cells with fibronectin in the capsule is likely the reason that the undifferentiated lens epithelial cells, as well as cells in the equatorial epithelium, are tightly adherent to the capsule.[19] Lens cells, as they differentiate, change their affinity for the capsule. The lens fiber cells, throughout their maturation, interact with, but are only loosely associated with, the posterior capsule.[19] Tenascin, sometimes classified as an antiadhesive protein, may be important in this process. Fibronectin is developmentally regulated, its expression decreasing between days 4 and 10 of development in the chick embryo. Microdissection of a 10-day lens into epithelial and fiber fractions reveals that fibronectin message, although present at a low level, is still being produced by the lens epithelial cells. However, no fibronectin message was detected in the lens fiber cells. A similar regulation of fibronectin was seen in lens cells undergoing differentiation in culture. At early times in culture, fibronectin message and protein are readily detected. At late culture times, after the formation of differentiated lentoid structures, the cells of which express features of lens fiber cells, fibronectin protein was still high, but fibronectin message had been dramatically downregulated. In both the embryonic chick lens and in a lens culture system, we have examined the expression of the integrin fibronectin receptor, α5β1, and have found that it also is regulated as a function of chick lens development and differentiation. α5 expression decreases between days 4 and 10 of chick embryo development. At 10 days, α5 is found primarily in the two epithelial fractions; however, a low level of α5 was still found associated with the peripheral fiber cells. Lens cultures also display a differentiation-dependent regulation of α5. These results indicate that in the lens, like in skeletal muscle and keratinocytes, α5β1 may loose its affinity for fibronectin before it is downregulated. The specific association of α5 and fibronectin with lens epithelial cells leaves them poised to play regulatory roles in lens development, not only in forming the close association between the lens epithelium and the lens capsule but in regulating proliferation that precedes the initiation of lens differentiation.

There are other changes in integrin expression that accompany lens cell differentiation. The integrin laminin receptor, α6Aβ1, is expressed at its highest levels in the equatorial epithelium and the peripheral fiber cells, both migratory populations. α6Aβ1 has been implicated in cell migration events in the differentiation of other cell types.[20] In contrast to α5 expression, α6A is maintained in the most differentiated fiber cells, the central fiber cells, although at a significantly lower level than in the peripheral fiber cells. Because laminin is uniformly distributed in the lens capsule, changes in α6 integrin expression are likely critical to the cell's ability to regulate its response to laminin in the matrix, as one might expect is necessary for migratory events in development.

Changes in the organization of cytoskeletal molecules in the lens are likely to reflect changes in integrin function and integrin signaling pathways specific to the differentiated state of the lens cell. The engagement of integrin receptors with cytoskeletal proteins has been implicated in altering receptor conformation, thereby changing receptor affinity for ligand interactions as well as stabilizing receptor interactions with counterreceptors.[3,21] Therefore, the association of integrins with the cytoskeletal apparatus can regulate both cell-substrate and cell-cell adhesion. We have examined changes in the association of proteins with the cytoskeleton in epithelial and fiber regions of the 10-day chick embryo lens by separating them into triton-soluble and insoluble (cytoskeletal associated) fractions. The results revealed that the organization of the cytoskeleton in the lens is highly regulated with differentiation and specific to each cytoskeletal molecule examined.

Talin is a molecule that associates with the cytoplasmic domain of β1 integrin and whose organization into focal adhesion structures has been used as a the hallmark of cell-substrate adhesion.[22–24] This cytoskeletal protein is expressed at much higher levels in lens epithelial cells than fiber cells. This is consistent with the tight association of the lens epithelial cells with the lens capsule. As is typical for this molecule, only a small percentage of talin is found in the triton-insoluble cytoskeletal fraction. α-actinin is a cytoskeletal protein that is found both at sites of cell-substrate[25] and cell-cell adhesion.[26] Like talin, it can bind to the cytoplasmic domain of β1 integrin[27] and is expressed at a much higher level in lens epithelial cells than in fiber cells. Its association with the cytoskeleton decreases in the fiber cell population. Vinculin is a cytoskeletal protein known to stabilize both cell-substrate and cell-cell interactions.[28,29] Unlike talin and α-actinin, expression of vinculin is dramatically upregulated with differentiation. In addition, there is a dramatic increase in the association of vinculin with the cytoskeleton of the differentiated lens fiber cells. This likely reflects the extensive cell-cell junctions that exist between the lens fiber cells.

There are other molecules associated with integrin adhesion structures that have been implicated in cell-signaling events. Paxillin is a vinculin-binding protein that has been shown to be regulated with development.[30,31] It has been implicated as a connector molecule in integrin signaling pathways.[32] In the lens, there is only a modest increase in the expression of paxillin with differentiation. However, its association with the cytoskeleton is dramatically increased in the fiber cell population. FAK is a tyrosine kinase that associates with the β1 integrin cytoplasmic domain and becomes phosphorylated upon the clustering of integrin molecules (necessary to obtain cell-substrate adhesion).[15,16] It phosphorylates downstream targets, such as paxillin, which can lead to changes in gene expression.[32] It is likely that by modifying the state of tyrosine phosphorylation of many of the cytoskeletal molecules discussed above, their association with adhesion structures is regulated. The expression and organization of FAK as a function of lens differentiation closely follows that of talin. Its overall expression is downregulated with differentiation, and only a small percentage is found associated with the cytoskeletal fraction.

The epithelial regions of the lens are in close contact with the lens capsule, migrate along the matrix components that constitute the capsule, and change their association with this capsule after they initiate their differentiation. In these regions of the lens, expression of the cytoskeletal proteins involved in cell-substrate interactions, talin, α-actinin, and the signaling proteins, are high. In the fiber-cell region of the lens, the cells establish stable cell-cell contacts over the long expanses of membrane interfaces between individual fiber cells. In this region, vinculin predominates and becomes highly associated with the cytoskeletal fraction.

The role of integrins in lens development is not only regulated by changes in the expression of different integrin receptors but is also closely correlated with the expression and organization of the molecules with which they associate. The events involved in lens differentiation involve cell migration, changes in cell shape and volume, and loss of nuclei, an apoptotic event. All of these characteristics, critical in forming a tissue whose primary function is the transmission and refraction of light, could be attributed to integrin-matrix interactions.

REFERENCES

1. HYNES, R. O. 1992. Integrins: versatility, modulation, and signaling in cell adhesion. Cell **69:** 11–25.
2. CHEN, Q., M. S. KINCH, T. H. LIN, K. BURRIDGE & R. L. JULIANO. 1994. Integrin-mediated cell adhesion activates mitogen-activated protein kinases. J. Biol. Chem. **269:** 26602–26605.
3. GINSBERG, M. H., X. DU & E. F. PLOW. 1992. Inside-out integrin signalling. [Review]. Curr. Opin. Cell Biol. **4:** 766–771.
4. LIN, C. Q. & M. J. BISSELL. 1993. Multi-faceted regulation of cell differentiation by extracellular matrix [see comments]. [Review]. FASEB J. **7:** 737–743.
5. MARTINS-GREEN, M. & M. J. BISSELL. 1995. Cell-ECM interactions in development. Semin. Dev. Biol. **6:** 149–159.
6. BISSELL, M. J., H. G. HALL & G. PARRY. 1982. How does extracellular matrix direct gene expression? J. Theor. Biol. **99:** 31–68.
7. STREULI, C. H., N. BAILEY & M. J. BISSELL. 1991. Control of mammary epithelial differen-

tiation: basement membrane induces tissue-specific gene expression in the absence of cell-cell interaction and morphological polarity. J. Cell Biol. **115:** 1383–1395.
8. KADOYA, Y., K. KADOYA, M. DURBEEJ, K. HOLMVALL, L. SOROKIN & P. EKBLOM. 1995. Antibodies against domain E3 of laminin-1 and integrin alpha 6 subunit perturb branching epithelial morphogenesis of submandibular gland, but by different modes. J. Cell Biol. **129:** 521–534.
9. SCHUGER, L., A. P. SKUBITZ, K. S. O'SHEA, J. F. CHANG & J. VARANI. 1991. Identification of laminin domains involved in branching morphogenesis: effects of anti-laminin monoclonal antibodies on mouse embryonic lung development. Dev. Biol. **146:** 531–541.
10. KLEIN, G., M. LANGEGGER, R. TIMPL & P. EKBLOM. 1988. Role of laminin A chain in the development of epithelial cell polarity. Cell **55:** 331–341.
11. SOROKIN, L., A. SONNENBERG, M. AUMAILLEY, R. TIMPL & P. EKBLOM. 1990. Recognition of the laminin E8 cell-binding site by an integrin possessing the alpha 6 subunit is essential for epithelial polarization in developing kidney tubules. J. Cell Biol. **111:** 1265–1273.
12. ADAMS, J. C. & F. M. WATT. 1990. Changes in keratinocyte adhesion during terminal differenti reduction in fibronectin binding precedes alpha 5 beta 1 in loss from the cell surface. Cell **63:** 425–435.
13. BOETTIGER, D., M. ENOMOTO-IWAMOTO, H. Y. YOON, U. HOFER, A. S. MENKO & R. CHIQUET-EHRISMANN. 1995. Regulation of integrin alpha 5 beta 1 affinity during myogenic differentiation. Dev Biol. **169:** 261–272.
14. LAUFFENBURGER, D. A. & A. F. HORWITZ. 1996. Cell migration: a physically integrated molecular process. [Review]. Cell **84:** 359–369.
15. KORNBERG, L., H. S. EARP, J. T. PARSONS, M. SCHALLER & R. L. JULIANO. 1992. Cell adhesion or integrin clustering increases phosphorylation of a focal adhesion-associated tyrosine kinase. J Biol Chem. **267:** 23439–23442.
16. GUAN, J. L., J. E. TREVITHICK & R. O. HYNES. 1991. Fibronectin/integrin interaction induces tyrosine phosphorylation of a 120-kDa protein. Cell Regul. **2:** 951–964.
17. SASTRY, S. K., M. LAKONISHOK, D. A. THOMAS, J. MUSCHLER & A. F. HORWITZ. 1996. Integrin alpha subunit ratios, cytoplasmic domains, and growth factor synergy regulate muscle proliferation and differentiation. J. Cell Biol. **133:** 169–184.
18. FITCH, J. M., R. MAYNE & T. F. LINSENMAYER. 1983. Developmental acquisition of basement membrane heterogeneit IV collagen in the Avian lens capsule. J. Cell Biol. **97:** 940–943.
19. RINAUDO, J. A. & P. S. ZELENKA. 1992. Expression of c-fos and c-jun mRNA in the developing chicken lens: relationship to cell proliferation, quiescence, and differentiation. Exp. Cell Res. **199:** 147–153.
20. JIANG, R. & L. B. GRABEL. 1995. Function and differential regulation of the alpha 6 integrin isoforms during parietal endoderm differentiation. Exp. Cell Res. **217:** 195–204.
21. RESZKA, A. A., Y. HAYASHI & A. F. HORWITZ. 1992. Identification of amino acid sequences in the integrin beta 1 cytoplasmic domain implicated in cytoskeletal association. J. Cell Biol. **117:** 1321–1330.
22. BURRIDGE, K. & L. CONNELL. 1983. A new protein of adhesion plaques and ruffling membranes. J. Cell Biol. **97:** 359–367.
23. BECKERLE, M. C. & R. K. YEH. 1990. Talin: role at sites of cell-substratum adhesion. [Review]. Cell Motil. Cytoskeleton **16:** 7–13.
24. HORWITZ, A. F., K. DUGGAN, C. A. BUCK, M. C. BECKERLE & K. BURRIDGE. 1986. Interaction of plasma membrane fibronectin receptor with talin-a transmembrane linkage. Nature **320:** 531–533.
25. PAVALKO, F. M., C. A. OTEY, K. O. SIMON & K. BURRIDGE. 1991. Alpha-actinin: a direct link between actin and integrins. Biochem. Soc. Trans. **19:** 1065–1069.
26. KNUDSEN, K. A., A. P. SOLER, K. R. JOHNSON & M. J. WHEELOCK. 1995. Interaction of alpha-actinin with the cadherin/catenin cell-cell adhesion complex via alpha-catenin. J. Cell Biol. **130:** 67–77.
27. OTEY, C. A., F. M. PAVALKO & K. BURRIDGE. 1990. An interaction between alpha-actinin and the beta 1 integrin subunit in vitro. J. Cell Biol. **111:** 721–729.
28. NACHMIAS, V. T. & R. GOLLA. 1991. Vinculin in relation to stress fibers in spread platelets. Cell Motil. Cytoskeleton **20:** 190–202.

29. OTTO, J. J. 1990. Vinculin. Cell Motil. Cytoskeleton **16:** 1–6.
30. TURNER, C. E., J. R. GLENNEY, JR. & K. BURRIDGE. 1990. Paxillin: a new vinculin-binding protein present in focal adhesions. J. Cell Biol. **111:** 1059–1068.
31. TURNER, C. E. 1991. Paxillin is a major phosphotyrosine-containing protein during embryonic development. J. Cell Biol. **115:** 201–207.
32. TURNER, C. E., M. D. SCHALLER & J. T. PARSONS. 1993. Tyrosine phosphorylation of the focal adhesion kinase pp125FAK during development: relation to paxillin. J. Cell Sci. **105:** 637–645.

Integrins and Matrix Molecules in Salivary Gland Cell Adhesion, Signaling, and Gene Expression

ROBERT M. LAFRENIE[a,c] AND KENNETH M. YAMADA[b]

[a]*Northeastern Ontario Regional Cancer Centre, Tumour Biology Research, Sudbury, Ontario, P3E 5J1, Canada*
[b]*Craniofacial Developmental Biology and Regeneration Branch, National Institute of Dental Research, National Institutes of Health, Bethesda, Maryland, 20892-4370 USA*

ABSTRACT: Integrins play crucial roles in embryonic and adult cell adhesion, migration, morphogenesis, growth, and differentiation in many cell systems, including human salivary gland cells. Integrins function by binding through their extracellular domain to a specific peptide recognition site in a ligand, and then transmitting information to the cytoplasm by way of their cytoplasmic tails. By this transmembrane signaling process, integrins can mediate assembly of adhesion sites and organization of the actin-containing cytoskeleton by forming supermolecular complexes of cytoskeletal and signaling molecules. The specific steps in the assembly of these complexes as well as novel mechanisms for synergy between integrin and growth factor signaling pathways are still being determined. Integrin-mediated interactions also have major effects on gene expression. For example, integrin-mediated adhesion to fibronectin by the HSG salivary gland cell line significantly alters the pattern of proteins synthesized and genes expressed. In fact, at least five transcription factors are activated, and over 30 genes (many of them novel) are found to be induced by such integrin-mediated interactions by salivary gland cells. The roles of integrins, in collaborative interactions with growth factors and signaling pathways, and in the induction of novel genes during salivary gland development, should provide fruitful areas of research for many years.

INTRODUCTION

Integrin adhesion molecules interact with the extracellular matrix and play critical roles in the differentiation of many tissues,[1,2] including salivary glands.[3,4] The HSG (human salivary gland) epithelial cell line provides an excellent model of salivary gland differentiation.[5,6] HSG cells were derived from a submandibular tumor and grow as an undifferentiated population with a phenotype similar to intercalated duct cells.[5] However, when HSG cells are cultured on Matrigel, a laminin- and growth factor–rich extracellular matrix preparation, they organize into structures that are morphologically similar to both ducts and acini.[7,8] Further, the expression of myoepithelial and acinar differentiation markers, including vimentin, cystatin SN, and α-amylase, is induced.[5,7,8] Similar upregulation of vimentin and cystatin SN expression occurs in response to culture of HSG cells on collagen I gels but not on fibronectin (Lafrenie and Yamada, unpublished). Adhesive interaction between the cells and extracellular matrix compo-

---

[c] Address correspondence to Dr. Robert M. Lafrenie, Northeastern Ontario Regional Cancer Centre, 41 Ramsey Lake Road, Sudbury, Ontario, P3E 5J1, Canada. Tel: (705) 522-6237 ext. 2702; fax: (705) 523-7326; e-mail: robert_lafrenie@cancercare.on.ca

nents is essential for this process. The addition of antibodies against the relevant extracellular components (laminin or collagen) or integrin adhesion molecules (*e.g.*, $\alpha_6\beta_1$) can block *in vitro* differentiation of HSG cells.[7,8]

The mechanisms underlying the adhesion-dependent effects on HSG cell differentiation are not understood, although several contributing factors have been suggested. For example, cell adhesion to extracellular matrix or to antiintegrin antibodies can activate signal transduction molecules of pathways that are proposed to control gene expression.[9–12] Integrin-dependent adhesion to the matrix also makes the cells more responsive to growth factors present in the environment, which can then control cell proliferation and gene expression.[13,14] Therefore, adhesion of HSG cells to extracellular matrix components by way of integrin adhesion molecules induces signals that are critical for initiating cellular differentiation.

SUPERMOLECULAR CYTOSKELETAL AND SIGNAL MOLECULE COMPLEXES

Interaction of cells with immobilized fibronectin or with anti-β_1 integrin antibodies that mimic ligand binding promotes the formation of a large multicomponent complex of cytoplasmic and transmembrane proteins at the site of adhesion (*i.e.*, focal contacts or close contacts).[15–17] The proteins found in these complexes include components of the actin cytoskeleton, a large number of different signal transduction molecules, including various *src*-related signal transduction molecules and growth factor receptors (Fig. 1). This response to adhesion is hierarchical depending on both integrin- and tyrosine phosphorylation–dependent events.[16] Aggregation of integrins with antibodies that do not bind near the ligand binding site coaggregates only tensin and focal adhesion kinase (FAK). Addition of soluble ligand or ligation with antibodies mimicking ligand in the absence of tyrosine phosphorylation (in the presence of phosphorylation inhibitors) also promotes the coaggregation of the cytoskeletal linker molecules, α-actinin, talin, and vinculin. Integrin ligation promotes a phosphorylation cascade, which results in the activation of MAP kinase and the recruitment of a large number of phosphorylated signal transduction molecules. These molecules include Ras, ERK, JNK, and Src, in addition to several tyrosine kinases and their substrates.[16,17]

Integrin aggregation and ligand occupation, therefore, allows the simultaneous activation of a large number of signal transduction cascades. A variety of signaling responses, including alterations in calcium influx, changes in cytoplasmic pH, changes in inositol phosphate metabolism, alterations in phospholipase activity, and changes in protein phosphorylation, have all been identified as metabolic consequences of adhesion to extracellular matrix or of ligation of integrin adhesion molecules.[9–12] Integrin-dependent adhesion activates multiple protein kinases, including focal adhesion kinase;[18,19] certain MAP kinases, specifically the extracellular regulated kinases (ERK1 and ERK2, which are linked to growth factor–responsive signal transduction pathways);[16,20,21] and Jun kinase[16] (which is activated by inflammatory cytokines or in response to cellular stresses[22]). In addition, integrin activation and tyrosine phosphorylation also promotes the aggregation of several growth factor receptors (*e.g.*, epidermal growth factor receptor and platelet-derived growth factor receptor).[14] Treatment of these cells with growth factors is well known to activate MAP kinase, and this activation is synergistic with the MAP kinase activation seen in response to integrin aggregation.[14] This finding suggests a mechanism for the collaboration between growth factor and adhesion-dependent signaling, which are both crucial for altering gene expression and mediating differentiation.

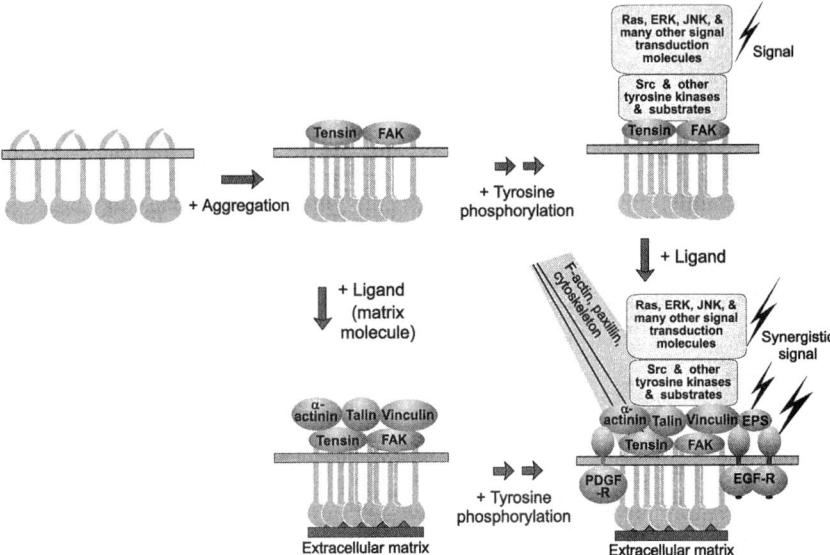

FIGURE 1. Stages and hierarchies of integrin-mediated responses. Aggregation of integrin adhesion molecules in the absence of ligand binding promotes coaggregation of tensin and FAK, whereas binding to ligand promotes additional coaggregation of several cytoskeletal molecules. In both cases, tyrosine phosphorylation permits the subsequent accumulation of a large array of signal transduction molecules. Combined integrin aggregation and ligand occupancy promotes the formation of a large complex of cytoskeletal molecules that interact with the actin cytoskeleton, the accumulation of at least 19 different signal transduction molecules, and transient coaggregation of growth factor receptors. The addition of growth factors to cells with such cytoskeletal and signaling complexes produces a synergistic signal. EPS, epidermal growth factor receptor substrate 8.

CHANGES IN HSG CELL GENE EXPRESSION FOLLOWING BINDING TO THE EXTRACELLULAR MATRIX

HSG cells undergo morphological differentiation and express differentiation markers (cystatin SN and α-amylase) when cultured for 3–5 days on extracellular matrix gels.[7,8] This differential regulation of gene expression following adhesion of cells to the extracellular matrix is likely mediated by activation of signal transduction pathways, thereby indicating that cell/matrix interaction is critical for promoting differentiation of this cell line. Adhesive interactions between HSG cells and the extracellular matrix are primarily mediated by β_1 integrin adhesion molecules; adhesion to collagen I is mediated by $\alpha_2\beta_1$ and $\alpha_3\beta_1$, and adhesion to fibronectin is mediated by $\alpha_5\beta_1$.[23] Because adhesion is required for changes in HSG cell gene expression, this pattern of integrin dependence suggests that the impact of the extracellular matrix on HSG cell function is mediated through specific integrin adhesion molecules.

We have characterized the integrin-mediated responses of HSG cells to extracellular matrix molecules in terms of specific alterations in gene expression and protein synthesis. We examined both the overall extent of the cellular biosynthetic response and identified specific molecular alterations. One of the striking findings was that a substantial proportion of cellular proteins was altered biosynthetically in response to cell interactions with specific matrix molecules[23] (Fig. 2). The adhesion of HSG cells to fibronectin and collagen I rapidly and substantially alters cellular biosynthesis. Two-dimensional electrophoresis of ^{35}S-methionine-labeled HSG cell proteins shows that the expression of 35% of total detected proteins are upregulated or downregulated by culture on collagen I gels or fibronectin.[23] Thirty-two different genes, including 20 previously unidentified genes, were shown to be upregulated by HSG cells adhering to fibronectin- or collagen I–coated substrates compared to uncoated substrates.[23] These genes were upregulated within 6 hours. Adhesion to fibronectin- or collagen I–coated substrates also enhanced the binding activity of five of seven transcription factors tested in mobility-shift assays.[23] Therefore, adhesion to collagen I or fibronectin resulted in fundamental changes in cellular biosynthetic control within hours. Further, changes in gene expression are likely a direct consequence of integrin-dependent adhesion inasmuch as expression of some genes was induced by treatment of HSG cells with anti-β_1 integrin antibodies that mimic ligand binding.[23]

The genes that are upregulated in 6 h by HSG cells cultured on fibronectin or collagen I gels have been isolated, sequenced, and classified[23] (Fig. 3). A particularly striking finding was that a majority of the genes that were identified as induced by integrin-mediated interactions with fibronectin or collagen were novel; that is, they were either not present in the GenBank DNA sequence database, or they were EST sequences. The latter "expressed sequence tags" are short DNA sequences derived from random sequencing of expressed mRNA molecules in genome projects, and their functions remain unknown. Further characterization of the 20 novel genes may lead to the poten-

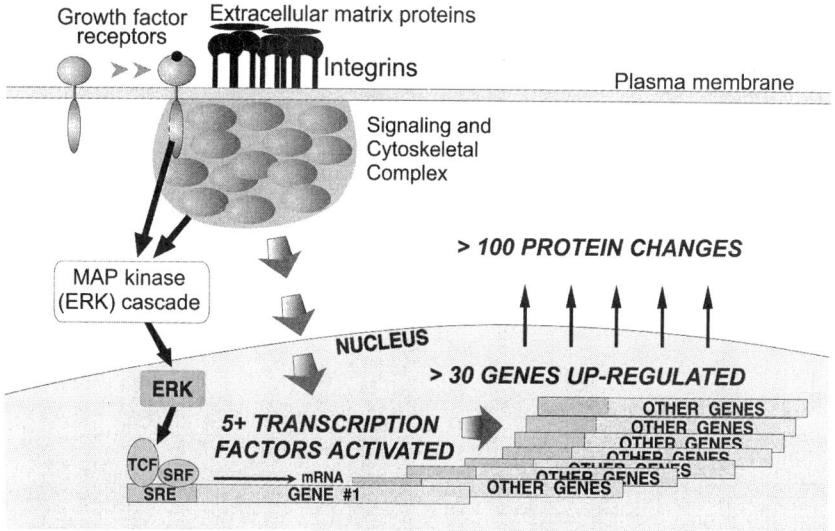

FIGURE 2. Stages and hierarchies of integrin response. Integrin-dependent adhesion of cells to extracellular matrix components promotes extensive alterations in cellular biosynthesis. The supermolecular signaling and cytoskeletal complex that forms in response to cell adhesion also results in activation of the MAP kinase cascade and in alterations in the expression of multiple genes and proteins. The expression of more than 100 different proteins is changed, more than 30 different genes are upregulated, and more than five different transcription factors are activated in response to HSG cell adhesion to fibronectin or collagen I. TCF, ternary complex factor; SRF, serum response factor; SRE, serum response element.

tial identification of important new regulators, mediators, or products of salivary gland cell responses to interaction with extracellular matrix molecules.

A number of the genes upregulated by adhesion to fibronectin or collagen I have been identified based on sequence analysis of the isolated clones. These induced genes include calnexin, 90 kDa heat shock protein, γ-actin, decorin, S-adenosylmethionine decarboxylase, five mitochondrial genes, and two different 40S ribosomal protein genes. Several of these genes have been previously implicated in adhesion- or differentiation-dependent processes, and their presence among the matched clones supports the utility of this approach in identifying genes important in adhesion-dependent processes. For example, S-adenosylmethionine decarboxylase is a key enzyme in the regulation of polyamine biosynthesis.[24] Because polyamine synthesis and the expression of a related enzyme, ornithine decarboxylase, is induced by cell adhesion and spreading[25] or treatment with growth factors,[26] expression of S-adenosylmethionine decarboxylase may be relevant to the adhesion-dependent regulation of function in HSG cells. The increased expression of some of the genes may be relevant to downstream cellular changes required for HSG differentiation. For example, increased mitochondrial gene expression has been correlated to differentiation of myoblasts and of some leukocytes, and inhibitors of mitochondrial protein expression inhibit differentiation in these model systems.[27–29] The endoplasmic reticulum chaperon, calnexin, can regulate the synthesis of cellular glycoproteins during differentiation.[30] For example, calnexin inhibits transport

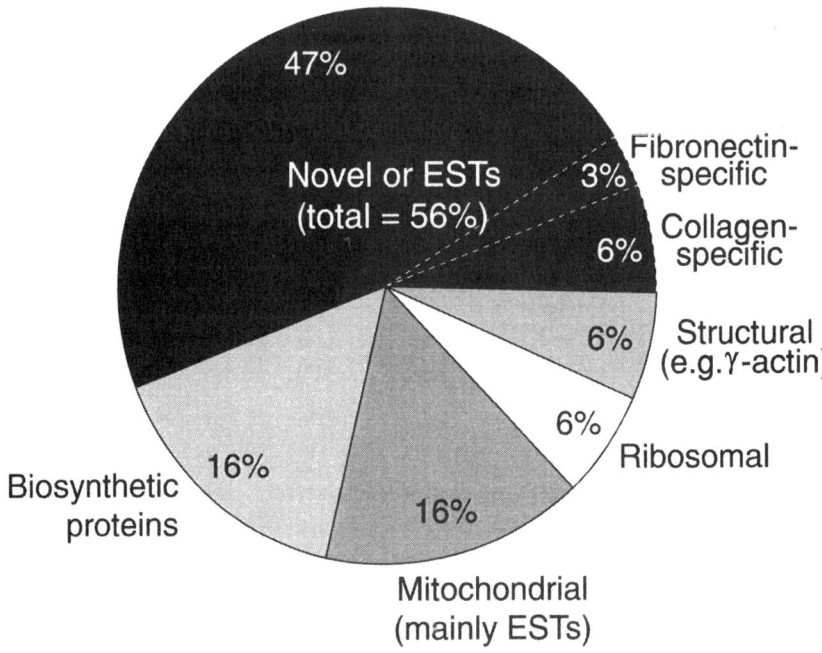

FIGURE 3. Identification of genes upregulated by HSG adhesion to extracellular matrix. There are at least 32 different genes upregulated by adhesion to fibronectin or collagen I, including "novel genes" (EST [expressed sequence tag] sequences or sequences not found in GenBank), mitochondrial genes, and genes encoding ribosomal proteins, structural proteins, and biosynthetic enzymes. A few genes are upregulated only on collagen I or on fibronectin but not on both substrates.

and downregulates expression of β_1 integrins in differentiating keratinocytes.[31] The induction of genes with assorted functions supports the requirement for numerous auxiliary and mediating effectors that are required to mediate cellular differentiation.

CONCLUSIONS

Integrin-dependent adhesion to fibronectin promotes aggregation of integrin adhesion molecules and of a host of signal transduction and cytoskeletal molecules. The formation of this supermolecular complex promotes the activation of several different signal transduction pathways, including MAP kinase, within minutes. Further, integrin-dependent adhesion also promotes aggregation of growth factor receptors into the supermolecular complex and is important in promoting growth factor–dependent signals such as MAP kinase activation. The accumulation of a large signaling complex in response to integrin-dependent cell adhesion suggests that adhesion could be important in the regulation of cellular biosynthesis. This is supported by the observation that the adhesion of HSG cells to extracellular matrix components for only 6 h promotes extensive alteration in cellular biosynthesis, altering the pattern of expression of more than 100 proteins and over 30 genes. Some of the genes upregulated by adhesion to extracellular matrix have been shown to be relevant to differentiation in other differentiation model systems. Inasmuch as integrin-dependent adhesion to the extracellular matrix has been shown to be crucial for differentiation in the HSG cell model, it is likely that the immediate changes in signal transduction activity and early changes in HSG cell expression could be related to the mechanism of differentiation. Further, the HSG cell model system could be used to examine the role of adhesion-dependent changes in signal transduction and gene expression in the process of salivary gland differentiation.

REFERENCES

1. ADAMS, J.C. & F.M. WATT. 1993. Regulation of development and differentiation by the extracellular matrix. Development (Camb.) **117:** 1183–1198.
2. HAY, E.D. 1991. Cell Biology of Extracellular Matrix, 2nd Ed. Plenum Press. New York.
3. CUTLER, L.S. 1990. The role of extracellular matrix in the morphogenesis and differentiation of salivary glands. Adv. Dent. Res. **4:** 27–33.
4. DURBAN, E.M. 1990 Mouse submandibular salivary epithelial cell growth and differentiation in long-term culture: Influence of the extracellular matrix. In Vitro Cell. Dev. Biol. **26:** 33–43.
5. OKURA, M., K. SHIRASUNA, T. HIRANUMA, H. YOSHIOKA, H. NAKAHARA, T. AIKAWA & T. MATSUYA. 1993. Characterization of growth and differentiation of normal human submandibular gland epithelial cells in serum-free medium. Differentiation **54:** 143–153.
6. SHIRASUNA, K., M. SATO & T. MIYAZAKI. 1981. A neoplastic epithelial duct cell line established from an irradiated human salivary gland. Cancer **48:** 745–752.
7. ROYCE, L.S., M.C. KIBBEY, P. MERTZ, H.K. KLEINMAN & B.J. BAUM. 1993. Human neoplastic submandibular intercalated duct cells express an acinar phenotype when cultured on a basement membrane. Differentiation **52:** 247–255.
8. HOFFMAN, M.P., M.C. KIBBEY, J.J. LETTERIO & H.K. KLEINMAN. 1996. Role of laminin-1 and TGF-β3 in acinar differentiation of a human submandibular gland cell line (HSG). J. Cell Sci. **109:** 2013–2021.
9. GIMOND, C. & M. AUMAILLEY. 1992 Cellular interactions with the extracellular matrix are coupled to diverse transmembrane signaling pathways. Exp. Cell Res. **203:** 365–373.
10. MCNAMEE, H.P., D.E. INGBER & M.A. SCHWARTZ. 1993. Adhesion to fibronectin stimulates inositol lipid synthesis and PDGF-induced inositol lipid breakdown. J. Cell Biol. **121:** 673–678.

11. LAFRENIE, R.M. & K.M. YAMADA. 1996. Integrin-dependent signal transduction. J. Cell. Biochem. **61:** 543–553.
12. SCHWARTZ, M.A., M.D. SCHALLER & M.H. GINSBERG. 1995. Integrins: Emerging paradigms of signal-transduction. Annu. Rev. Cell Dev. Biol. **11:** 549–599.
13. CHEN, Q., M.S. KINCH, T.H.E. LIN, K. BURRIDGE & R.L. JULIANO. 1994. Integrin-mediated cell adhesion activates mitogen-activated protein kinases. J. Biol. Chem. **269:** 26602–26605.
14. MIYAMOTO, S., H. TERAMOTO, J.S. GUTKIND & K.M. YAMADA. 1996. Integrins can collaborate with growth factors for phosphorylation of receptor tyrosine kinases and MAP kinase activation: Roles of integrin aggregation and occupancy of receptors. J. Cell Biol. **135:** 1633–1642.
15. MIYAMOTO, S., S.K. AKIYAMA & K.M. YAMADA. 1995. Synergistic roles for receptor occupancy and aggregation in integrin transmembrane function. Science **267:** 883–885.
16. MIYAMOTO, S., H. TERAMOTO, O.A. COSO, J.S. GUTKIND, P.D. BURBELO, S.K. AKIYAMA & K.M. YAMADA. 1995. Integrin function: Molecular hierarchies of cytoskeletal and signalling molecules. J. Cell Biol. **131:** 791–805.
17. PLOPPER, G.E., H.P. MCNAMEE, L.E. DIKE, K. BOJANOWSKI & D.E. INGBER. 1995. Convergence of integrin and growth factor receptor signaling pathways within the focal adhesion complex. Mol. Biol. Cell **6:** 1349–1365.
18. AKIYAMA, S.K., S.S. YAMADA, K.M. YAMADA & S.E. LAFLAMME. 1994. Transmembrane signal transduction by integrin cytoplasmic domains expressed in single-subunit chimeras. J. Biol. Chem. **269:** 15961–15964.
19. GUAN, J.-L., J.E. TREVITHICK & R.O. HYNES. 1991. Fibronectin/integrin interaction induces tyrosine phosphorylation of a 120 kDa protein. Cell Regul. **2:** 951–964.
20. MORINO, N., T. MIMURA, K. HAMASAKI, K. TOBE, K. UEKI, K. KINUCHI, K. TAKEHARA, T. KADOWAKI, Y. YAZAKI & Y. NOJIMA. 1994. Matrix/integrin interaction activates the mitogen-activated protein kinase, p44erk1 and p42erk2. J. Biol. Chem. **270:** 269–273.
21. MARSHALL, C.J. 1995. Specificity of receptor tyrosine kinase signaling: Transient versus sustained extracellular signal-regulated kinase activation. Cell **80:** 179–185.
22. DERIJARD, B., M. HIBI, I.H. WU, T. BARRETT, B. SU, T. DENG, M. KARIN & R.J. DAVIS. 1994. JNK1: A protein kinase stimulated by UV light and Ha-ras that binds and phosphorylates c-Jun activation domain. Cell **76:** 1025–1037.
23. LAFRENIE, R.M., S.M. BERNIER & K.M. YAMADA. 1998. Adhesion to fibronectin or collagen I gel induces rapid biosynthetic alterations in epithelial cells by multiple mechanisms. J. Cell. Physiol. **175.** In press.
24. MARIC, S.C., A. CROZAT & O.A. JANNE. 1992. Structure and organization of the human S-adenosylmethionine decarboxylase gene. J. Biol. Chem. **267:** 18915–18923.
25. MORRISON, R.F. & E.R. SEIDEL. 1995. Cell spreading and the regulation of ornithine decarboxylase. J. Cell Sci. **108:** 3787–37974.
26. GAWEL-THOMPSON, K.J. & R.M. GREENE. 1989. Epidermal growth factor: Modulator of murine embryonic palate mesenchymal cell proliferation, polyamine biosynthesis, and polyamine transport. J. Cell. Physiol. **140:** 359–370.
27. KAGAWA, Y. & S. OHTA. 1990. Regulation of mitochondrial ATP synthesis in mammalian cells by transcriptional control. Int. J. Biochem. **22:** 219–229.
28. KANEKO, T., T. WATANABE & M. OISHI. 1988. Effect of mitochondrial protein synthesis inhibitors on erythroid differentiation of mouse erythroleukemia cells. Mol. Cell. Biol. **8:** 3311–3315.
29. ROCHARD, P., I. CASSAR-MALEK, S. MARCHAL, C. WRUTNIAK & G. CABELLO. 1996. Changes in mitochondrial activity during avian myoblast differentiation: Influence of triiodothyronine or v-erb A expression. J. Cell. Physiol. **168:** 239–247.
30. WILLIAMS, D.B. 1995. Calnexin: a molecular chaperone with a taste for carbohydrate. Biochem. Cell Biol. **73:** 123–132.
31. HOTCHIN, N.A., A. GANDARILLAS & F.M. WATT. 1995. Regulation of cell surface β1 integrin levels during keratinocyte terminal differentiation. J. Cell Biol. **128:** 1209–1219.

Expression of *Rhizobium* Chitin Oligosaccharide Fucosyltransferase in Zebrafish Embryos Disrupts Normal Development[a]

CARLOS E. SEMINO,[b,d] MIGUEL L. ALLENDE,[b] JEROEN BAKKERS,[c] HERMAN P. SPAINK,[c] AND PHILLIPS P. ROBBINS[b]

[b]*Center for Cancer Research, Building E17, Room 125, Massachusetts Institute of Technology, 77 Massachusetts Avenue, Cambridge, Massachusetts 02139, USA*
[c]*Institute for Molecular Plant Sciences, Leiden University, Wassenaarseweg 64, 2333 Al Leiden, the Netherlands*

ABSTRACT: In this report we present data about the effect of the *Rhizobium* NodZ enzyme on zebrafish development. We injected zebrafish embryos with a plasmid expressing NodZ protein, and we confirmed that the enzyme is active and has chitin oligosaccharide fucosyltransferase (NodZ) activity *in vitro*. In addition, the embryos injected with the NodZ-expressing plasmid, but not with a control plasmid, showed malformations or bends in the tail, and in some cases shunted tail structures and fused somites. These results clearly indicate that the likely substrates for this enzyme, chitin oligosaccharides and free *N*-glycans, have essential functions during early vertebrate embryogenesis.

INTRODUCTION

The symbiotic relationship between bacteria of the genera *Rhizobium* and legumes results in the formation of a nitrogen-fixing root organ, the nodule.[1] The bacteria respond to specific compounds secreted by the plant roots (flavonoids) by production and excretion of lipochitin oligosaccharides (modified chitin oligosaccharides, also known as Nod factors), signaling molecules that act as plant morphogens promoting root infection and the consequent nodulation.[2,3,6] The backbone of the Nod factors consists of an oligomer of 3 to 5 residues of *N*-acetylglucosamine, *N*-acylated on the nonreducing end. This backbone is synthesized by three enzymes, NodA, NodB, and NodC. NodC is the first enzyme in this pathway and is responsible for the synthesis of chitin oligosaccharides.[4,5,7] Additional gene products, such as NodZ, a chitin oligosaccharide fucosyltransferase, are involved in chemical modifications that have been shown to determine host specificity.[8]

Polymeric chitin has been found in the epidermal cuticle of teleost fish,[22] and more recently chitin oligosaccharides have been isolated from *Xenopus laevis* and zebrafish embryos.[10,11] In addition, genes highly homologous to NodC have been cloned from *X. laevis*, zebrafish, and mouse (DG42, ZDG42, and MDG42, respectively[9,10,13]). In *Xenopus* and zebrafish, these genes are expressed during a short window of time during de-

---

[a] This work was supported by Grant GM31318 (to P. P. Robbins). M. L. Allende was supported by a Public Health Service fellowship (HD 07818).
[d] Tel: (617) 258-8057; fax: (617) 258-8315; e-mail: seminoraimon@wccf.mit.edu.

velopment, between the gastrula and neurula stages.[9–11] We are interested in investigating the possible biological function of chitin oligosaccharides during vertebrate embryogenesis, in particular to learn whether chitin oligosaccharides act as signaling molecules as they do during the nodulation process in plants.

Previously, using a cell-free *in vitro* transcription/translation system, we showed that the DG42 protein is able to catalyze synthesis of chitin oligosaccharides that vary in chain length from three to six residues of *N*-acetylglucosamine, as well as polymeric chitin.[14] We have also demonstrated that when cell extracts from frog and zebrafish embryos of the appropriate developmental stage are used it is possible to obtain *in vitro* synthesis of chitin oligosaccharides.[10] In these extracts, chitin oligosaccharide synthase activity, but not hyaluronate (HA) synthase activity, can be inactivated with a specific anti-DG42 antibody.[10] Similar results have also been found in carp embryos.[15]

In this report we present data that support our previous observations on the effect of the NodZ enzyme on zebrafish development. We injected zebrafish embryos with a plasmid expressing NodZ, and we confirmed that the enzyme is active and has chitin oligosaccharide fucosyltransferase activity *in vitro*. The embryos injected with the NodZ-expressing plasmid, but not with a control plasmid, show defects similar to those seen when purified NodZ protein was injected.[15]

RESULTS AND DISCUSSION

NodZ-expressing Embryos Show Chitin Oligosaccharide Fucosyltransferase Activity

The NodZ enzyme transfers a fucose residue from the sugar donor GDP-β-L-fucose (GDP-Fuc) to the C-6 position of the GlcNAc residue at the reducing end of chitin oligosaccharides.[8] Previously, we have shown that injection of the purified NodZ enzyme into early embryos induces abnormalities visible at 24 hours of development[15] and that the effect is similar to that produced by injection of a chitinase[11] or an anti-DG42 protein antibody.[11,15] We were interested in determining whether the recombinant NodZ enzyme was able to elicit the same effect, which would confirm the specificity of the prior results.

The *NodZ* gene of *Bradyrhizobium japonicum* was cloned into the expression vector pcDNA3 downstream of the cytomegalovirus (CMV) promoter, which is able to direct high levels of RNA expression in zebrafish embryos.[21] Fertilized zebrafish embryos at the one-cell stage were injected with this construct (pcDNA3-BJ-NodZ) or with the parental plasmid pcDNA3 as a control (see legend of FIG. 1). After injection, the embryos were raised under standard conditions.[12] At 12 hours (early somite stage) NodZ enzyme activity was assayed. NodZ is specific for chitin oligosaccharides of 2–6 residues of *N*-acetylglucosamine. We incubated cell extracts from the two groups of injected embryos in the presence of GDP[^{14}C]-Fuc, Mg^{2+}, Ca^{2+}, Mn^{2+}, ATP and chitin pentaose (see legend to FIG. 1). After incubation, the water soluble and neutral material was applied to a thin-layer chromatography (TLC) plate. The embryos injected with the plasmid pcDNA3-BJ-NodZ (FIG. 1, lane A), but not the control embryos (FIG. 1, lane B), show fucosyltransferase activity. The [^{14}C]fucosylated compound has a mobility identical to fucosylated chitin pentaose by both TLC (FIG. 1, lane A), and HPLC (data not shown). This result clearly indicates that the embryos express functional NodZ enzyme, with the same properties found before with the *E. coli*–expressed protein.[15]

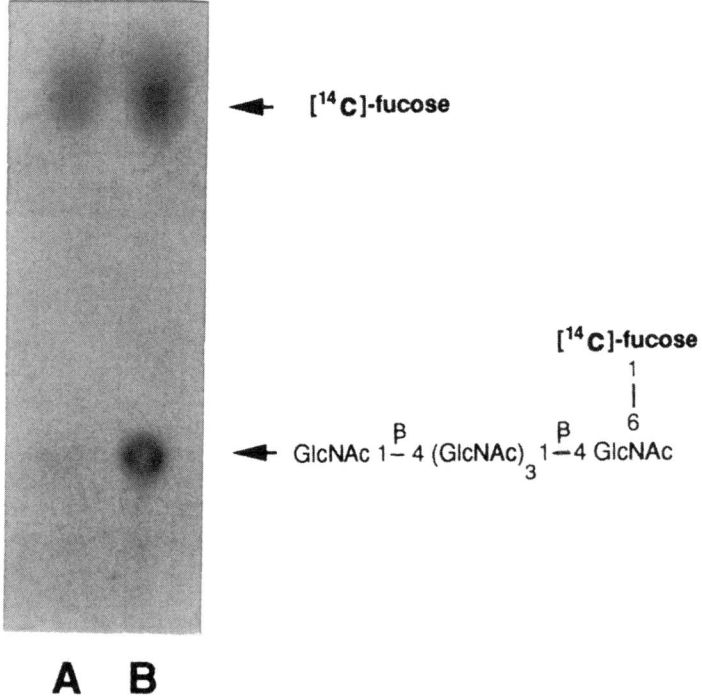

FIGURE 1. Chitin oligosaccharide fucosyltransferase activity in NodZ-expressing embryos. The plasmid pMP2452, containing the *NodZ* gene,[23] was digested with Xba I and Bam HI, and the 950 bp *NodZ* fragment was cloned into pB SK (+/−) (Stratagene). The resulting construct, pB SK(+/−)-Bj-NodZ, was digested with Sac I and Xho I, and the 1 Kb insert encoding *NodZ* was subcloned into pcDNA3 (Invitrogen). This construct, pcDNA3-Bj-NodZ, has the *NodZ* gene under the control of the human cytomegalovirus (CMV) enhancer-promoter sequence. 5 to 8 nL of the plasmids pcDNA3-Bj-NodZ or pcDNA3 (0.2 mg/mL in 0.2 M KCl) were microinjected into one cell–stage zebrafish embryos (40–50 per experiment), which were raised to 12 hours of development and used to prepare cell extracts, as described before.[10] The cell extracts (50 μL) were incubated as described[23] at room temperature for 30 minutes with 1 mM of ATP; 5 mM of Mg^{2+}, Ca^{2+} and Mn^{2+}; 50 nCi of GDP-β-[^{14}C]-L-fucose (272 mCi / mmol) (DuPont, NEN); and 1 mM chitin pentaose standard (penta-*N*-acetyl-D-chitopentaose) (Seikagaku America, FL). The reaction was stopped by adding 100 μL water and boiling for two minutes. The sample was centrifuged at 14,000 rpm for 10 minutes, and the supernatant was loaded onto a mixed ion-exchange column (400 μL of Rexyn I-300 H-OH, Fisher Scientific Co.) prepared in a Pasteur pipette. The column was washed twice with 200 μL of water. The water-soluble material eluted from the column (neutral) was concentrated and loaded on a thin-layer chromatography (TLC) plate. The TLC was performed on silica gel G plates (5 × 10 cm) (Merck) in *n*-butanol / ethanol / water, 5 : 4 : 3 (vol/vol). The external standards used were [^{14}C]fucosylated chitin oligosaccharides from 2 to 6 residues of *N*-acetylglucosamine obtained after incubation of chitin oligosaccharides in the presence of GDP [^{14}C]fucose and pure NodZ enzyme expressed in *E. coli*.

The FIGURE shows the chromatographic mobility of free [^{14}C]fucose and also the molecular structure of the fucosyl β(1–6)-chitopentaose. **A:** Embryos microinjected with pcDNA3; **B:** embryos microinjected with pcDNA3-Bj-NodZ plasmid.

Embryos Expressing the NodZ Enzyme Develop an Abnormal Phenotype

Embryos microinjected with the NodZ-expressing (pcDNA3-Bj-NodZ) plasmids and the control (pcDNA3) plasmids were raised and visually inspected at 6, 12, 24, and 48 hours postfertilization. Among the embryos injected with the control plasmid (FIG. 2A), approximately 5% showed abnormalities (n–112), which were comparable to the background defects normally found associated with the injection procedure. On the other hand, by 24 hours, embryos injected with the NodZ-expressing plasmid presented a phenotype that was similar to that seen previously when purified NodZ enzyme,[15] anti-DG42 antibody,[15] or chitinase[11] were injected. Approximately 70% (n=145) of embryos in this group were affected, although with varying severity. Moderately affected individuals showed slight malformations or bends in the tail (FIG. 2B). The more severely affected individuals had shunted or absent tail structures and often showed fused somites (FIG. 2C).

It was recently shown that the DG42 protein is involved in synthesis of HA,[16,17] and it was proposed that chitin oligosaccharides may function *in vivo* as primers for this process.[18] Preliminary data from our group suggests that the chitin oligomers produced by the DG42 protein can, in fact, act as a template for HA biosynthesis but that free

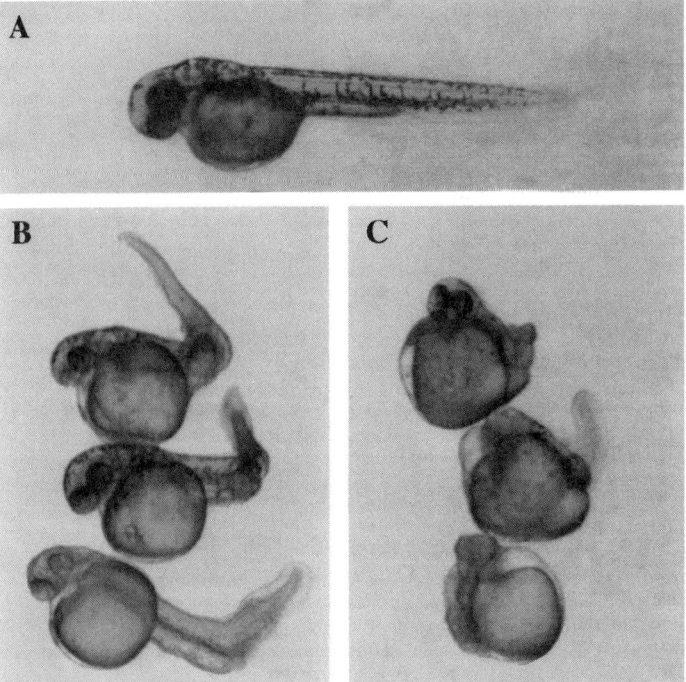

FIGURE 2. Phenotype of embryos expressing *Rhizobium* NodZ enzyme. Zebrafish embryos microinjected with pcDNA3 and pcDNA3-Bj-NodZ (see legend to FIG. 1) were cultured under standard conditions and raised to 48 hours postfertilization.[12] Photographs show embryos injected with (**A**) pcDNA3 and (**B**) pcDNA3-Bj-NodZ, showing moderate phenotype; **C**, same as **B**, presents a more severe phenotype.

chitin oligosaccharides are also generated.[19] These free oligomers could have an additional biochemical function.[2,3,6] Injection of anti-DG42 antibody into zebrafish embryos inhibits chitin synthase activity *in vitro* as well as *in vivo* and causes abnormal embryonic development: the formation of the posterior trunk and tail of the embryo are severely affected.[11,15] Consistent with this, a similar effect was obtained after injecting embryos with purified NodZ, a chitin oligosaccharide-modifying enzyme that transfers a fucose residue from GDP-β-L-fucose to the C-6 position of the reducing end of chitin oligosaccharides.[15] Chitinase-63 from *Streptomyces plicatus*, which has high affinity for chitin oligosaccharides, also produces this phenotype.[11] This suggests that *in vivo* modification of the chitin oligosaccharide structure (by adding a new fucose residue or by degradation) may functionally inactivate the molecule and generate a visible effect on embryonic development.[11,15]

The NodZ enzyme has a high affinity for chitin oligosaccharides, their natural substrates, with a K_m of 0.12 mM.[23] N-glycans carrying an N,N'-chitobiosyl structure at their reducing termini are also substrates for the enzyme, but with higher K_m.[23] N-glycanase activity has been reported in the early embryos of *Oryzias latipes* (Medaka fish),[20] suggesting that free N-glycan chains with the chitobiose at the reducing end are present in Medaka fish embryos cells; this may also be the case in zebra fish embryos. Fucosylation by NodZ may modify these oligosaccharides to an extent that causes an inhibition of their cellular function in early embryos, which leads to a visible phenotype. The glycans and/or their fucosylated derivatives should, therefore, be evaluated as alternative signaling molecules. However, it appears clear that in teleosts and amphibians, chitin oligosaccharides and free N-glycans have essential functions during embryogenesis.

ACKNOWLEDGMENT

We thank Nancy Hopkins for the use of laboratory facilities and zebrafish.

REFERENCES

1. LONG, S.R. 1989. *Rhizobium*-legume nodulation: Life together in the underground. Cell **56**: 203–214.
2. DENARIE, J., F. DEBELLE & J.C. PROME. 1996. *Rhizobium* lipo chitooligosaccharide nodulation factors: Signaling molecules mediating recognition and morphogenesis. Annu. Rev. Biochem. **65**: 503–535.
3. LEROUGE, P., P. ROUCHE, C. FAUCHER, F. MAILLET, G. TRUCHET, J.C. PROME & J. DENARIE. 1990. Symbiotic host-specificity of *Rhizobium meliloti* is determined by a sulphated and acylated glucosamine oligosaccharide signal. Nature (Lond.) **344**: 781–784.
4. GEREMIA, R.A., P. MERGAET, D. GEELAN, M. VAN MONTAGU & M. HOLSTERS. 1994. The NodC protein of *Azorhizobium caulinodans* is an N-acetyl glucosaminyltransferase. Proc. Natl. Acad. Sci. USA **91**: 2669–2673.
5. SEMINO, C.E. & M.A. DANKERT. 1994. The *in vitro* biosynthesis of functional nodulation factors (Nod Rm) produced by *Rhizobium meliloti* 1021. Cell. Mol. Biol. **40**: 1029–1037.
6. SPAINK, H. 1995. The molecular basis of infection and nodulation by rhizobia: The ins and outs of sympathogenesis. Annu. Rev. Phytopatol. **33**: 345–368.
7. SPAINK, H.P., A.H.M. WIJFJES, G.M. VAN DER DRIFT, J. HAVERKAMP, J.E. THOMAS-OATES & B.J.J. LUGTENBERG. 1994. Structural identification of metabolites produced by the NodB and NodC proteins of *Rhizobium leguminosarum*. Mol. Microbiol. **13**: 821–831.
8. LOPEZ-LARA, I.M., L. BLOKTIP, C. QUINTO, M.L. GARCIA, G. STACEY, G.V. BLOEMBERG, G.E.M. LAMERS, B.J.J. LUGTENBERG, J.E. THOMASOATES & H. P. SPAINK. 1996. NodZ of *Bradyrhizobium* extends the nodulation host range of *Rhizobium* by adding a fucosyl residue to nodulation signals. Mol. Microbiol. **21** (2): 397–408.

9. ROSA, F., T.D. SARGENT, M.L. REBBERT, G.S. MICHAELS, M. JAMRICH, H. CRUZ, E. JONAS, J.A. WINKLES & I.B. DAWID. 1988. Accumulation and decay of DG42 gene products follow a gradient pattern during *Xenopus* embryogenesis. Dev. Biol. **129:** 114–123.
10. SEMINO, C.E., C.A. SPECHT, A. RAIMONDI & P.W. ROBBINS. 1996. Homologs of the *Xenopus* developmental gene *DG42* are present in zebrafish and mouse and are involved in the synthesis of Nod-like chitin oligosaccharides during early embryogenesis. Proc. Natl. Acad. Sci. USA **93:** 4548–4553.
11. SEMINO, C.E., M.L. ALLENDE & P.W. ROBBINS. 1998. Temporal synthesis and degradation of chitin oligosaccharides during embryonic zebrafish development. Submitted.
12. WESTERFIELD, M. 1994. The Zebrafish Book. A Guide for the Laboratory Use of Zebrafish *(Brachydario rerio)*. University of Oregon Press.
13. BULAWA, C.E. & W. WASCO. 1991. Chitin and nodulation. Nature (Lond.) **353:** 710.
14. SEMINO, C.E. & P.W. ROBBINS. 1995. Synthesis of "Nod"-like chitin oligosaccharides by the *Xenopus* developmental protein DG42. Proc. Natl. Acad. Sci. USA **92:** 3498–3501.
15. BAKKERS, J., C.E. SEMINO, H. STROBAND, P.W. ROBBINS, J.W. KIJNE & H.P. SPAINK. 1997. An important developmental role for oligosaccharides during early embryogenesis of cyprinid fish. Proc. Natl. Acad. Sci. USA **94:** 7982–7986.
16. MEYER, M.F. & G. KREIL. 1996. Cells expressing the DG42 gene from early *Xenopus* embryos synthesize hyaluronan. Proc. Natl. Acad. Sci. USA **93:** 4543–4547.
17. DEANGELIS, P.L. & A.M. ACHYUTHAN. 1996. Yeast-derived recombinant DG42 protein of Xenopus can synthesize hyaluronan *in vitro*. J. Biol. Chem. **271:** 23657–23660.
18. VARKI, A. 1996. Does DG42 synthesize hyaluronan or chitin? A controversy about oligosaccharides in vertebrate development. Proc. Natl. Acad. Sci. USA **93:** 4523–4525.
19. SEMINO, C.E. & P.W. ROBBINS. 1997. *Xenopus* developmental protein DG42 expressed in yeast synthesize variable ratios of hyaluronate and chitin oligosaccharides *in vitro* depending on incubation conditions. Submitted.
20. SUZUKI, T., A. SEKO, K. KITAJIMA, Y. INOUE & S. INOUE. 1994. Purification and enzymatic properties of peptide:*N*-glycanase from C3H mouse-derived L-929 fibroblast cells. J. Biol. Chem. **269:** 17611–17618.
21. GIBBS, P.D.L., A. PEEK & G. THOROGAAD. 1994. An *in vivo* screen for the luciferase transgene in zebrafish. Mol. Mar. Biol. Biotech. **3:** 307–316.
22. WAGNER, G.P., J. LO, R. LAINE & ALMEDER. 1993. Chitin in the epidermal cuticle of a vertebrate (*Paralipophrys triglodites*, Blenniidae, Teleostei). Experientia **49:** 317–319.
23. QUINTO, C., A.H.M. WIJFJES, G.V. BLOEMBERG, L. BLOK-TIP, I.M. LOPEZ-LARA, B.J.J. LUGTENBERG, J.E. THOMAS-OATES & H.P. SPAINK. 1997. Proc Natl. Acad. Sci. USA **94:** 4336–4341.

Regulation and Formation of the *Drosophila* Salivary Glands[a]

DEBORAH J. ANDREW[b]

Department of Cell Biology and Anatomy, The Johns Hopkins University School of Medicine, 725 North Wolfe Street, Baltimore, Maryland 21205-2196, USA

ABSTRACT: The homeotic gene, *Sex combs reduced (Scr)*, is a master regulator of *Drosophila* salivary gland formation. Embryos in which *Scr* function is missing do not form salivary glands, and embryos in which SCR protein is expressed everywhere form extra salivary glands. However, other known proteins, including the homeotic protein Abdominal-B, the unusual zinc finger protein Teashirt, and the secreted signaling molecule Decapentaplegic (a TGF-β family member), limit the recruitment of SCR-expressing cells to salivary glands. To learn the molecular details of how salivary gland gene expression is controlled and as a first step toward understanding how the SCR transcription factor controls salivary gland morphogenesis, we screened for genes expressed in the developing salivary gland. Among our best candidates for potential direct downstream targets of SCR in the salivary gland are the genes *trachealess (trh)*, *dCREB-A*, *jalapeño*, and *Semaphorin II (SemaII)*. Our genetic studies suggest distinct and important roles for each of these genes in salivary gland morphogenesis. Current work includes studying the molecular interactions between SCR and these downstream target genes and asking how target genes coordinate their activities to effect the cell biological changes required to build functional salivary glands.

HOMEOTIC GENES CONTROL THE DEVELOPMENT OF SPECIFIC TISSUES IN DIFFERENT BODY SEGMENTS

How do organs form during development? What controls the size, placement, morphology, and function of a specific tissue? If we ask these questions in human terms, we ask what the factors are that control, for example, whether or not you have a liver, where in your body the liver forms, the number and types of cells that contribute to the liver, and finally, what controls the distinctions between a liver cell and any other cell in the body with respect to which structural proteins and enzymes are synthesized in the mature organ. We know from genetic studies that master regulators, such as those encoded by the homeotic genes, determine which structures form in the different body segments. Homeotic genes are expressed in limited domains along the anterior-posterior body axis, and mutations in homeotic genes cause structures within a particular segment or segments to be replaced by structures normally found elsewhere (for example, eyes to wings or legs to antennae). In *Drosophila,* many of the homeotic genes are organized within two major complexes, the bithorax complex (BX-C) and the Antennapedia complex (ANT-C).[1,2] The BX-C includes the *Ultrabithorax (Ubx)*, the *abdominal-A (Abd-A)*, and the *Abdominal-B (Abd-B)* genes whose functions are required for correct development of the posterior thoracic and abdominal segments. The ANT-C

---

[a] Our work has been supported by NIH Grant #RO1 GM51311, an American Cancer Society Institutional Research Grant, a JHU Institutional Research Grant, and by the Council for Tobacco Research, Grant #4275R1.

[b] Tel: (410) 614-2722; fax: (410) 955-4129; e-mail: debbie__andrew@qmail.bs.jhu.edu.

genes important for segment identity include *labial (lab)*, *proboscipedia (pb)*, *Deformed (Dfd)*, *Sex combs reduced (Scr)*, and *Antennapedia (Antp)*. Products of the ANT-C genes specify structures in the head and anterior thoracic segments. Transcription of the ANT-C and BX-C genes is precisely regulated; the spatial and temporal expression patterns of the homeotic genes ultimately specify which structures are made in each segment of the fly.

Similar homeotic gene complexes exist in other organisms, including mammals. The *Drosophila* and mammalian homeotic complexes are similar in both protein sequence homologies and the organization of genes within the complexes.[3] However, unlike in flies where two separate homeotic complexes exist, the mammalian homeotic genes, the HOX genes, are organized within a single complex (although there are four copies of the complex in the genome). As in flies, mutations in mammalian homeotic genes cause specific and dramatic developmental effects. Moreover, the mammalian genes, when ectopically expressed in flies, cause the same developmental abnormalities as the homologous fly genes. The similarity in gene sequence, organization, and function suggests that what is learned about the role of homeotic genes in *Drosophila* organogenesis will be directly relevant to developmental studies in all mammals, including humans.

Each of the BX-C, ANT-C, and HOX genes encodes one or more related DNA-binding transcription factors.[4,5] Thus, homeotic genes control cell fate by regulated transcription of downstream target genes. What are these target genes? Despite a concerted effort in the past several years, very few target genes have been identified.[6] The largest group of genes known to be controlled by homeotics are the homeotic genes themselves.[7–16] The few additional target genes include two genes expressed in the embryonic midgut that overlap the expression patterns of one or more homeotic genes;[14,17–19] *connection*, a gene expressed in the central nervous system that is either regulated by *Ubx* or *Antp*;[20,21] *Distal-less*, which itself may be a transcriptional regulator;[22,23] *unplugged*, a gene controlling segment-specific tracheal branching;[24] *centrosomin*, a gene whose expression is regulated by different homeotic proteins in different tissues;[25] three transcription factors expressed in the salivary gland, *trachealess*, *fork head (fkh)* and *dCREB-A*;[26–29] and a few less-well-characterized genes.[30–32] Only in the embryonic midgut and in the larval salivary gland is a picture emerging of how homeotic target genes function during tissue morphogenesis.

SALIVARY GLAND FORMATION IS A SIMPLE SYSTEM FOR STUDYING HOW HOMEOTIC GENES CONTROL TISSUE MORPHOGENESIS

My laboratory focuses on how the homeotic gene *Scr* controls the formation of a relatively simple organ, the larval salivary gland. Larval salivary glands provide a simple developmental system to study how early-acting regulatory molecules control the assembly of multicellular organs. Salivary glands start out as two ventrolateral plates of approximately 100 cells each, in the region of the presumptive posterior head.[33] No additional cell divisions occur during salivary gland differentiation. Instead, the salivary glands increase in size simply by increasing the volume of individual cells. Thus, all of the changes that occur during differentiation take place within and between existing cells. This greatly simplifies the analysis of organ development, because we need not be concerned with the regulated control of cell division, the potential unequal partitioning of cellular factors during mitosis, or programmed cell death. As embryogenesis proceeds, the salivary gland cells undergo a number of simple and interesting events. The nuclei move from the surface of the embryo to a more basal position within each cell, and the salivary gland secretory cells change shape from cuboidal to columnar. The cells then initiate multiple rounds of DNA replication that create the giant polytene chromosomes needed to accommodate the increased size of each cell.[34] Later, the salivary gland secretory cells invaginate and move dorsally and posteriorly, led by the cells near the lateral edge of each plate. With this movement, the salivary glands become internalized. Lumen-specific antigens can be detected as soon as invagination begins (FIG. 1).[28] By late embryogenesis, the salivary gland cells have migrated to their most posterior location, reaching to the middle of the third thoracic segment dorsolateral to the ventral nerve cord. The salivary duct cells, which derive from the most ventral cells of the salivary gland primordia, are the last to invaginate. These tube-forming cells, which form both the lateral individual ducts and the central common duct, connect the secretory cells of the salivary glands to the larval mouth. The developing salivary gland thus provides a simple system for study of the transition from euploidy to polyteny, control of organelle position, cell shape changes, cell migration, tube formation, and tissue-specific gene regulation.

IDENTIFICATION OF GENES EXPRESSED IN THE SALIVARY GLAND

To identify genes expressed in the embryonic salivary gland, we screened several different "enhancer-trap" stock collections. Enhancer-traps are created by the insertion of transposable elements containing the *E. coli* β-galactosidase (β-gal) gene fused to a relatively inactive promoter. Insertion of the transposons within or near enhancers for different genes often results in the expression of β-gal in patterns that mirror the expression of those genes.[35–39] Thus we can sample a large portion of the genome for genes expressed in various tissues simply by assaying β-gal expression in different lines harboring a single transposable element inserted at essentially random positions. The transposable elements have several features that allow easy molecular and functional characterization of the genes into which they insert. Selected genes can be mapped by *in situ* hybridization to polytene chromosomes using the original transposon DNA as a molecular probe. The genes can be easily cloned because of the presence of the *E. coli* origin of replication and the drug resistance gene within the transposon. Mutations in selected genes can be made simply by mobilizing the transposons and selecting for imprecise excisions. Thus the enhancer-trap lines provide molecular as well as mutational access to genes selected solely on the basis of their expression within a particular tissue.

We identified 36 different lines in which β-gal was expressed in the embryonic salivary gland from enhancer-trap collections available through the Scott/Fuller laboratories, the Spradling laboratory, and the Goodman/Rubin laboratories. We mapped the 36 lines to 20 different sites in the genome. All lines that mapped to the same chromosomal position either have identical or overlapping patterns of expression, suggesting that the multiple independent insertions are sampling enhancers of the same genes. A few of the enhancer traps are insertions in genes known previously to be expressed in embryonic salivary glands, including *Toll (Tl)*, *hückebein (hkb)*, and *dCREB-A*. All 20 of the lines show β-gal expression late in salivary gland development; however, seven of the genes are also expressed very early in the primordial cells of the embryonic salivary gland, making them good candidates for direct control by *Scr*. Some or all of the thirteen late genes may, in turn, be regulated by the early genes. Many of these late genes show complex expression patterns and are therefore good markers for salivary gland differentiation.

In our screen for salivary gland–expressed enhancer-trap lines, not a single line was identified that results in β-gal expression exclusively in the salivary gland; each salivary gland line also displays β-gal expression in a subset of other embryonic tissues. For example, an insert in the *jalapeño (jal)* gene is expressed in the salivary gland secretory cells, the embryonic fat body, a subset of cells in the pharynx, the apodemes (cells that function as muscle attachment sites in the epidermis), and, in later stages, in the epi-

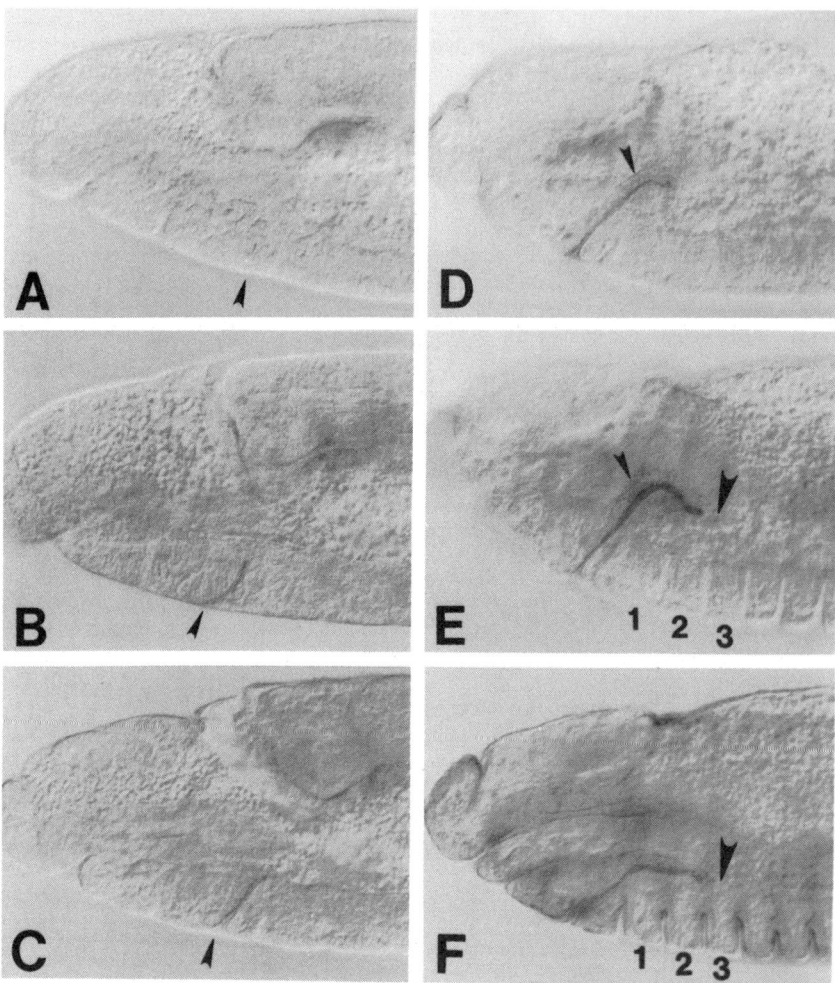

FIGURE 1. Salivary gland morphogenesis. Salivary gland cells begin to express the lumen-specific antigen, D3, when the salivary gland cells first invaginate (panel A). Using the D3 antibody it is possible to track the movements of the salivary gland cells. The cells first move at a 45° angle dorsally and posteriorly (panels B and C). By the end of germ-band retraction, the salivary gland cells turn and move posteriorly (panel D). The salivary gland cells extend to the middle of the third thoracic segment by the end of embryogenesis (panel F). The small arrowheads in each figure point to the invaginating salivary gland. The large arrowheads in E and F indicate the most posterior extent of the salivary gland. 1, 2, and 3 refer to the first, second, and third thoracic segments, respectively.

dermis itself (R. Yochem, B. Abella, and D.J.Andrew, unpublished results). Another candidate target gene, *dCREB-A*, is expressed in the salivary gland secretory cells, the proventriculus, the epidermis, and in the dorsal trunk cells of the trachea.[29] Based on the observation that multiple genes are coordinately expressed early in the salivary gland primordia and the apparent absence of genes expressed exclusively in the salivary gland, we propose that salivary glands form because of the activation of a unique set of genes whose combined activities coordinate the morphogenesis of this tissue. By studying how these genes function in nonsalivary gland tissues, we will obtain further clues about their roles in salivary gland development.

Scr IS A MASTER REGULATOR OF SALIVARY GLAND GENES

We first tested whether *Scr* regulates expression of the salivary gland genes identified in the above screen. This was done by assaying expression of these genes in both loss-of-function *Scr* mutants and in animals where SCR protein is expressed everywhere using an induced HS-SCR (an *Scr* cDNA under the control of a *h*eat *s*hock-inducible promoter) transgene. With all of the genes examined so far, expression in the salivary gland depends on *Scr*. In *Scr*⁻ animals, there is no expression of *dCREB-A, jal, hkb, fkh*, two salivary gland genes in 85D, or *trh* in the region where the salivary gland would have normally formed, although expression of each of these genes in other tissues is unaffected. In animals expressing *Scr* protein ubiquitously, additional expression of each gene occurs in cells anterior to the normal salivary gland.[26,28,40] Ectopically, each gene is expressed in cells in the same dorsal/ventral position as the normal salivary gland–forming cells (FIG. 2). We were a little surprised that although SCR is expressed everywhere with the HS-SCR construct, the new cells that express the salivary gland markers are found almost exclusively in regions anterior to the normal salivary gland. This result is different from that observed by Panzer *et al.*[28] in studies with *fork head (fkh)*, another gene expressed in the salivary gland. Using a *fkh* antibody and a *fkh-lacZ* transgene, Panzer *et al.*[28] detected ectopic expression in segments both anterior and posterior to the normal salivary gland. Thus, although each of the tested salivary gland genes responds to ectopic expression of *Scr*, the genes respond differentially.

We were curious why most salivary gland genes are expressed ectopically in only anterior segments when SCR protein is made everywhere. This curiosity led to the experiments demonstrating that two very different transcription factors block expression of salivary gland genes in posterior segments, an unusual zinc finger protein encoded by the trunk gene *teashirt (tsh)* and a homeotic protein encoded by *Abdominal-B (Abd-B)* (FIG. 3).[28] Thus, although *Scr* is absolutely required for salivary gland formation and is capable of inducing salivary gland fates in cells that do not normally express *Scr*, the recruitment of *Scr*-expressing cells to form salivary glands is limited by known genes. Along the dorsal-ventral axis, a TGF-β homologue, *decapentaplegic (dpp)*, limits the number of cells that can form salivary glands.[26,27] In future studies of salivary gland target genes, we expect that each gene will be activated by SCR but that activation may be blocked by other regulatory molecules such as those encoded by *dpp, tsh,* and *Abd-B*.

THE *trachealess* GENE IS A GOOD CANDIDATE FOR DIRECT REGULATION BY *Scr* IN THE DEVELOPING SALIVARY GLAND

Among the earliest expressed enhancer-trap lines identified in our screen was an insert in the *trachealess (trh)* gene.[41,42] As with every gene identified in our screen, *trh* ex-

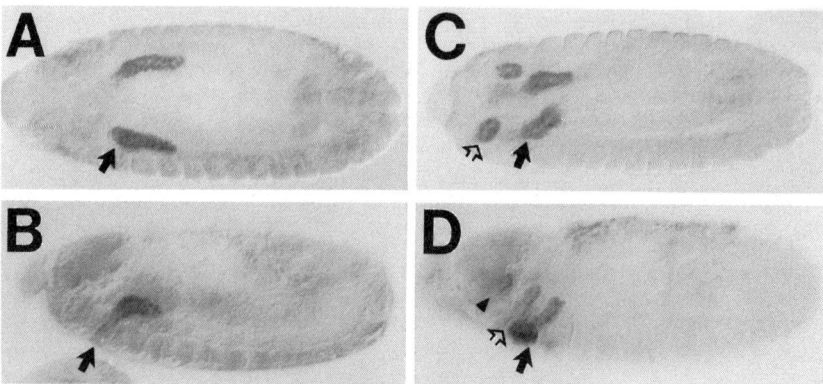

FIGURE 2. Global production of SCR induces salivary gland formation in new places. Using the HS-SCR construct to produce SCR protein everywhere in the embryo, it is possible to induce extra salivary glands in new places. However, with most of the salivary gland markers we have tested, salivary gland formation is induced only anterior to the normal salivary gland–forming segment, known as parasegment 2. Panels A and B show salivary gland marker staining in wild-type embryos. Panels C and D show salivary gland marker staining in HS-SCR animals. Note the position and morphology of the extra salivary gland cells. Top panels are ventral views and lower panels are lateral views. The filled arrows point to the salivary glands that derive from parasegment 2. The open arrows point to ectopic salivary glands that derive from parasegment 1. The arrowhead points to an ectopic salivary gland that derives from parasegment 0.

pression is not limited to the salivary gland; *trh* is also expressed in the trachea, filzkörper, and a subset of cells in the central nervous system. However, *Scr* affects *trh* expression in only the salivary gland primordia and not in these other tissues. In *Scr*⁻ embryos, *trh* expression is absent in the region of the salivary gland primordia, and, in embryos expressing the SCR protein everywhere, ectopic *trh* expression occurs in more anterior segments. Because *trh* is a good candidate for a direct downstream target gene of *Scr*, we initiated a phenotypic and molecular characterization of the *trh* gene.[26]

PHENOTYPIC CHARACTERIZATION OF *trachealess*

The enhancer-trap insertion in cytological region 61C, isolated because of its corresponding β-gal expression in the entire salivary gland primordia, created a loss-of-function allele of *trh*. This conclusion is based on complementation tests between the insertion allele and a *trh* ethylmethane sulfonate (EMS) allele, and excision experiments demonstrating that the *trh*⁻ phenotype and corresponding lethality are reversed when the enhancer-trap insertion is cleanly excised. The excision experiments also yielded five new alleles of *trh*, including both weak and strong loss-of-function alleles.

FIGURE 3. TSH and ABD-B block SCR induction of salivary glands. Panels A, B, and C are embryos stained with antibodies to the *Drosophila* dCREB-A (darker staining) and antibodies to the ENGRAILED protein (lighter segmentally repeated staining). Engrailed (EN) is detected in the most anterior cells of each parasegment. Panel A is a wild-type embryo showing dCREB-A salivary gland staining in cells limited to parasegment 2. Panel B shows dCREB-A and EN staining in an embryo expressing SCR protein everywhere (using an induced heat-shock pro-

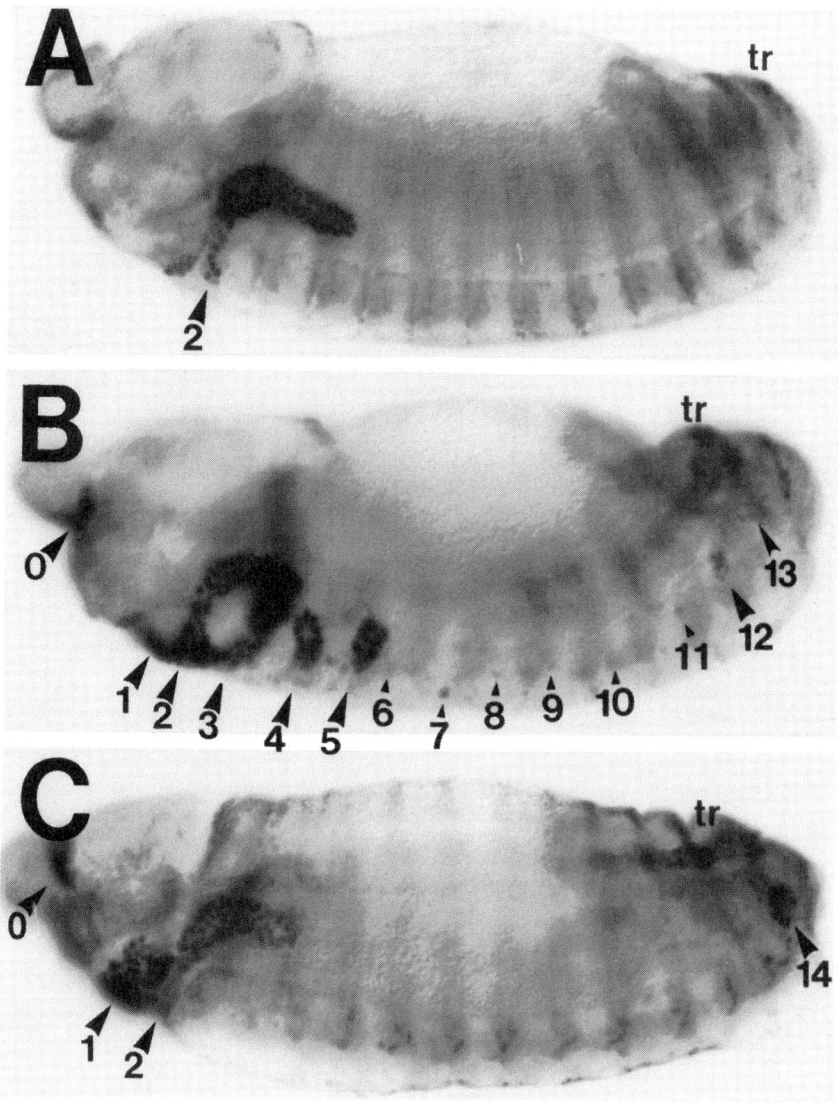

moter fused to an *SCR* cDNA) and simultaneously missing function of the *teashirt (tsh)* gene. In addition to the normal staining in parasegment 2, strong ectopic salivary gland staining of dCREB-A is observed in cells that derive from parasegments 0, 1, 3, 4, and 5, with fewer cells expressing dCREB-A in parasegments 6–13. Higher levels of SCR expression result in more cells in all parasegments from 0–1 and 3–13 expressing the dCREB-A salivary marker protein.[28] Panel C shows dCREB-A and EN staining in an embryo that expresses SCR protein everywhere (using an induced heat-shock promoter fused to an SCR cDNA) and is deficient for genes in the Bithorax complex. In addition to the normal parasegment 2 staining, strong ectopic salivary gland staining of dCREB-A is observed in cells that derive from parasegments 0, 1, and 14. Similar expression patterns are observed in embryos expressing SCR protein everywhere and simply missing a function of the *Abdominal-B* gene of the Bithorax complex.

From the phenotypes of seven *trh* alleles (an EMS allele, the insertion allele, and five excision alleles), we know that *trh* is required for tube formation in three different tissues: the salivary gland duct, the trachea, and the filzkörper. In loss-of-function *trh* mutants, the salivary gland duct cells remain on the embryo surface and fail to invaginate to form tubes (FIG. 4), the tracheal cells also remain on the embryo surface and fail to invaginate, and the cells that form the filzkörper remain clustered and do not organize into tubes. Scanning electron micrographs of the surface of *trh* mutants indicate that even the invaginations that lead to tracheal pit formation fail to occur, suggesting that *trh* is required for the earliest stages of tube formation.[26] *trh* is expressed in the trachea throughout embryogenesis and in third instar larvae, suggesting that *trh* function may be required continuously. In *trh* mutants, the tracheal precursor cells that remain on the embryo surface express at least three tracheal markers, the POU-homeodomain protein encoded by the *drifter* gene,[43] the CRUMBS (CRB) protein,[44] and *trh*-β-gal, strongly suggesting that the tracheal cells in *trh* mutants have not lost their identity, but instead have simply lost their ability to invaginate and organize tubes. Similarly, although the filzkörper do not form the tubular chambers that function as air filters for the trachea, these cells nevertheless secrete the high levels of cuticle that normally line the filzkörper in wild-type embryos (FIG. 5). Based on these results we hypothesize that *trh* is not required to specify the identity of any of the cell types but instead functions specifically in the cell biological changes of tube formation.

EMBRYONIC EXPRESSION OF *tracheless*

We cloned the genomic DNA surrounding the *trh* insertion and isolated corresponding cDNAs. Whole-mount *in situ* hybridization with either genomic or cDNA clones indicate that *trh* is expressed in all of the cells that require its function. In the sali-

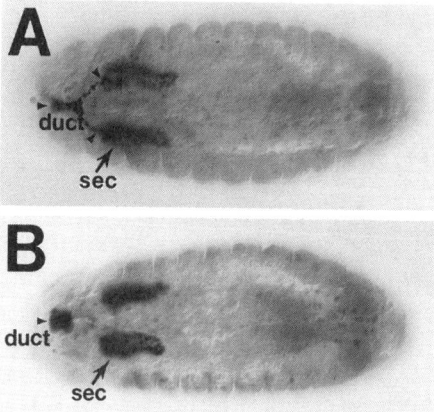

FIGURE 4. In *trh* mutants, the salivary duct cells fail to invaginate to form the tubes that normally connect the salivary gland secretory cells to the foregut. Panels A and B are embryos (wild-type embryo, panel A; *trh* mutant embryo, panel B) stained with a nuclear marker expressed in the salivary gland duct and secretory cells. The arrowheads point to the salivary gland duct cells. The arrows point to the salivary gland secretory cells. Notice that in the *trh* mutant embryo (B) the duct cells fail to invaginate and remain at their site of origin in the ectoderm. The morphology of the secretory cells (sec) appears normal in *trh* mutants.

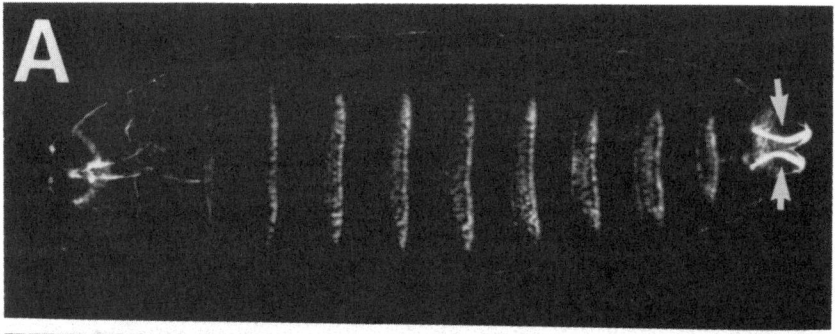
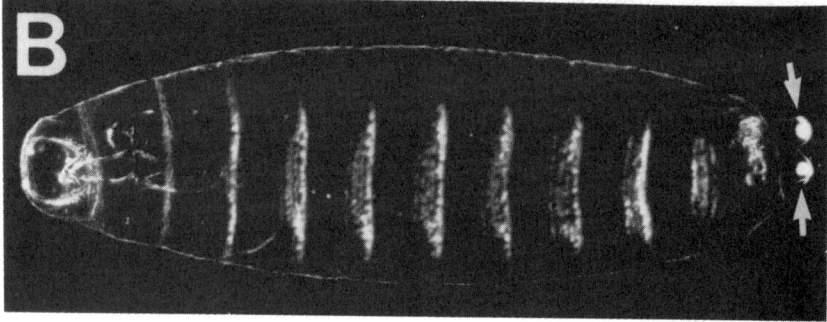

FIGURE 5. Filzkörper do not elongate in *trh* mutants. Panels A and B are dark field micrographs of cuticle preparations from wild-type (A) and *trh* mutant (B) first-instar larvae. The larval cuticle is relatively normal in both animals, except the filzkörper (arrows) fail to elongate in the *trh* mutant larva (B). Note that the cuticular threads that line the filzkörper (which appear as dense white material in these dark field images) are synthesized in both wild-type and *trh* mutant larvae.

vary gland, *trh* is initially expressed in the entire primordia, in both duct and secretory cells. At later stages, *trh* expression in the secretory cells disappears and expression persists in the duct cells, the only cells of the salivary gland affected by *trh* mutations. *trh* is expressed in all tracheal cells from embryonic stage 8 throughout embryogenesis. The onset of *trh* expression in the trachea precedes by at least one hour the first morphological indications of tube formation, the formation of the tracheal placodes. *trh* expression in the filzkörper primordia is first detectable during germ band extension and is then present throughout embryogenesis. The only other cells that express detectable levels of *trh* mRNA are a subset of cells in the central nervous system (CNS), where a function for *trh* has not yet been determined.

REGULATION OF *trachealess* IN THE SALIVARY GLAND

trh expression in the salivary gland is controlled by at least four different regulators[26]: Expression in the salivary gland is absolutely dependent on *Scr*. In loss-of-function *Scr* mutants, *trh* expression is never detected in parasegment 2 (PS2), the region where salivary glands normally arise. In induced HS-SCR embryos, ectopic *trh* expression is seen in regions corresponding to PS0 and PS1, an expression profile similar to most other tested salivary gland genes. Expression of *trh* is prevented by TSH in posterior segments. In *tsh⁻* embryos, *trh* expression expands into PS3, concomitant with the expansion of the *Scr* expression domain in *tsh* mutant embryos. Expression of *trh* on the dorsal side of the embryo is prevented by DPP. In *dpp⁻* embryos, *trh* expression in the salivary gland and tracheal precursors expands into the entire dorsal surface of the embryo. Expression of *trh* is limited to the duct cells by FKH. *trh* mRNA is normally detected in the entire salivary gland primordia but very quickly becomes limited to the duct cells. In *fkh⁻* embryos, *trh* expression in the secretory cells persists.

trachealess ENCODES A TRANSCRIPTION FACTOR CLOSELY RELATED TO PROTEINS ENCODED BY THE *DROSOPHILA single-minded* AND HUMAN *hypoxia-inducible factor 1*-α GENES

Conceptual translation of the single large open reading frame indicates that *trh* encodes a protein with homologies to known transcription factors.[26,45] The two proteins with greatest similarity to *trh* are those encoded by the *Drosophila single-minded (sim)* gene and the human *hypoxia-inducible factor-1*α *(HIF-1*α*)* gene. sim is required for the development of neurons, glia, and other nonneuronal cells that derive from the midline of the embryonic CNS.[46,47] HIF-1α is a protein required for transcriptional activation of the erythropoietin gene in response to low oxygen tension.[48] All three genes, *trh, sim,* and *HIF-1*α*,* encode proteins with the following features: an extreme N-terminal basic helix-loop-helix (bHLH) DNA-binding protein-dimerization domain, followed by what is known as a PAS domain (The name PAS is based on other proteins that also contain this domain: P for the PER protein, encoded by the *period (per)* gene, which controls the periodicity of *Drosophila* behavior; A for a protein that forms part of the aromatic hydrocarbon receptor complex, which is also a bHLH protein; and S for the SIM protein), and finally a region C-terminal to the PAS domain, the HST domain, a 50 amino acid region that is uniquely conserved (so far) to HIF-1α, SIM, and TRH. At least two genes require *trh* for expression in the salivary duct, *breathless (btl)* and *Serrate (Ser).*[49]

THE *fork head* AND *dCREB-A* GENES ARE ALSO GOOD CANDIDATES FOR DIRECT REGULATION BY *Scr* IN THE DEVELOPING SALIVARY GLAND

fork head was the first gene to be identified as a potential downstream target gene for SCR regulation in the salivary gland.[27] *fkh* expression in the salivary gland is absent in *Scr⁻* embryos, and when SCR is expressed ubiquitously, ectopic *fkh* expression is observed not only in more anterior segments but in every segment of the embryo. By all other criteria, the ectopic expression of *fkh* in these more posterior segments does not recruit cells to form salivary glands, thus *fkh* alone is insufficient to induce salivary gland fates. These results suggest that although *fkh* is positively regulated by SCR in the salivary gland, activation of *fkh* by SCR is not blocked by TSH or ABD-B, as are the majority of salivary gland genes so far tested. *fkh* expression is blocked dorsally by DPP and ventrally by the *"spitz*-group" genes, thus limiting expression of *fkh* to the salivary gland secretory cell population.[27]

In embryos homozygous for loss-of-function mutations in *fkh,* the secretory cells fail to invaginate, remain on the embryo surface, and eventually disappear, a phenotype analogous to that of *trh* in the salivary duct cell population.[26,50] Although *fkh* is not required for the initial expression of any of several salivary gland genes we have tested, it is required to maintain its own expression as well as the later expression of another salivary gland gene, *dCREB-A* (J. Aishima and D.J.Andrew). *fkh* is also required to shut off expression of *trh* in the salivary gland secretory cells.[26,49] Because *fkh* encodes a "winged-helix" DNA-binding protein, it is likely that FKH regulates salivary gland gene expression directly.[51] *fkh* is required not only for an early event in salivary gland morphogenesis, invagination of the secretory cells, but FKH appears to directly regulate expression of at least two salivary-specific structural protein genes, *Salivary gland secretion protein 3 (Sgs3)*[52] and *Salivary gland secretion protein 4 (Sgs4)*.[53] These "glue" proteins are expressed in the salivary gland near the end of larval life when they are secreted to form a sticky matrix to which the larva adheres in preparation for pupariation.

In our salivary gland expression screen, we identified two independent insertions in *dCREB-A* (CREB = Cyclic AMP Response Element Binding protein), a gene previously known only because of its DNA-binding properties[54] and its regulation by SCR.[28] *dCREB-A* is expressed in epithelial tissues, including the salivary gland, the trachea, and the epidermis, which will secrete the larval cuticle. The most obvious defect observed with loss of function mutations in *dCREB-A* is a weakening and lateralization of the larval cuticle; only lateral epidermal structures develop around the entire circumference of each segment. In the salivary gland the morphological effects of loss of *dCREB-A* function are relatively mild. *dCREB-A* mutant embryos have crooked salivary glands, a phenotype that overlaps that of wild-type embryos.[29] The salivary gland defect could be related to the epidermal defects; both tissues are composed of polarized secretory epithelial cells, and both tissues respond to extracellular dorsal-ventral patterning cues. Thus, *dCREB-A* may control the synthesis of secreted gene products shared by both tissues, and/or *dCREB-A* may be required to respond to extracellular patterning information.

REGULATORY INTERACTIONS AMONG THE EARLY SALIVARY GLAND GENES

We and others have made exciting discoveries about the regulation and morphogenesis of the developing salivary gland in *Drosophila* (FIG. 6).[26–29,49,51,52] SCR and the genes that limit SCR activation of salivary gland genes determine where salivary glands will form and the number of cells recruited to salivary gland fates.[27,28] These early studies also reveal what controls the distinction between the two major cell populations of the salivary gland: SCR alone recruits cells to secretory cell fates, and SCR in combination with the SPITZ-group proteins recruits cells to a duct cell fate.[26,49] Among the earliest known genes expressed in the secretory cell population are (1) *fkh*, a gene required for the invagination of the secretory cells, regulation of other early salivary gland genes, and expression of salivary-specific structural proteins made at later stages;[26,29,50–52] (2) *dCREB-A*, a gene required for the structural integrity of the secretory cells;[29] (3) *jalapeño*, a gene required to organize and/or maintain the polarized epithelium of the secretory cell population (R. Yochem, B. Abella, and D.J.Andrew, unpublished observations); and (4) *Semaphorin II*, a gene required for positioning the salivary gland (K. Henderson, A. Kolodkin, and D.J.Andrew, unpublished observations). The duct cells express *trh*, a gene required for duct cell invagination and tube formation. In turn, *trh* regulates expression of *btl*, a fibroblast growth factor receptor family member,[45,49,55] and *Ser*, a ligand in the *Notch* signaling pathway.[29,56,57] Future work will reveal the molecular details of how each salivary gland gene is regulated, and,

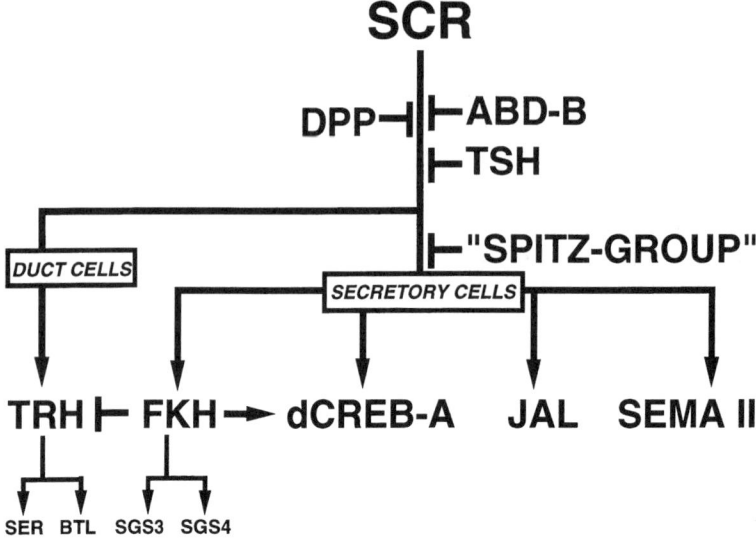

FIGURE 6. Regulatory interactions in the developing salivary gland. The homeotic gene *Scr* is the only known positive inducer of salivary glands. In the absence of *Scr*, salivary glands do not form, and when SCR is expressed in new places, salivary glands form in new places. However, every cell that expresses SCR is not recruited to a salivary fate. Cells that also express either DPP, ABD-B, or TSH do not contribute to salivary glands. One of the two major cell types in the salivary glands are the duct cells that express the *trh* gene as well as two genes downstream of *trh*, the *Ser* and *btl* genes;[26,49] *trh* has been shown to autoregulate.[45] The other major salivary gland cell type is the secretory cell population that expresses the genes *fkh, dCREB-A, jal* and *SemaII*; *fkh* has been shown to positively regulate its own expression and expression of *dCREB-A*[50] (J. Aishima and D.J.Andrew, unpublished results.) *fkh* shuts off *trh* expression in the secretory cells[26] and positively regulates expression of the salivary gland–secreted proteins, SGS3 and SGS4.[53,52] The distinction between duct and secretory cells arises early and is dependent on the *spitz*-group genes. The *spitz*-group blocks expression of the secretory cell–specific gene *fkh* (and probably other secretory-specific genes) while not affecting expression of the duct-specific gene *trh*.[27,49]

in turn, how each gene controls the specific salivary gland functions for which it is required.

ACKNOWLEDGMENTS

I thank all of the people who have been involved in our contributions to this work, including especially the past and present members of my laboratory (J. Aishima, A. Baig, P. Bhanot, K. Henderson, D. Isaac, C. Machado, B. Miller, P. Seshaiah, and R. Yochem) and contributing members of the laboratory at Stanford University, where this work was initiated (M. Horner, M. Petitt, and M. Scott). I thank P. Bradley and D. Isaac for their comments on the manuscript. I thank the members of the laboratory of S. Beckendorf who have contributed substantially to our current understanding of salivary gland regulation. I thank A. Spradling, G. Rubin, C. Goodman, M. Scott, and M. Fuller who made their enhancer-trap stocks available.

REFERENCES

1. DUNCAN, I.M. 1987. The bithorax complex. Annu. Rev. Genet. **21:** 285–319.
2. KAUFMAN, T.C., M.A. SEEGER & G. OLSEN. 1990. Molecular and genetic organization of the Antennapedia gene complex of *Drosophila melanogaster.* Adv. Genet. **27:** 309–362.
3. MCGINNIS, W. & R. KRUMLAUF. 1992. Homeobox genes and axial patterning. Cell **68:** 283–302.
4. LEVINE, M. & T. HOEY. 1988. Homoebox proteins as sequence-specific transcription factors. Cell **55:** 537–540.
5. SCOTT, M.P., J.W. TAMKUN & G.W. HARTZELL III. 1989. The structure and function of the homeodomain. BBA Rev. Cancer **989:** 25–48.
6. ANDREW, D.J. & M.P. SCOTT. 1992. Downstream of the homeotic genes. New Biol. **4:** 5–15.
7. HAFEN, E., M. LEVINE & W.J. GEHRING. 1984. Regulation of *Antennapedia* transcript distribution by the bithorax complex in *Drosophila*. Nature **307:** 287–289.
8. HARDING, K., C. WEDEEN, W. MCGINNIS & M. LEVINE. 1985. Spatially regulated expression of homeotic genes in Drosophila. Science **229:** 1236–1242.
9. STRUHL, G. & R.A. WHITE. 1985. Regulation of the *Ultrabithorax* gene of Drosophila by other bithorax complex genes. Cell **43:** 507–519.
10. CARROLL, S.B., R.A. LAYMON, M.A. MCCUTCHEON, P.D. RILEY & M.P. SCOTT. 1986. The localization and regulation of *Antennapedia* protein expression in *Drosophila* embryos. Cell **47:** 113–122.
11. RILEY P.D., S.B. CARROLL & M.P. SCOTT. 1987. The expression and regulation of *Sex combs reduced* protein in Drosophila embryos. Genes & Dev. **1:** 716–730.
12. BIENZ, M. & G. TREMML. 1988. Domain of *Ultrabithorax* expression in Drosophila visceral mesoderm from autoregulation and exclusion. Nature **333:** 576–578.
13. KUZIORA, M.A. & W. MCGINNIS. 1988. Autoregulation of a Drosophila homeotic selector gene. Cell **55:** 477–485.
14. REUTER, R., G.E.F. PANGANIBAN, F.M. HOFFMAN & M.P. SCOTT. 1990. Homeotic genes regulate the spatial expression of putative growth factors in the visceral mesoderm of *Drosophila* embryos. Development **110:** 1031–1040.
15. RILEY, G.R., E.M. JORGENSEN, R.K. BAKER & R.L. GARBER. 1991. Positive and negative control of the Antennapedia promoter P2. Development **112:** 177–185.
16. IRVINE, K.D., J. BOTAS, S. JHA, R.S. MANN & D.S. HOGNESS. 1993. Negative autoregulation by Ultrabithorax controls the level and pattern of its expression. Development **117:** 387–399.
17. IMMERGLUCK, K., P.A. LAWRENCE & M. BIENZ. 1990. Induction across germ layers in Drosophila mediated by a genetic cascade. Cell **62:** 261–268.
18. PANGANIBAN, G.E.F., R. REUTER, M.P. SCOTT & F.M. HOFFMANN. 1990. A Drosophila growth factor homolog, *decapentaplegic,* regulates homeotic gene expression within and across germ layers during midgut morphogenesis. Development **110:** 1041–1050.
19. MATHIES, L.D., S. KERRIDGE & M.P. SCOTT. 1994. Role of the *teashirt* gene in *Drosophila* midgut morphogenesis: Secreted proteins mediate the action of homeotic genes. Development **120:** 2799–2809.
20. GOULD, A.P., J.J. BROOKMAN, D.I. STRUTT & R.A.H. WHITE. 1990. Targets of homeotic gene control in Drosophila. Nature **348:** 308–312.
21. GOULD, A.P. & R. WHITE. 1992. *Connectin,* a target of homeotic gene control in *Drosophila.* Development **116:** 1163–1174.
22. COHEN, S.M., G. BRONNER, F. KUTTNER, G. JURGENS & H. JACKLE. 1989. Distal-less encodes a homoeodomain protein required for limb development in Drosophila. Nature **338:** 432–434.
23. VACHON, G., B. COHEN, C. PFEIFLE, M.E. MCGUFFIN, J. BOTAS & S.M. COHEN. 1992. Homeotic genes of the bithorax complex repress limb development in the abdomen of the Drosophila embryo through the target gene *Distal-less.* Cell **71:** 437–450.
24. CHIANG, C., K.E. YOUNG & P.A. BEACHY. 1995. Control of *Drosophila* tracheal branching by the novel homeodomain gene *unplugged,* a regulatory target for genes of the bithorax complex. Development **121:** 3901–3912.
25. HEUER, J.G., K. LI & T.C. KAUFMAN. 1995. The *Drosophila* homeotic target gene *centro-*

somin (cnn) encodes a novel centrosomal protein with leucine zippers and maps to a genomic region required for midgut morphogenesis. Development **121**: 3861–3876.
26. ISAAC, D.D. & D.J. ANDREW. 1996. Tubulogenesis in Drosophila: A requirement for the *trachealess* gene product. Genes & Dev. **10**: 103–117.
27. PANZER, S., D. WEIGEL & S.K. BECKENDORF. 1992. Organogenesis in Drosophila melanogaster. Embryonic salivary gland determination is controlled by homeotic and dorsoventral patterning genes. Development **114**: 49–57.
28. ANDREW, D.J., M.A. HORNER, M.G. PETITT, S.M. SMOLIK & M.P. SCOTT. 1994. Setting limits on homeotic gene function: Restraint of *Sex combs reduced* activity by *teashirt* and other homeotic genes. EMBO J. **13**: 1132–1144.
29. ANDREW, D.J., A. BAIG, P. BHANOT, S.M. SMOLIK & K.D. HENDERSON. 1997. The *Drosophila dCREB-A* gene is required for dorsal/ventral patterning of the larval cuticle. Development **124**: 181–193.
30. GRABA, Y., D. ARAGNOL, P. LAURENTI, V. GARZINO, D. CHARMOT, H. BERENGER & J. PRADEL. 1992. Homeotic control in Drosophila: The *scabrous* gene is an *in vivo* target of *Ultrabithorax* proteins. EMBO J. **11**: 3375–3384.
31. HINZ, U., A. WOLK & R. RENKAWITZ-POHL. 1992. *Ultrabithorax* is a regulator of beta-3 tubulin expression in the *Drosophila* visceral mesoderm. Development **116**: 543–554.
32. MASTICK, G.S., R. MCKAY, T. OLIGINO, K. DONOVAN & A.J. LOPEZ. 1995. Identification of target genes regulated by homeotic proteins in *Drosophila melanogaster* through genetic selection of *Ultrabithorax* protein-binding sites in yeast. Genetics **139**: 349–363.
33. CAMPOS-ORTEGA, J. A. & V. HARTENSTEIN. 1985. The Embryonic Development of *Drosophila melanogaster*. Springer-Verlag. Berlin.
34. SMITH, A. V. & T.L. ORR-WEAVER. 1991. The regulation of the cell cycle during *Drosophila* embryogenesis: The transition to polyteny. Development **112**: 997–1008.
35. BELLEN, H.J., C. O'KANE, C. WILSON, U. GROSSNIKLAUS, R.K. PEARSON & W.J. GEHRING. 1989. P-element-mediated enhancer detection: A versatile method to study development in *Drosophila*. Genes & Dev. **3**: 1288–1300.
36. BIER, E., H. VAESSIN, S. SHEPHERD, K. LEE, K. MCCALL, S. BARBEL, L. ACKERMAN, R. CARRETTP, T. UEMURA, E. GRELL, L.Y. JAN & Y.N. JAN. 1989. Searching for pattern and mutation in the *Drosophila* genome with a P-*lacZ* vector. Genes & Dev **3**: 1273–1287.
37. GROSSNIKLAUS, U., H.J. BELLEN, C. WILSON & W.J. GEHRING. 1989. P-element-mediated enhancer detection applied to the study of oogenesis in *Drosophila*. Development **107**: 189–200.
38. O'KANE, C.J. & W.J. GEHRING. 1987. Detection *in situ* of genomic regulatory elements in Drosophila. Proc. Natl. Acad. Sci. USA **84**: 9123–9127.
39. WILSON, C., R.K. PEARSON, H.J. BELLEN, C.J. O'KANE, U. GROSSNIKLAUS & W.J. GEHRING. 1989. P-element-mediated enhancer detection: An efficient method for isolating and characterizing developmentally regulated genes in *Drosophila*. Genes & Dev. **3**: 1301–1313.
40. ZENG, W., D.J. ANDREW, L.D. MATHIES, M.A. HORNER & M.P. SCOTT. 1993. Ectopic expression and function of the *Antp* and *Scr* homeotic genes: The N terminus of the homeodomain is critical to functional specificity. Development **118**: 339–352.
41. JURGENS, G., E. WIESCHAUS, C. NUSSLEIN-VOLHARD & H. KLUDING. 1984. Mutations affecting the pattern of the larval cuticle in *Drosophila melanogaster*. II. Zygotic loci on the third chromosome. Wilhelm Roux's Arch. Dev. Biol. **193**: 283–295.
42. YOUNOSSI-HARTENSTEIN, A. & V. HARTENSTEIN. 1993. The role of tracheae and musculature during pathfinding of *Drosophila* embryonic sensory axons. Dev. Biol. **158**: 430–437.
43. ANDERSON, M.G., G.L. PERKINS, P. CHITTICK, R.J. SHRIGLEY & W.A JOHNSON. 1995. *drifter,* a *Drosophila* POU-domain transcription factor, is required for correct differentiation and migration of tracheal cells and midline glia. Genes & Dev. **9**: 123–137.
44. TEPA, U., C. THERES & E. KNUST. 1990. *crumbs* encodes an EGF-like protein expressed on apical membranes of Drosphila epithelial cells and required for organization of the epithelia. Cell **61**: 787–799.
45. WILK, R., I. WEIZMAN & B.-Z. SHILO. 1996. *trachealess* encodes a bHLH-PAS protein that is an inducer of tracheal cell fates in *Drosophila*. Genes & Dev. **10**: 93–102.
46. NAMBU, J.R., R.G. FRANKS, S. HU & S.T. CREWS. 1990. The *single-minded* gene of

Drosophila is required for the expression of genes important for the development of CNS midline cells. Cell **63**: 63–75.
47. NAMBU, J.R., J.O. LEWIS, K.A.J. WHARTON & S.T. CREWS. 1991. The Drosophila *single-minded* gene encodes a helix-loop-helix protein that acts as a master regulator of CNS midline development. Cell **67**: 1157–1167.
48. WANG, G.L., B.-H. JIANG, E.A. RUE & G.L. SEMENZA. 1995. Hypoxia-inducible factor 1 is a basic-helix-loop-helix-PAS heterodimer regulated by cellular O_2 tension. Proc. Natl. Acad. Sci. USA **92**: 5510–5514.
49. KUO, Y.M., N. JONES, B. ZHOU, S. PANZER, V. LARSON & S.K. BECKENDORF. 1996. Salivary duct determination in *Drosophila:* Roles of the EGF receptor signaling pathway and the transcription factors Fork head and Trachealess. Development **122**: 1909–1917.
50. WEIGEL, D., H. BELLEN, G. JURGENS, F. KUTTNER, E. SEIFERT & H. JACKLE. 1989. Primordium-specific requirement of the homeotic gene *fork head* in the developing gut of the *Drosophila* embryo. Wilhelm Roux's Arch. Dev. Biol. **198**: 201–210.
51. KAUFMANN, E., E. HOCH & H. JACKLE. 1994. The interaction of DNA with the DNA-binding domain encoded by the *Drosophila* gene *fork head.* Eur. J. Biochem. **223**: 329–337.
52. MACH, V., K. OHNO, H. KOKUBO & Y. SUZUKI 1996. The *Drosophila* Fork head factor directly controls larval salivary gland-specific expression of the glue protein gene *Sgs3.* Nucleic Acids Res. **12**: 2387–2394.
53. LEHMANN, M. & G. KORGE. 1996. The *fork head* product directly specifies the tissue-specific hormone responsiveness of the *Drosophila Sgs-4 gene.* EMBO J. **18**: 4825–4834.
54. SMOLIK, S.M., R.E. ROSE & R.H. GOODMAN. 1992. A cyclic AMP-responsive element-binding transcriptional activator in Drosophila melanogaster, dCREB-A, is a member of the leucine zipper family. Mol. Cell. Biol. **12**: 4123–4131.
55. KLAMBT, C., L. GLAZER & B.-Z. SHILO. 1992. *breathless,* a Drosophila FGF receptor homolog, is essential for migration of tracheal and specific midline glial cells. Genes & Dev. **6**: 1668–1678.
56. FLEMING, R.J., T.N. SCOTTGALE, R.I. DIEDERICH & S. ARTAVANIS-TSAKONAS. 1990. The gene *Serrate* encodes a putative EGF-like transmembrane protein essential for proper ectodermal development in *Drosophila melanogaster.* Genes & Dev. **4**: 2188–2201.
57. THOMAS, U., S.A. SPEICHER & E. KNUST. 1991. The *Drosophila* gene *Serrate* encodes an EGF-like transmembrane protein with a complex expression pattern in embryos and wing discs. Development **111**: 749–761.

Salivary Gland Nucleotide Receptors

Changes in Expression and Activity Related to Development and Tissue Damage[a]

JOHN T. TURNER,[b] MINJUNG PARK, JEAN M. CAMDEN, AND GARY A. WEISMAN

Department of Pharmacology and Biochemistry, University of Missouri School of Medicine, 1 Hospital Drive, Columbia, Missouri 65212, USA

ABSTRACT: Experiments were performed to document the presence of G protein-coupled P2Y nucleotide receptors in rat salivary glands and to examine changes in receptor expression during development and under conditions in which gland architecture is altered. The results indicate that, as opposed to mature rat submandibular gland (SMG), immature glands express functional $P2Y_1$ receptors. $P2Y_1$ receptor activity was highest at birth and declined over the next four weeks to undetectable levels. $P2Y_1$ receptor mRNA levels remained constant over this time course, suggesting that receptor activity is regulated at some point other than transcription.

Conversely, short-term culture of cells from the three major salivary glands resulted in upregulation of functional $P2Y_2$ receptors. Responses to the $P2Y_2$-selective agonist, UTP, were obtained after 3 h in culture and were maximal by 72 hours. This increase was paralleled by increased steady-state $P2Y_2$ receptor mRNA levels. Upregulation of $P2Y_2$ receptors also occurred *in vivo* following ligation of the main excretory duct of the SMG. These studies suggest that nucleotide receptors are dynamically regulated during development and as a result of perturbations to gland architecture.

INTRODUCTION

There is clear evidence of a role for ligand-gated ion channel P2X nucleotide receptors in the regulation of salivary gland functions, including ion transport.[9] Conversely, there is little evidence in intact salivary glands or in freshly dispersed cells isolated from the glands for the presence of functional G protein-coupled P2Y nucleotide receptors. This observation is in contrast to results obtained in a number of transformed cell lines of salivary origin, in which functional $P2Y_2$-subtype receptors have been identified.[2,6,7,10] The goal of the present study was to examine P2Y receptor expression and activity in normal cells isolated from immature rat salivary glands and in salivary cells from immature and adult animals following short-term culture. In addition, P2Y receptor expression following *in vivo* ligation of the main submandibular gland excretory duct was examined. Our results indicate that the expression and activity of multiple P2Y receptor subtypes change in normal salivary gland cells during development and in response to alterations of gland architecture.

---

[a] This work was supported by NIH/NIDR Grant DE07389.
[b] Tel: (573) 882-2479; fax: (573) 884-4558; e-mail: pharmjt@showme.missouri.edu

METHODS

Preparation of Dispersed Cell Aggregates from Rat Salivary Gland

Cell aggregates were prepared from the submandibular gland/sublingual gland complex of 1-day-old to 4-week-old, as well as adult, Sprague-Dawley rats, as described previously.[5] Gland complexes were removed under anesthesia, minced, and placed in Dulbecco's modified Eagle medium/Ham's F12 (DMEM/F12) containing 2.7 units of collagenase and 10 unis of hyaluronidase per milligram of tissue. Cell aggregates were further dispersed with passage through 10 mL pipettes at 20 min, 30 min, and 40 min of incubation. Dispersed cell aggregates were washed in acini buffer (120 mM NaCl, 4 mM KCl, 1.2 mM KH_2PO_4, 1.2 mM $MgSO_4$, 1 mM $CaCl_2$, 10 mM glucose, 15 mM HEPES (pH 7.4), and 1% (w:v) bovine serum albumin (BSA)) and filtered through nylon mesh. The cells were washed twice and resuspended in acini buffer containing 0.1% BSA for assay.

Short-term Culture of Dispersed Salivary Gland Cells

Dispersed SMG cell aggregates from 1 or 2 rats were placed in 75 cm^2 Falcon Primeria flasks in DMEM/F12 containing 50 µg/mL gentamicin, 0.1 µM retinoic acid, 80 ng/mL epidermal growth factor, 2 nM triiodothyronine, 5 mM glutamine, 8.4 ng/mL cholera toxin, 0.4 µg/mL hydrocortisone, 5 µg/mL insulin, 5 µg/mL transferrin, 5 ng/mL sodium selenite, and 2.5% (v/v) fetal bovine serum. Cultures were maintained in a humidified 95% air:5% CO_2 incubator at 37°C for 3 to 144 hours.

Duct Ligation in Vivo

Unilateral ligation of the SMG was performed as described previously.[5] Briefly, rats were anesthetized, and the SMG main excretory duct was dissected and tied 7 mm distal to the gland hilum, then the incision was closed. Three days postsurgery, the animals were sacrificed, and SMG were removed for the preparation of dispersed cell aggregates for immediate assay. In each case, the contralateral, nonligated gland served as the control.

Intracellular Calcium Measurements

Changes in the intracellular free calcium concentration ($[Ca^{2+}]_i$) in dispersed salivary gland cells were measured with Fura-2/AM in a Spex CM1T111 dual-excitation spectrofluorometer (SPEX Industries, Edison, NJ) by the method of Grynkiewicz et al.,[3] as described previously for salivary gland aggregates.[8] Nucleotides and other agonists were added after baseline fluorescence was established, and changes in $[Ca^{2+}]_i$ were determined.

Semiquantitative Reverse Transcription-Polymerase Chain Reaction (RT-PCR)

Total RNA was prepared from cell aggregates from each age group, followed by treatment with RNase-free DNase. cDNA was synthesized from 2 µg of total RNA and oligo-d(T)$_{18}$ primer using a first-strand cDNA Synthesis Kit. Ten percent of the cDNA was then used as template in the PCR reaction. Primer sets specific for the P2Y$_1$

and $P2Y_2$ receptor also were used to construct exogenous DNA fragments using a PCR MIMIC Construction Kit. The mimic fragments (0.02 amol) were used as the internal standard in the PCR reactions, which were performed with 3 units of Vent (exo⁻) DNA polymerase, 0.25 units of Vent DNA polymerase, and 20 pmol of each primer in a 50 μL reaction volume. The PCR conditions were denaturation at 94 °C for 1 min, annealing at 60 °C for 1 min, and extension at 72 °C for 1 min, for 35 cycles, followed by a 7-min extension at 72 °C. The resultant amplified PCR products were resolved on a 2% agarose gel. Wild-type and $P2Y_1$ or $P2Y_2$ receptor mRNA-transfected 1321N1 astrocytoma cells[1] were used as negative and positive control mRNA sources for RT-PCR, respectively. Bands were visualized with UV light. Amplified bands were excised and purified with the Wizard PCR Prep DNA purification system prior to DNA sequencing, using internal P2Y receptor subtype-specific primers and fluorescent chain terminator dNTPs on an Applied Biosystems sequencer. Relative densities of the P2Y receptor bands were quantified by densitometry and normalized to the intensity of the mimic bands.

RESULTS AND DISCUSSION

As shown in FIGURE 1, the increase in $[Ca^{2+}]_i$ in response to a maximally effective concentration (100 μM) of the $P2Y_1$ receptor ligand, 2-methylthio-ATP (2MeSATP), was greatest in salivary gland cells isolated from 1-day-old rats. The $[Ca^{2+}]_i$ increase di-

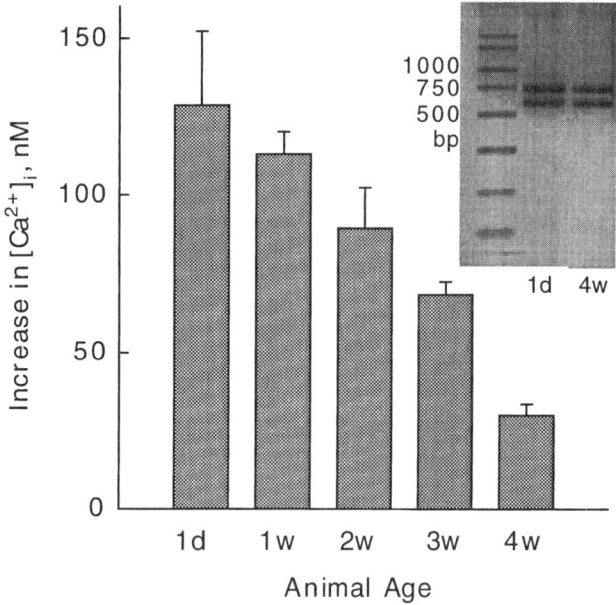

FIGURE 1. Calcium-mobilizing effect of 2MeSATP in dispersed SMG cell aggregates from rats of various ages. Cell aggregates were prepared as described in METHODS, loaded with Fura-2/AM, and then exposed to 100 μM 2MeSATP. The maximal increases in $[Ca^{2+}]_i$ over basal are shown. The values shown are the mean ± SEM of 3 experiments. Inset: $P2Y_1$ receptor mRNA in SMG from 1-day-old and 4-week-old rats, as detected by RT-PCR.

minished as a function of animal age, such that only a slight effect was seen in cells from 4-week-old animals. The EC_{50} value for 2MeSATP-stimulated increases in $[Ca^{2+}]_i$ (approximately 0.3 µM) was similar at all animal ages studied, and the pharmacological profile for the response (2MeSATP > ADP > ADPβS = ATP) was consistent with the involvement of $P2Y_1$ receptors (data not shown). RT-PCR experiments with $P2Y_1$ receptor-specific primers confirmed the presence of mRNA for this receptor subtype (FIG. 1 inset). However, there was little apparent change in the steady state level of the $P2Y_1$ mRNA in salivary gland cells from animals of different ages, suggesting that regulation of $P2Y_1$ receptor activity occurs at a step other than transcription.

When dispersed salivary gland cell aggregates from adult rats are immediately assayed for calcium mobilization responses to the $P2Y_2$ receptor agonist, UTP, no effects are observed. However, as shown in FIGURE 2, placing the dispersed cell aggregates in

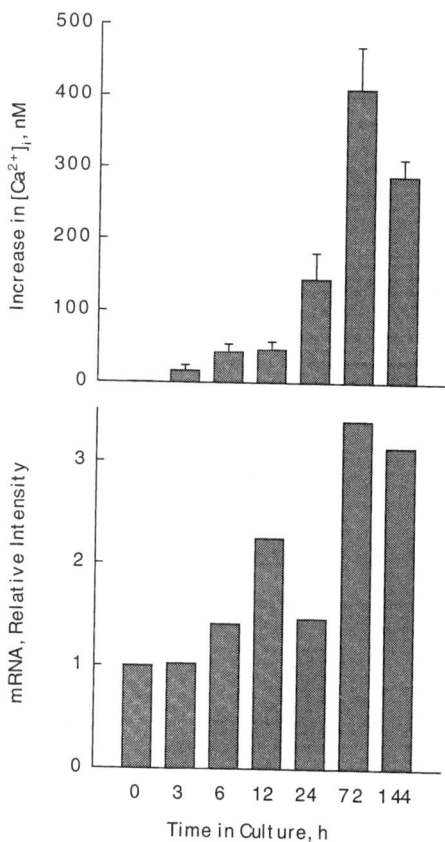

FIGURE 2. Changes in UTP-induced increases in $[Ca^{2+}]_i$ and $P2Y_2$ receptor mRNA levels in dispersed rat SMG cells as a function of time in culture. Cells were isolated as described and either assayed immediately (zero time point) or placed in culture for the indicated times. Upper panel: Cells were loaded with Fura-2/AM and then exposed to 100 µM UTP; changes in $[Ca^{2+}]_i$ were determined. Lower panel: Cellular RNA was isolated, and the relative abundance of $P2Y_2$ receptor mRNA was determined by semiquantitative RT-PCR.

TABLE 1. Effect of Unilateral SMG Duct Ligation on Calcium Mobilization Responses to the Muscarinic Cholinergic and P2Y$_1$ Nucleotide Receptor Agonists, Carbachol and UTP[a]

	Increase in $[Ca^{2+}]_i$, nM	
	Carbachol (100 μM)	UTP (100 μM)
Control gland	213 ± 67	0
Ligated gland	34 ± 7	44 ± 1

[a]For each condition, n=3.

culture for as little as 3 h resulted in the increased ability of UTP to increase $[Ca^{2+}]_i$ in these cells. As is also shown in FIGURE 2, there is a concomitant increase in P2Y$_2$ receptor mRNA levels, indicating a pronounced upregulation of receptor expression as a result of culturing. We have also observed a similar increase in receptor mRNA and activity when serum and the other additives are removed from the culture medium. P2Y$_2$ receptor upregulation is blocked in the presence of inhibitors of transcription (actinomycin D) or translation (cycloheximide), whereas muscarinic cholinergic receptor activity is unchanged (data not shown).

P2Y$_2$ receptor upregulation also occurs *in vivo* as a consequence of unilateral ligation of the main excretory duct of the rat SMG. As shown in TABLE 1, the previously documented[4] decrease in muscarinic cholinoceptor activity following duct ligation is accompanied by the acquisition of a response in cells from the ligated gland to UTP, whereas the contralateral, unligated gland demonstrates neither change. These findings suggest that multiple G protein–coupled P2Y nucleotide receptors may have important roles during salivary gland development as well as in the gland response to damage or disease. Thus, both the P2X ligand-gated ion channels[9] and the P2Y G protein–coupled nucleotide receptors may be involved in the regulation of salivary gland functions.

REFERENCES

1. ERB, L., R. C. GARRAD, Y. WANG, T. QUINN, J. T. TURNER & G. A. WEISMAN. 1995. Site-directed mutagenesis of P$_{2U}$ purinoceptors. Positively charged amino acids in transmembrane helices 6 and 7 affect agonist potency and specificity. J. Biol. Chem. **270:** 4185–4188.
2. GIBB, C. A., S. SINGH, D. I. COOK, P. PORONNIK & A. D. CONIGRAVE. 1994. A nucleotide receptor that mobilizes Ca^{2+} in the mouse submandibular salivary cell line ST$_{885}$. Br. J. Pharmacol. **111:** 1135–1139.
3. GRYNKIEWICZ, G., M. POENIE & R. Y. TSIEN. 1985. A new generation of Ca^{2+} indicators with greatly improved fluorescence properties. J. Biol. Chem. **260:** 3440–3450.
4. HUMPHREYS-BEHER, M. G. 1993. Control of cell growth and proliferation. In Biology of the Salivary Glands. K. Dobrosielski-Vergona, Ed.: 239–262. CRC Press. Boca Raton, FL.
5. MARTINEZ, J. R. & N. CASSITY. 1985. ^{36}Cl fluxes in dispersed rat submandibular acini: Effects of acetylcholine and transport inhibitors. Eur. J. Pharmacol. **403:** 50–54.
6. QUISSELL, D. O., K. A. BARZEN, R. S. REDMAN, J. M. CAMDEN & J. T. TURNER. 1998. Development and characterization of SV40 immortalized rat parotid acinar cell lines. *In Vitro* Cell. Dev. Biol. **34:** 58–67.
7. QUISSELL, D. O., K. B. BARZEN, D. C. GRUENERT, R. S. REDMAN, J. M. CAMDEN & J. T. TURNER. 1997. Development and characterization of SV40 immortalized rat submandibular acinar cell lines. *In Vitro* Cell. Dev. Biol. **33:** 164–173.
8. SEAGRAVE, J. C., S. BARKER, A. M. MARTINEZ & J. R. MARTINEZ. 1993. Muscarinic signaling pathway in submandibular cells of adult and early postnatal rats. Proc. Soc. Exp. Biol. Med. **203:** 490–500.

9. SOLTOFF, S. P., M. K. MCMILLIAN, E. J. CRAGOE, L. C. CANTLEY & B. R. TALAMO. 1990. Effects of extracellular ATP on ion transport systems and $[Ca^{2+}]_i$ in rat parotid acinar cells. J. Gen. Physiol. **95:** 319–346.
10. YU, H. & J. T. TURNER. 1991. Functional studies in the human submandibular duct cell line, HSG-PA, suggest a second salivary gland receptor subtype for nucleotides. J. Pharmacol. Exp. Ther. **259:** 1344–1350.

The Role of the Insulin-like Growth Factor I Receptor in Transformation and Apoptosis

MARIANA RESNICOFF[a] AND RENATO BASERGA

Kimmel Cancer Institute, Thomas Jefferson University, 606 Bluemle Life Sciences Building, 233 South Tenth Street, Philadelphia, Pennsylvania 19107-5541, USA

> ABSTRACT: The insulin-like growth factor I receptor (IGF-IR) regulates cell proliferation by at least three different mechanisms: (1) it is mitogenic; (2) it is required for the establishment and maintenance of the transformed phenotype; and (3) it protects cells from apoptosis both *in vitro* and *in vivo*.

Targeting the IGF-IR in C6 rat glioblastoma cells by antisense strategies, we have shown that there is a correlation between a decrease in IGF-IR levels and the extent of apoptosis in vivo. Tumorigenesis in nude mice is, in turn, correlated to the fraction of cells escaping apoptosis. In syngeneic rats, the apoptotic effect is accompanied by the induction of an antitumor response in the animals, leading to complete inhibition of tumorigenesis. This antitumor response, characterized so far as a CD8-dependent immune response, can protect the animals from subsequent tumor challenge, even when the challenge takes place three months after immunization or at distant sites (in opposite flanks or intracranially). Moreover, it can cause complete regression of established subcutaneous or intracranial tumors, with no recurrence observed for more than six months. Our findings have potential implications for therapeutic intervention in human glioblastomas.

THE INSULIN-LIKE GROWTH FACTOR I RECEPTOR

The insulin-like growth factor I receptor (IGF-IR) belongs to the tyrosine kinase growth factor receptor family, and it shares 70% homology with the insulin receptor.[1] It is formed by two alpha subunits and two beta subunits, linked by disulfide bonds. The alpha subunit is entirely extracellular and contains the ligand-binding domain. The beta subunit has a transmembrane domain and contains the ATP binding site and the tyrosine kinase catalytic domain, which are entirely intracellular. When activated by its ligands (IGF-I, IGF-II, or insulin at supraphysiological concentrations), the IGF-IR transmits a signal to its two major substrates, IRS-1 and Shc,[2,3] which is subsequently transduced by way of the common signal-transducing pathway, through ras and raf, all the way to the nucleus.[4,5]

An activated IGF-IR regulates cell proliferation by at least three different mechanisms: (1) it is mitogenic; (2) it is required for the establishment and maintenance of the transformed phenotype; and (3) it protects cells from apoptosis, both *in vitro* and *in vivo*. For a review, see reference 6.

THE IGF-IR IN CELL GROWTH

For many years, an activated IGF-IR has been known to be mitogenic in cells in culture; however, in growth-regulated cells (like 3T3 cells or human diploid fibroblasts),

---

[a] Tel: (215) 503 4519; fax: (215) 923 0249; e-mail: resnico1@jeflin.tju.edu

IGF-I alone cannot sustain growth of cells in serum-free medium but needs the cooperation of other growth factors, like platelet-derived growth factor (PDGF), which by itself also fails to induce cellular proliferation. The importance of the IGF-IR in cell growth has been recently confirmed *in vivo* by the finding that mouse embryos, with a targeted disruption (by homologous recombination) of the IGF-IR genes and the IGF-II gene, have a size at birth that is only 30% the size of wild-type littermates.[7,8] This finding is the formal demonstration that the IGF-IR and its ligands are required *in vivo*, where they control 70% of murine embryonal growth. 3T3-like cells were subsequently derived from the knockout mouse embryos as well as from their wild-type littermates and designated, respectively, R⁻ cells and W cells.[9] Using these cells, Sell *et al.*[10] were able to define the role of the IGF-IR in cell growth: (1) cells lacking the IGF-IR (R⁻ cells) fail to grow in serum-free medium supplemented with the growth factors that sustain the growth of W cells or other 3T3 cells; (2) in 10% serum, R⁻ cells grow at a slower rate than W cells, indicating that the IGF-IR is not an absolute requirement for growth, although it is required for optimal cell growth; (3) in R⁻ cells all phases of the cell cycle are elongated, suggesting a requirement for IGF-I in all phases of the cell cycle;[10,11] (4) the growth deficits of R⁻ cells are abrogated if the cells are stably transfected with a wild-type (but not a mutant) IGF-IR cDNA,[9,12] unequivocally showing that the growth phenotype of R⁻ cells is specifically due to the absence of the IGF-IR.

THE IGF-IR IN TRANSFORMATION

Cells derived from mouse embryos with a targeted disruption of the IGF-IR genes (R⁻ cells) cannot be transformed by the SV40 T antigen, by an activated and overexpressed Ha-ras, by a combination of both, or by overexpressed growth factor receptors, such as the epidermal growth factor receptor[12] and the platelet-derived growth factor receptor,[13] all of which transform very efficiently the corresponding W cells or other 3T3 cells.[9,10] This resistance of R⁻ cells to transformation is also abolished if a plasmid expressing a wild-type (but not a mutant) human IGF-IR cDNA is stably transfected into R⁻ cells (with or without the T antigen), indicating that the defect in transformation is specifically due to the lack of IGF-IR.[9,12]

If the absence of an IGF-IR precludes the establishment of transformation, then interference with the IGF-IR in tumor cells should reverse the transformed phenotype. For this purpose, several laboratories have used different strategies: antisense strategies to target IGF-IR, using of expression plasmids or oligodeoxynucleotides;[14–18] antisense strategies to IGF-I[19,20] or IGF-II;[21] antibodies directed against IGF-IR;[22,23] or expression of dominant negative mutants of IGF-IR.[24–28] All of these experiments have unequivocally shown that interference with IGF-IR in a variety of tumor cell lines results in reversal of the transformed phenotype, as measured by colony formation in soft agar. The tumor cell lines tested so far include T98G human glioblastoma, C6 rat glioblastoma, FO-1 human melanoma, B1792-F10 mouse melanoma, CaOV-3 and OVCAR-3 human ovarian carcinoma, CALA-6 human small cell lung carcinoma, and MCF-7 human breast carcinoma.

TUMORIGENESIS IN SYNGENEIC ANIMALS

In *in vivo* tumorigenesis, the most dramatic effects were observed with C6 rat glioblastoma cells expressing an antisense IGF-IR RNA. These cells were no longer tumorigenic in syngeneic rats, and they were able to elicit an antitumor response in the animals, protecting them from subsequent tumor challenge and causing regression of established C6 wild-type tumors.[15] In order to verify whether the protective effect was specifically associated with expression of antisense IGF-IR RNA or with nonproliferating or nonviable cells, C6 wild-type, sense and antisense cells were irradiated with 5000 rads of ^{60}Co prior to subcutaneous injection. Irradiated cells were nontumorigenic in syngeneic rats, but only irradiated antisense cells were able to protect the rats from subsequent tumor challenge, demonstrating that the protective effect was specifically associated with expression of antisense IGF-IR RNA and was not lost after irradiation. Irradiated antisense cells were also able to induce regression of established subcutaneous tumors, but complete regression took a week longer than with nonirradiated antisense cells.

THE IGF-IR IN CELL SURVIVAL

The abrogation of tumorigenicity observed in C6 cells expressing an antisense IGF-IR RNA suggested that these cells were dying *in vivo*. In order to demonstrate this, we decided to encapsulate the cells in a diffusion chamber prior to implantation in the subcutaneous tissue of the animals. The diffusion chambers are constructed with 14 mm. Lucite rings and 0.1 μm pore-sized membranes that allow the passage of soluble factors excluding the entry or exit of intact cells.[29] The chambers are sterilized with ethylene oxide prior to use. Cells behave in the diffusion chamber precisely as they do when injected in the subcutaneous tissue of the animals: only anchorage-independent cells will grow in either condition. A major advantage of using this device resides in the fact that the chambers can be removed from the animals at different intervals, the cell number can be accurately determined, and the recovered cells can then be used for several studies, including cell culture because all the procedures are performed under sterile conditions. Using this device, we were able to demonstrate that tumor cells expressing an antisense IGF-IR RNA undergo massive apoptosis within 24 hr *in vivo*, whereas wild-type or sense-transfected tumor cells double in cell number under the same conditions.[30,31] The rapidity in the onset of apoptosis *in vivo* allowed us to test even non-syngeneic cells (such as human cells) using this device. Moreover, we have shown that the extent of apoptosis *in vivo* is correlated to the decrease in the number of IGF-IRs. Tumorigenesis in nude mice is, in turn, correlated to the fraction of surviving cells. In syngeneic rats, an antitumor response is elicited in the host, leading to complete inhibition of tumorigenesis when the fraction of surviving cells is about 1%, that is, 100,000 cells. When 30% or more cells survive, the tumors appear, but the host response causes the tumors to regress.[31]

CHARACTERIZATION OF THE ANTITUMOR RESPONSE ELICITED BY C6 CELLS EXPRESSING AN ANTISENSE IGF-IR RNA IN SYNGENEIC RATS

In order to characterize the antitumor response elicited by C6 cells expressing an antisense IGF-IR RNA in syngeneic rats, several parameters of immune function were analyzed. These studies are described in detail in reference 32.

Initial attempts focused on the nature of this response, to establish whether it is humoral or cellular. No antibodies directed against C6 cells could be detected in the serum from rats injected with C6 antisense cells. Therefore, we have no evidence for a humoral response.

In order to analyze the contribution of a cellular response, lymphoproliferative assays were performed using splenic lymphocytes isolated from rats injected with C6 antisense cells. We observed lymphocyte proliferation in response to irradiated C6 cells;

this proliferative response was due to a doubling in the number of CD8+ cells, whereas the CD4+ cell population was not affected. No proliferative response was observed with lymphocytes isolated from control rats (untreated or injected with C6 sense cells). Cytotoxic assays demonstrated a 2- to 4-fold increase in cytotoxicity of lymphocytes isolated from rats injected with C6 antisense cells compared to controls. In athymic nude mice, the protective effect was not observed: the nude mice were not protected from subsequent tumor challenge, and established tumors did not regress. In summary, the antitumor response elicited by C6 cells expressing an antisense IGF-IR RNA in syngeneic rats has been characterized so far as a CD8-dependent immune response.

EFFICACY OF THIS STRATEGY ON BRAIN TUMORS

We have also evaluated the efficacy of this strategy on C6 brain tumors. For this purpose, 2.5×10^5 C6 cells were implanted intracerebrally (ic) using a stereotactic apparatus. C6 cells expressing a sense or antisense IGF-IR RNA were implanted subcutaneously in a diffusion chamber (5×10^5 cells per chamber) for 24 hours, either a week before or a day after the ic injection. The rats were monitored for survival. By day 8, 80% of the controls (which received only the ic injection) and 56% of all sense-treated rats were dead. Histological analysis performed in the brain samples from these rats showed a relatively well demarcated hypercellular glioblastoma, confirming that these animals died due to the brain tumor. None of these groups of rats survived after three weeks, whereas 100% of the antisense-treated rats were still alive and without symptoms of apparent disease. Long-term survival of the rats (for more than seven months) was observed in 100% of the rats that received the antisense cells a week before and in 25% of the rats that received the antisense cells a day after the ic injection. After 221 days, these animals were sacrificed in order to analyze their brains. Histological analysis performed in the brain samples of the antisense-treated rats showed cystic cavities in the right cerebral hemispheres that corresponded to the location of the tumor mass in control rats; deposits of hemosiderin and residual inflammatory infiltrates were present focally, and minimal gliosis was detected in the wall at the cystic cavity. These observations are compatible with brain tumor regression, confirming that the cells expressing an antisense IGF-IR RNA, placed in a diffusion chamber for only 24 hours in the subcutaneous tissue of the rats, were able to elicit an antitumor response in the brain, leading to long-term survival of the rats.[33]

In another set of experiments, primary cultures of human glioblastoma grade IV were pretreated with antisense oligodeoxynucleotides targeting the IGF-IR DNA for 24 hours before being placed in diffusion chambers and implanted in the subcutaneous tissue of the rats. Twenty-four hours later, the chambers were removed from the animals and the cells were quantitatively recovered. These primary cultures of human glioblastoma grade IV underwent massive apoptosis *in vivo* following treatment with antisense oligodeoxynucleotides targeting the IGF-IR DNA for 24 hours at a dose of 19 µM, whereas treatment with control oligodeoxynucleotides (random sequences) did not have any effect. The extent of apoptosis measured after 24 hours *in vivo* was more than 99%; this effect was comparable to the one reported for the several tumor cell lines tested so far.[30]

CONCLUDING REMARKS

Targeting the IGF-IR in tumor cells by a variety of strategies (antisense, dominant negatives, or antibodies) results in inhibition of tumorigenesis. This effect is achieved by induction of apoptosis *in vivo* together with an immune response elicited in the animals that eliminates the residual surviving cells. This strategy seems to discriminate between normal and tumor cells. We have preliminary evidence indicating that WI-38 human diploid fibroblasts are not affected by high doses of antisense oligodeoxynucleotides targeting the IGF-IR DNA. Taken together, our findings have potential implications for therapeutic intervention in human glioblastoma. The fact that the cells, pretreated with antisense oligodeoxynucleotides targeting the IGF-IR DNA, are encapsulated in diffusion chambers that impede the exit or entry of intact cells renders this procedure much safer for human testing without affecting the treatment efficacy.

REFERENCES

1. ULLRICH, A., A. GRAY, A.W. TAM, T. YANG-FENG, M. TSUBOKAWA, C. COLLINS, W. HENZEL, T. LE BON, S. KAHURIA, E. CHEN, S. JAKOBS, U. FRANCKE, J. RAMACHANDRAN & Y. FUJITA-YAMAGUCHI. 1986. Insulin-like growth factor I receptor primary structure: Comparison with insulin receptor suggests structural determinants that define functional specificity. EMBO J. **5:** 2503–2512.
2. MYERS, M.G., X.J. SUN, B. CHEATHAM, B.R. JACHNA, E.M. GLASHEEN, J.M. BACKER & M.F. WHITE 1993. IRS-1 is a common element in insulin and insulin-like growth factor I signaling to the phosphatidylinositol 3′ kinase. Endocrinology **132:** 1421–1430.
3. WHITE, M.F. & C.R. KAHN. 1994. The insulin signaling system. J. Biol. Chem. **269:** 1–4.
4. CREWS, C.M. & R.L. ERIKSON. 1993. Extracellular signals and reversible protein phosphorylation: What to MEK of it all. Cell **74:** 215–217.
5. HILL, C.S. & R. TREISMAN. 1995. Transcriptional regulation by extracellular signals: Mechanisms and specificity. Cell **80:** 199–211.
6. BASERGA, R. 1995. The IGF-I receptor: A key to tumor growth? Cancer Res. **55:** 249–252.
7. LIU, J.P., J. BAKER, A.S. PERKINS, E.J. ROBERTSON & A. EFSTRATIADIS. 1993. Mice carrying null mutations of the genes encoding insulin-like growth factor I (igf-1) and type I IGF receptor (igf 1 r). Cell **75:** 59–72.
8. BAKER, J., J.P. LIU, E.J. ROBERTSON & A. EFSTRATIADIS. 1993. Role of insulin-like growth factors in embryonic and postnatal growth. Cell **75:** 73–82.
9. SELL, C., M. RUBINI, R. RUBIN, J.P. LIU, A. EFSTRATIADIS & R. BASERGA. 1993. Simian virus 40 large tumor antigen is unable to transform mouse embryonic fibroblasts lacking type I IGF receptor. Proc. Natl. Acad. Sci. USA **90:** 11217–11221.
10. SELL, C., G. DUMENIL, C. DEVEAUD, M. MIURA, D. COPPOLA, T. DE ANGELIS, R. RUBIN, A. EFSTRATIADIS & R. BASERGA. 1994. Effect of a null mutation of the type I IGF receptor gene on growth and transformation of mouse embryo fibroblasts. Mol. Cell. Biol. **14:** 3604–3612.
11. VALENTINIS, B., P.L. PORCU, K. QUINN & R. BASERGA. 1994. The role of the insulin-like growth factor I receptor in the transformation by simian virus 40 T antigen. Oncogene **9:** 825–831.
12. COPPOLA, D., A. FERBER, M. MIURA, C. SELL, C. D'AMBROSIO, R. RUBIN & BASERGA. 1994. A functional insulin-like growth factor I receptor is required for the mitogenic and transforming activities of the epidermal growth factor receptor. Mol. Cell. Biol. **14:** 4588–4595.
13. DE ANGELIS, T., A. FERBER & R. BASERGA. 1995. Insulin-like growth factor I receptor is required for the mitogenic and transforming activities of the platelet-derived growth factor receptor. J. Cell. Physiol. **164:** 214–221.
14. RESNICOFF, M., D. AMBROSE, D. COPPOLA & R. RUBIN. 1993. Insulin-like growth factor I and its receptor mediate the autocrine proliferation of human ovarian carcinoma cell lines. Lab. Invest. **69:** 756–760.
15. RESNICOFF, M., C. SELL, M. RUBINI, D. COPPOLA, D. AMBROSE, R. BASERGA & R. RUBIN. 1994. Rat glioblastoma cells expressing an antisense RNA to the insulin-like growth factor I (IGF-I) receptor are non-tumorigenic and induce regression of wild-type tumors. Cancer Res. **54:** 2218–2222.
16. RESNICOFF, M., D. COPPOLA, C. SELL, R. RUBIN, S. FERRONE & R. BASERGA. 1994. Growth

inhibition of human melanoma cells in nude mice by antisense strategies to the type 1 insulin-like growth factor receptor. Cancer Res. **54:** 4848–4850.
17. AMBROSE, D., M. RESNICOFF, D. COPPOLA, C. SELL, M. MIURA, S. JAMESON, R. BASERGA & R. RUBIN. 1994. Growth regulation of human glioblastoma T98G cells by insulin-like growth factor 1 and its receptor. J. Cell. Physiol. **159:** 92–100.
18. SHAPIRO, D.N., B.G. JONES, L.H. SHAPIRO, P. DIAS & P.J. HOUGHTON. 1994. Antisense-mediated reduction in insulin-like growth factor I receptor expression suppresses the malignant phenotype of a human alveolar rhabdomyosarcoma. J. Clin. Invest. **94:** 1235–1242.
19. TROJAN, J., B.K. BLOSSEY, T.R. JOHNSON, S.D. RUDIN, M. TYKOCINSKI, J. ILAN & J. ILAN. 1992. Loss of tumorigenicity of rat glioblastoma directed by episome-based antisense cDNA transcription of insulin-like growth factor I. Proc. Natl. Acad. Sci. USA **89:** 4874–4878.
20. TROJAN, J., T.R. JOHNSON, S.D. RUDIN, J. ILAN, M.L. TYKOCINSKI & J. ILAN. 1993. Treatment and prevention of rat glioblastoma by immunogenic C6 cells expressing antisense insulin-like growth factor 1 RNA. Science **259:** 94–97.
21. CHRISTOFORI, G., P. NAIK & D. HANAHAN. 1994. A second signal supplied by insulin-like growth factor II in oncogene-induced tumorigenesis. Nature **369:** 414–418.
22. ARTEAGA, C.L. & C.K. OSBORNE. 1989 Growth inhibition of human breast cancer cells *in vitro* with an antibody against the type 1 somatomedin receptor. Cancer Res. **49:** 6237–6241.
23. KALEBIC, T., M. TSOKOS & L.J. HELMAN. 1994. *In vivo* treatment with antibody against IGF-1 receptor suppresses growth of human rhabdomyosarcoma and down-regulates p34 cdc2. Cancer Res. **54:** 5531–5534.
24. LI, S., A. FERBER, M. MIURA & R. BASERGA. 1994. Mitogenicity and transforming activity of the insulin-like growth factor I receptor with mutations in the tyrosine kinase domain. J. Biol. Chem. **269:** 32558–32564.
25. LI, S., M. RESNICOFF & R. BASERGA. 1996. Effect of mutations at serines 1280–1283 on the mitogenic and transforming activities of the insulin-like growth factor I receptor. J. Biol. Chem. **271:** 12254–12260.
26. PRAGER, D., H.L. LI, S. ASA & S. MELMED. 1994. Dominant negative inhibition of tumorigenesis *in vivo* by human insulin-like growth factor I receptor mutant. Proc. Natl. Acad. Sci. USA **91:** 2181–2185.
27. BURGAUD, J-L., M. RESNICOFF & R. BASERGA. 1995. Mutant IGF-1 receptors as dominant negatives for growth and transformation. Biochem. Biophys. Res. Commun. **214:** 475–481.
28. D'AMBROSIO, C., A. FERBER, M. RESNICOFF & R. BASERGA. 1996. A soluble insulin-like growth factor I receptor that induces apoptosis of tumor cells *in vivo* and inhibits tumorigenesis. Cancer Res. **56:** 4013–4020.
29. ABRAHAM, D., A.M. LANGE, W. YUTANAVIBOONCHAI, M. TRPIS, J.W. DICKERSON, B. SWENSON & M.L. EBERHARD. 1993. Survival and development of larval *Onchocerca volvulus* in primate and rodent hosts. J. Parasit. **79:** 571–582.
30. RESNICOFF, M., D. ABRAHAM, W. YUTANAWIBOONCHAI, H.L. ROTMAN, J. KAJSTURA, R. RUBIN, P. ZOLTIC & R. BASERGA. 1995. The insulin-like growth factor I receptor protects tumor cells from apoptosis *in vivo*. Cancer Res. **55:** 2463–2469.
31. RESNICOFF, M., J.-L. BURGAUD, H. ROTMAN, D. ABRAHAM & R. BASERGA. 1995. Correlation between apoptosis, tumorigenesis and levels of insulin-like growth factor I receptors. Cancer Res. **55:** 3739–3741.
32. RESNICOFF, M., W. LI, S. BASAK, D. HERLYN, R. BASERGA & R. RUBIN. 1996. Mechanisms of rat C6 glioblastoma tumor growth inhibition by expression of insulin-like growth factor I receptor antisense mRNA. Cancer Immunol. Immunother. **42:** 64–68.
33. RESNICOFF, M., J. TJUVAJEV, H.L. ROTMAN, D. ABRAHAM, M. CURTIS, R. AIKEN & R. BASERGA. 1996. Regression of C6 rat brain tumors by cells expressing an antisense insulin-like growth factor I receptor RNA. J. Exp. Ther. Oncol. **1:** 385–389.

Apoptosis: A Modulator of Cellular Homeostasis and Disease States

MARY J. DELONG[a]

Department of Environmental Health, Rollins School of Public Health, Emory University, 1518 Clifton Road, Atlanta, Georgia 30322, USA

> ABSTRACT: In normal epithelial tissue, a homeostatic balance is maintained between cell replication and apoptosis. Disruption of this balance has serious pathological consequences in disease states, such as Sjögren's syndrome, salivary gland degeneration, and cancers. Apoptosis may be modulated by cytokine endogenous factors and exogenous factors. A vast array of environmental compounds, such as differentiating agents and microconstituents found in the diet, initiate apoptosis through a redox signal mechanism. In addition to increasing apoptosis, these redox signals and transient or permanent changes in cellular redox status elevate detoxification enzymes known to protect against many disease states. Clearly a further understanding of the regulation of apoptosis and protective enzyme elevation by exogenous redox signals will lead to the development of future therapeutic strategies against disease.

IMPORTANCE OF APOPTOSIS

Apoptosis, also known as programmed cell death, is a highly regulated process of selective cell deletion involved in normal cell turnover, development, cell-mediated immunity, and tumor regression. It is also the end stage of cellular differentiation. Dysfunction of the normal cellular homeostatic machinery is likely to have serious pathological consequences. These include disorders of autoimmunity, such as Sjögren's syndrome (SS); oncogenesis, such as oral and other cancers; and degenerative diseases, such as Alzheimer's disease. Apoptosis is characterized by a series of morphological and biochemical cellular alterations. These appear as condensation of chromatin, compaction of cytoplasmic organelles, blebbing of the cell surface, and DNA fragmentation into oligomers of 180–200 bp. These alterations terminate in the formation of membrane-enclosed structures termed "apoptotic bodies" that are extruded into the extracellular space.[1,2] Uptake of apoptotic bodies is carefully controlled. Phagocytic macrophages specifically recognize and clear these apoptotic bodies, allowing cell death to occur without inflammation.[2]

Apoptosis exerts a homeostatic function in tissue. A balance between cell replication and cell death achieves a steady state of continuously renewed tissue.[3] Normally, epithelial cells that constitute the lining of the digestive tract, from the oral mucosal lining and salivary gland epithelium to the large bowel, are constantly dividing, differentiating, and undergoing apoptosis. As mature, differentiated cells are shed by apoptosis, signals are generated for stem cells to divide in order to replenish cell number. This maintains cellular homeostasis. Cellular proliferation, differentiation, and apoptosis of epithelial cells are mediated by an endogenous family of proteins called cytokines. In addition, exogenous environmental factors, such as smoke, alcohol, or dietary sources (such as vitamins A and D), differentiating agents, and nonnutritive compounds, mod-

---

[a] Tel: (404) 727-3697; fax: (404) 727-8744; e-mail: delong@sph.emory.edu

ulate normal cellular homeostasis and apoptosis in the oral cavity as well as throughout the body.

CELLULAR MECHANISMS OF APOPTOSIS

Evidence indicates that apoptosis is regulated by signal transduction pathways similar to others previously identified in physiological responses. These responses include alterations of intracellular Ca^{2+} distribution, activation of protein kinases and phosphatases, change in cellular pH, and cellular changes associated with oxidative stress. Interestingly, signals that promote apoptosis in one cellular system can suppress it in another. This indicates that cellular responses are determined by the intrinsic programming of the specific cell type and tissue.[4] Signaling mechanisms of cellular apoptosis that are directly related to salivary gland function and disease are both endogenous and exogenous. Two endogenous factors are the Fas receptor and ligand associated with immune cells, and the cytokines tumor necrosis factor-alpha (TNF-α) and interferon-gamma (INF-γ) present in the salivary gland environment. An exogenous factor, oxidative stress, is produced by a vast array of common pharmaceuticals and dietary constituents.

Fas Receptor and Ligand

The Fas receptor and the Fas ligand, a type II membrane protein, are especially important in the regulation of apoptosis in immunological systems.[5] The cell-surface receptor, Fas (FasR, Apo-1, CD95), and its ligand (FasL), are mediators of apoptosis that have been shown to be implicated in peripheral deletion of autoimmune cells, activation-induced T-cell death, and one of the two major cytolytic pathways mediated by $CD8^+$ cytolytic T cells.[6] Fas signaling mechanisms include the hematopoietic cell phosphatase (HCP) and sphingomyelinase, whereas TCR-signaling mechanisms modulate expression of FasL.

The inhibition or loss of lymphocytic Fas-initiated apoptosis has been observed in patients with SS, in the salivary gland, and lymphatic disease.[7] Infiltrating lymphocytes in the focal lesions of the salivary glands of patients with SS are blocked in their ability to commit to apoptosis, even though they may express Fas. The presence of Bcl-2 in these cells may explain their inability to undergo apoptosis. By contrast, the acinar epithelial cells may undergo Fas-mediated apoptosis, suggesting that the Fas-death pathway may be an important mechanism leading to the glandular destruction found in SS.[7]

The observed lymphocytopenia in SS patients has also been associated with an abnormal balance between Fas and Bcl-2 expression in subsets of peripheral blood lymphocytes.[8] The rate of Fas^+ CD4 peripheral blood lymphocyte formation was significantly elevated in SS patients compared to normal controls as well as to Fas^+ $CD3^+$ and Fas^+ $D8^+$ cells. These, and other studies, suggest that the increased expression of Fas may result in enhanced susceptibility to apoptosis and lymphocytopenia commonly observed in SS patients. Molecular and genetic analysis of Fas and FasL indicates that the mouse lymphoproliferation mutation (lkpr) and generalized lymphoproliferative disease (gld) are mutations of Fas receptor and FasL, respectively.[9]

TNF-α and IFN-γ

Cytokines elevated in the salivary gland microenvironment of SS patients are TNF-α and IFN-γ. In the cultured human salivary gland (HSG) cell line treated with long-term IFN-γ ± TNF-α, cells are growth inhibited with a decrease in cell number to below that initially plated. Cells treated with both TNF-α and INF-γ exhibited 58% degradation in 12 days. Thus, long-term exposure of HSG epithelial cells to INF-γ ± TNF-α leads to increased DNA degradation and cell death and suggests a potential mechanism for SS based on exposure to apoptotic cytokine signals in the salivary gland environment.[8,10]

Based on morphological analysis, TNF-α-induced cell death resembles necrosis, whereas Fas-mediated cell killing resembles apoptosis, evidenced by the appearance of membrane blebbing, nuclear condensation, and nonrandom DNA degradation. It is known that TNF-α cytotoxicity is mediated by reactive oxygen intermediates generated during mitochondrial respiration. However, these mediators are not significantly involved in Fas-mediated cell death, as shown by the lack of protective effect of mitochondrial inhibitors or antioxidants on Fas-stimulated apoptosis.[11]

Bcl-2

Bcl-2 balances the apoptotic-inducing effects of Fas, and TNF-α and INF-γ. Bcl-2 has a unique function as a negative regulator of and protector against apoptosis.[12] Apparently, its primary role is to maintain *in vivo* survival of specific cell types of developing and adult organisms. A large portion of Bcl-2 is located on mitochondrial and microsomal membranes, suggesting its importance in oxidant and Ca^{2+} regulation.[13] Bcl-2 is protective against oxidative stress in mammalian cells and can be replaced by antioxidants in a factor-deprivation model of apoptosis. These results are consistent with a model of apoptotic death involving oxidative stress in a central pathway. The recent discovery of several Bcl-2-related genes, some of which also inhibit apoptosis, and others that unexpectedly promote apoptosis, has shed new light on several aspects of the action of Bcl-2.[14]

Two other emerging cytokine families that are important in inhibiting apoptosis are the interleukin-1 beta-converging enzyme family of cysteine proteases and those related to Bcl-2. The understanding of the interaction of these molecules in autoimmune disease may lead to more specific therapies for immunosuppression disease and apoptosis defects that are present in SS.[15]

CELLULAR REDOX CHANGES AS INITIATORS OF APOPTOSIS

The maintenance of cellular redox status appears to play a key role in apoptosis. Production of oxidative stress, leading to apoptosis, can result from either an increase in the rate of oxidant production or a reduction in the removal rate of radical species. DNA, transcription factors, proteins, and Ca^{2+} homeostasis regulators are all potential targets of oxidative stress alteration during apoptosis.[16]

Mounting evidence supports the involvement of reactive oxygen species or oxidative stress in apoptotic cell death.[17] Exogenous molecules, including redox-active quinones and peroxides, as well as xenobiotics that can be metabolized to oxidant compounds, trigger apoptosis in diverse cellular systems.[14,17–21] In general, low concentrations of oxidant induce apoptosis, whereas higher levels trigger necrotic cell death.[19] The importance of redox stress and its effect on cellular thiols, especially glutathione (GSH), is further demonstrated by the use of a variety of antioxidants and thiol-generating compounds (for example, *N*-acetyl cysteine, ascorbate, vitamin E, and citrate). These have been shown to block apoptosis.[14,21–23] Evidence that the apoptosis suppressors, Bcl-2 and Bcl-x1, inhibit apoptosis through effects on intracellular redox underscores the importance of this mechanism.[14,24,25] It is also important to note that hypoxia-induced cell death can involve apoptosis, which brings into question the mandatory role of oxygen radicals in this response.[26–28] Recent findings that demonstrate no correlation between high levels of oxidative stress and apoptosis indicate a need for further research on this topic.[29]

Though the mechanism underlying oxygen radical production in apoptotic cells is still not clear, recent research has demonstrated changes in mitochondrial membrane and function.[30] Mitochondrial membrane potential (delta psi mito) drops precipitously preceding the formation of superoxide radicals. This drop in delta psi mito can be prevented by inhibitors of interleukin-converting-enzyme (ICE)-like proteases and Bcl-2.[31–36] In addition, the release of cytochrome C from mitochondria is postulated to be the primary site for Bcl-2 regulation of apoptosis.[37,38] A role for mitochondria in apoptosis is reasonable, due to its importance in Ca^{2+} regulation and the relation of intracellular acidification with mitochondrial dysfunction.[30] Furthermore, it has been demonstrated that mitochondrial protein cytochrome C release promotes apoptosis and endonuclease activation.[4] Recently, it has been demonstrated that the critical thiols determining cell fate after apoptotic signaling by glucocorticoids or DNA damage are located in the mitochondrial matrix[39] and constitute a crucial sensor of the cellular redox potential, but not by Fas/CD95 cross-linking. Because apoptosis is a crucial mechanism regulating cell survival *in vivo,* manipulation of intracellular thiols may represent a novel therapeutic target for the regulation of cellular function.

REDOX SIGNALS AS PREVENTORS OF DISEASE THROUGH APOPTOSIS AND ELEVATION OF DETOXIFICATION ENZYMES

In contrast to endogenously controlled cellular apoptosis signals, a vast array of environmental factors increase the rate of apoptosis by increasing the rate of epithelial differentiation that terminates in apoptosis. A number of these differentiating compounds are found within the human diet (for example, sodium butyrate in the gut from fermentation of fiber, vitamin A, conjugated linoleic acid, and genistein). These agents have been associated with prevention of disease, including cancer, by human and animal epidemiological studies. Although the mechanism of action of these protective factors may differ among cell type, a common feature of all differentiating agents is their ability to inhibit cell growth and increase the rate of apoptosis. This facilitates the loss of potentially injured or defective cells that may lead to pathology, such as autoimmune disease and cancer.

In the salivary gland, a lowered risk of carcinoma has been associated with the consumption of dietary foods that contain differentiating agents, such as vitamin A, the antioxidant enzymes vitamins C and E,[40] and the consumption of leafy, dark-yellow vegetables.[41] Findings from our laboratory show that, in addition to vitamins, yellow/green vegetables contain numerous microconstituents, such as isothiocyanates, indoles, dimethyl fumarate (DMF), and allyl sulfide (AS). By producing a redox signal, these compounds enhance apoptosis and simultaneously elevate levels of detoxification enzymes. Through the redox signal, as demonstrated by changes in reduced to oxidized ratios of glutathione (GSH/GSSG), critical changes in the mitochondrial membrane trigger apoptosis. In addition, due to the same redox signal, stress-activated protein kinase (SAPK), also known as Jun kinase (JNK), activates the transcription factor c-Jun and increases levels of detoxification enzymes[42–44] (Fig. 1). The redox signal generated by dietary microconstituents also results in the reduction of the cysteinyl residues of c-Jun, increasing AP-1 binding in the antioxidant response element (ARE) site in the promoter region of these genes. An extensive body of research has accumulated on the effectiveness of the elevation of the detoxification enzymes, glutathione S-transferase (GST) and NAD(P)H:quinone reductase (QR). By elevating these enzymes, dietary microconstituents may prevent toxicity and cancer. Elevation of QR, also known as DT diaphorase, protects against redox cycling of quinones and similar metabolites, that produce oxygen radical species, by a mandatory two-electron transfer. The family of GSTs, through conjugation with the nucleophile GSH, eliminates a vast array of xenobiotic and carcinogenic toxicants, from epoxides to chlorinated compounds. Further transcriptional transactivation of the QR and GST genes by dietary-generated redox signals is through the activation of JNK, which results in the phosphorylation of c-Jun at Ser 63 and 73 (FIG. 1).

In our laboratory, we have used human colon HT-29 cells that exhibit the normal processes of division, differentiation, and apoptosis. We have investigated the redox control of apoptosis and GST and QR induction. The growth and maturation of HT-29 cells in culture mimics *in vivo* differentiation. *In vivo,* dividing stem cells at the bottom of the colon crypt differentiate as they rise to the surface of the colonic lumen and slough off by apoptosis.[45] To demonstrate the relationship of apoptosis to redox signals generated by common dietary signals, the extent of apoptosis was measured as a function of cell lifting, propidium iodide staining, and the TUNEL method. The condensed chromatin structure, characteristic of apoptotic cells, rapidly stains with propidium iodide. The TUNEL method employs specific binding of terminal deoxynucleotidyl transferase (TdT) to 3'-OH ends of DNA used to incorporate a biotinylated probe at the site of DNA breaks.

HT-29 cells were treated with the dietary constituents AS (from garlic), dimethyl fumarate (from apples), and benzyl isothiocyanate (from cruciferous vegetables). These produced a transient decrease in GSH for up to 4 h, with a compensatory rise in GST

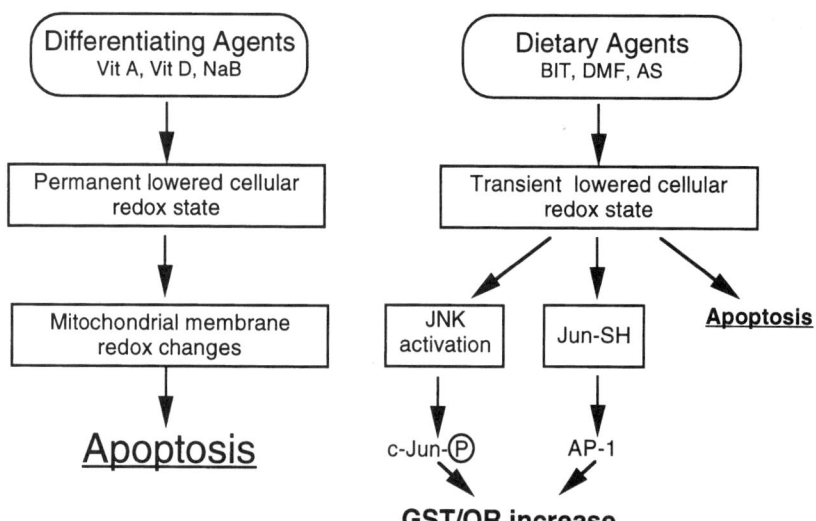

FIGURE 1. Exogenous redox signals producing protective cellular effects. Abbreviations: BIT=benzylisothiocyanate, DMF=dimethyl fumarate, AS=allyl sulfide, NaB=sodium butyrate, JNK=Jun N-terminal kinase, AP-1=activator protein-1, GST=glutathione-S-transferase, QR=NAD(P)H:quinone reductase. Jun-SH=reduced Jun transcription factor.

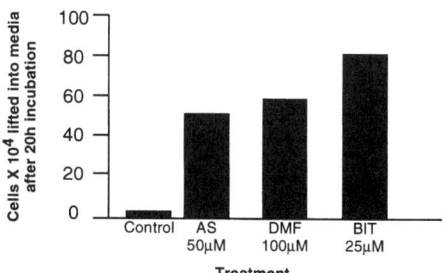

FIGURE 2. Effects of dietary inducers of GST/QR on HT-29 apoptosis. HT-29 cells lifting into the media after a 20-h incubation with indicated inducers.

to above normal levels at 24 hours. Addition of these compounds to HT-29 cells for 24 h resulted in apoptosis (FIG. 2), with a parallel elevation of QR and GST from 130% to 180% above control values.

Treatment of HT-29 cells with the differentiating agent, sodium butyrate (NaB), 5 mM for 72 h, differentiates cells, as measured by alkaline phosphatase levels, and increases apoptosis 100-fold (FIG. 3). Cells treated with NaB have a +46 mV change to a more oxidized state, as calculated using the Nernst equation. Treating differentiated cells with benzylisothiocyanate (BIT) caused even more cell lifting in a synergistic manner to 350-fold over control values. A synergistic increase of enzyme levels was seen when differentiated cells were treated with BIT. The percentage of DNA fragmentation as measured by the TUNEL method (FIG. 4) supported an apoptotic process in cells treated by BIT or NaB and dramatically increased if the HT-29 cells were first differentiated with sodium butyrate and then treated with BIT.

SUMMARY

Apoptosis is an important process in the normal cellular homeostasis of cells. Dysfunction of normal apoptosis may result in disease states, such as Sjörgren's syndrome, cancer, and cellular degeneration. Apoptosis may be regulated by endogenous signals,

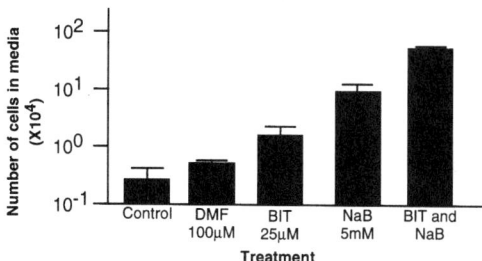

FIGURE 3. Apoptotic cell number in HT-29 cells treated with dietary inducers DMF, BIT, and differentiating agent, NaB. The combination of inducer and differentiating agent yields the greatest amount of lifting in HT-29 cells.

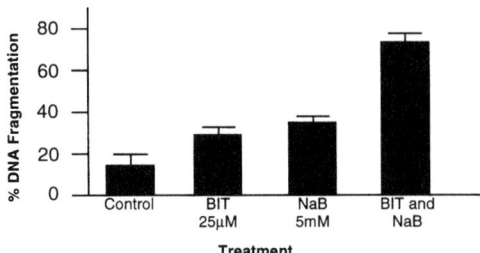

FIGURE 4. Treatment-dependent DNA fragmentation of HT-29 apoptotic cells. Most fragmentation occurred with BIT and NaB treatment.

such as cytokines, exogenous compounds found in the diet, medications, and the environment. Such compounds generate a redox signal and protect cells by increasing apoptosis of potentially damaged cells and increasing detoxification enzymes. This protects against disease, including cancer. The redox signal acts through GSH/GSSG changes, which decrease mitochondrial membrane potential, increase AP-1 binding, and activates Jun kinase. Therefore, regulating the redox signals given to the cell or adding preventive thiols may be protective and have therapeutic value in salivary gland diseases associated with dysfunctional apoptosis.

REFERENCES

1. WYLLIE, A.H., J.F. KEER & A.R. CURRIE. 1980. Cell death: the significance of apoptosis Int. Rev. Cytol. **68:** 251–305.
2. SAVILL, J. et al. 1993. Phagocytic recognition of cells undergoing apoptosis. Immunol. Today. **14:** 131–136.
3. GAVRIELI, Y., Y. SHERMAN, S.A. BEN-SASSON. 1992. Identification of programmed cell death in situ via specific labeling of nuclear DNA fragmentation. J.Cell. Biol. **119:** 493–501.
4. MCCONKEY, D.J. & S. ORRENIUS. 1996. Signal transduction pathways in apoptosis. Stem Cells **14:** 619–631.
5. NAGATA, S. 1996. Fas-mediated apoptosis. Adv. Exp. Med. Biol. **406:** 119–124.
6. FRENCH, L.E., & J. TSCHOPP. 1996. Constitutive Fas ligand expression in several non-lymphoid mouse tissues: implications for immune-protection and cell turnover. Behring Inst. Mitt. **97:** 156–160.
7. KONG, L., N. OGAWA, T. NAKABAYASHI. 1997. Fas and Gas ligand expression in the salivary glands of patients with primary Sjogren's syndrome Arthritis Rheum. **40:** 87–97.
8. ICHIKAWA, Y., K. ARIMORI, M. YOSHIDA et al. 1995. Abnormal expression of apoptosis-related antigens, Fas and Bcl-2 on circulating T-lymphocyte subsets in primary Sjogren's syndrome. Clin. & Exp. Rheumatol. **13:** 307–313.
9. NAGATA, S. 1996. Apoptosis mediated by the Fas system. Prog. Mol. Subcell. Biol. **16:** 87–103.
10. WU, A.J., Z.J. CHEN et al. 1996. Interferon-gamma induced cell death in a cultured human salivary gland cell line. J. Cell. Physiol. **167:** 297–304.
11. SCHULZE-OSTHOFF, K., P.H. KRAMMER & W. DROGE. 1994. Divergent signaling via AP-1/Fas and the TNF-α receptor, two homologous molecules involved in physiological cell death. EMBO J. **13:** 4587–4596.
12. KORSMEYER, S.J., X.M. YIN, Z.N. OLTVAI et al. 1995. Reactive oxygen species and the regulation of cell death by the Bcl-2 gene family. Biochim. Biophys. Acta **127:** 63–66.
13. HOCKENBERRY, D.M., G. NUNEZ, C. MILLIMAN et al. 1990. Bcl-2 is an inner mitochondrial membrane protein that blocks programmed cell death. Nature (Lond.) **348:** 334–336.

14. HOCKENBERRY, D.M., Z.N. OLTVAI, X.M. YIN et al. 1993. Bcl-2 functions in an antioxidant pathway to prevent apoptosis. Cell **75:** 241–251.
15. MOUNTZ, J.D., T. ZHOU, T. SU et al. 1996. Autoimmune disease results from multiple interactive defects in apoptosis induction molecules and signaling pathways. Behring Inst. Mitt. **97:** 200–219.
16. POWIS, G., M. BRIEHL & J. OBLONG. 1995. Redox signaling and control of cell growth and death. Pharmacol. & Ther. **68:** 149–173.
17. BUTTKE, T.M. & P.A. SANDSTROM. 1995. Redox regulation of programmed cell death in lymphocytes. Free Radical Res. Commun. **22:** 389–397.
18. MCCONKEY, D.J., P. HARTZELL, P. NICOTERA et al. 1988. Stimulation of endogenous endonuclease activity in hepatocytes exposed to oxidative stress. Toxicol. Lett. **42:** 123–130.
19. LENNON, S.V., S.J. MARTIN, T.G. COTTER. 1990. Induction of apoptosis (programmed cell death) in tumor cells by widely diverging stimuli. Biochem. Soc. Trans. **18:** 343–345.
20. FERNANDEZ, A., J. KIEFER, L. FOSDICK et al. 1995. Oxygen radical production and thiol depletion are required for Ca+2-mediated endogenous endonuclease activation in apoptotic thymocytes. J. Immunol. **155:** 5133–5139.
21. SLATER, A.F., C.S. NOBEL, S. ORRENIUS. 1995. The role of intracellular oxidants in apoptosis. Biochim. Biophys. Acta **127:** 59–62.
22. WOLFE, J.T., D. ROSS & G.M. COHEN. 1994. A role for metals and free radicals in the induction of apoptosis in thymocytes. FEBS Lett. **352:** 58–62.
23. MAYER, M. & M. NOBLE. 1994. N-acetyl-L-cysteine is a pluripotent protector against cell death and enhancer of trophic factor-mediated cell survival *in vivo.* Proc. Natl. Acad. Sci. USA **91:** 7496–7500.
24. KANE, D.J., T.A. SARAFIAN, R. ANTON et al. 1993. Bcl-2 inhibition of neural death: decreased generation of reactive oxygen species. Science **262:** 1274–1277.
25. FANG, W., J.J. RIVARD, J.A. GANSER et al. Bcl-xl rescues WEHI231B lymphocytes from oxidant mediated death following diverging apoptotic stimuli. J. Immunol. **155:** 66–75.
26. JACOBSON, M.D. & M.C. RAFF. 1995. Programmed cell death and Bcl-2 protection in very low oxygen. Nature **374:** 814–816.
27. SHIMIZU, S., Y. EGUCHI, H. KOSAKA et al. 1995. Prevention of hypoxia-induced cell death by Bcl-2 and Bcl-xl. Nature **374:** 811–813.
28. YAO, K.S., M. CLAYTON & P.J. O'DWYER. 1995. Apoptosis in human adenocarcinoma HT-29 cells induced by exposure to hypoxia. J. Natl. Cancer Inst. **87:** 117–122.
29. KAZZAZ, J.A., J. XU, T.A. PALAIA et al. 1996. Cellular oxygen toxicity. Oxidant injury without apoptosis. J. Biol. Chem. **271:** 15182–15186.
30. RICHTER, C. 1993. Pro-oxidants and mitochondrial Ca+2: their relationship to apoptosis and oncogenesis. FEBS Lett. **325:** 104–107.
31. ZAMAZMI, N., P. MARCHETTI, M. CASTEDO et al. 1995. Sequential reduction of mitochondrial transmembrane potential and generation of reactive oxygen species in early programmed cell death. J. Exp. Med. **182:** 367–377.
32. ZAMZAMI, N., P. MARCHETTI, M. CASTEDO et al. 1995. Reduction in mitochondrial potential constitutes an early irreversible step of programmed lymphocyte death in vivo. J. Exp. Med. **181:** 1661–1672.
33. PETIT, P.X., S.A. SUSIN, N. ZAMZAMI et al. 1996. Mitochondria and programmed cell death: back to the future. FEBS Lett. **396:** 7–13.
34. CASTEDO, M., T. HIRSCH, S.A. SUSIN et al. 1996. Sequential acquisition of mitochondrial and plasma membrane alterations during early lymphocyte apoptosis. J. Immunol. **157:** 512–521.
35. CASTEDO, M., A. MACHO, N. ZAMZAMI et al. 1995. Mitochondrial perturbations define lymphocytes undergoing apoptotic depletion *in vivo.* Eur. J. Immunol. **25:** 3277–3284.
36. RAO, L. & E. WHITE. 1997. Bcl-2 and the ICE family of apoptotic regulators: making a connection. Curr. Opin. Gen. & Dev. **7:** 52–58.
37. KLUCK, R.M., E. BOSSY-WETZEL, D.R. GREEN et al. 1997. The release of cytochrome C from mitochondria: a primary site for Bcl-2 regulation of apoptosis. Science **275:** 1132–1136.
38. YANG, J., S. LIUU, K. BHALLA et al. 1997. Prevention of apoptosis by Bcl-2: release of cytochrome C from mitochondria blocked. Science **275:** 1129–1132.

39. MARCHETTI, P., D. DECAUDIN, A. MACHO *et al.* 1997. Redox regulation of apoptosis: impact of thiol oxidation status on mitochondrial function. Eur. J. Immunol. **27:** 289–296.
40. ENWONWU, C.O., & V.I. MEEKS. 1995. Bionutrition and Oral Cancer in Humans. Cri. Rev. Oral. Biol. Med. **6:** 5–17.
41. ZHENG, W., X.O. SHU, B.T. JI *et al.* 1996. Diet and risk factors for cancer of the salivary glands: a population-based case-control study. Int. J. Cancer **67:** 194–198.
42. BERGELSON, S., R. PINKUS & V. DANIEL. 1994. Intracellular glutathione levels regulate Fos/Jun induction and activation of glutathione S-transferase gene expression. Cancer Res. **54:** 36–40.
43. MEYER, M., H.L. PAHL & P.A. BAEUERLE. 1994. Regulation of the transcription factors NF-kappa B and AP-1 by redox changes. Chem. Biol. Interact. **91:** 91–100.
44. SHERTZER, H.G., V. VASILIOU, R-M. LIU *et al.* 1995. Enzyme induction by L-butathionine (S,R) sulfoximine in cultured mouse hepatoma cells. Chem.Res. Toxcicol. **8:** 431–436.
45. WHITFIELD, J.F. 1992. Calcium signals and cancer. Crit. Rev. Oncog. **3:** 55–90.

Nucleotide Sugars, Nucleotide Sulfate, and ATP Transporters of the Endoplasmic Reticulum and Golgi Apparatus[a]

PATRICIA BERNINSONE AND CARLOS B. HIRSCHBERG[b]

Department of Biochemistry and Molecular Biology, University of Massachusetts Medical Center, Worcester, Massachusetts 01655, USA

> ABSTRACT: The lumina of the endoplasmic reticulum and Golgi apparatus are the subcellular sites where glycosylation, sulfation, and phosphorylation of secretory and membrane-bound proteins, proteoglycans, and lipids occur. Nucleotide sugars, nucleotide sulfate, and ATP are substrates in the above reactions and must first be translocated from the cytosol into the lumen of these organelles. Translocation of these nucleotide derivatives is mediated by highly specific transporters, which are antiporters with the corresponding nucleoside monophosphate, as shown by genetic and biochemical approaches in mammals and yeast. Studies with mammalian, yeast, and protozoa mutants have shown that a defect in a specific translocator results in selective impairments of glycosylation of proteins, lipids and proteoglycans *in vivo*. Several of these transporters have been purified, cloned, and found to encode very hydrophobic proteins with multitransmembrane domains. Experiments with yeast and mammalian cells demonstrate that these transporters play a regulatory role in posttranslational modifications.

Membrane and secretory proteins are made on membrane-bound polysomes and translocated as nascent polypeptides into the lumen of the endoplasmic reticulum.[1–4] Here ATP and UDP-glucose are substrates in reactions to maintain properly folded proteins.[5–8] Following budding of vesicles from the endoplasmic reticulum and fusion with elements of the Golgi apparatus, some of the above proteins, as well as glycolipids and proteoglycans, are glycosylated, sulfated, and phosphorylated in the lumen of the Golgi apparatus. Nucleotide sugars, nucleotide sulfate, and ATP are substrates for these reactions; they are not synthesized in the lumen of the Golgi apparatus but in the cytosol, except for cytidine monophosphate (CMP)-sialic acid, which is synthesized in the nucleus and ATP, most of which is synthesized in mitochondria.[9] All of these nucleotides and nucleotide derivatives enter the Golgi lumen by way of specific carrier proteins (see below).

CHARACTERISTICS OF NUCLEOTIDE SUGAR, PAPS, AND ATP TRANSPORT INTO VESICLES FROM THE GOLGI APPARATUS AND ENDOPLASMIC RETICULUM

Assays *in vitro* have been developed to measure the transport of the above nucleotides and nucleotide derivatives into the lumen of vesicles derived from the Golgi apparatus and endoplasmic reticulum. For these studies, vesicles must be reasonably

---

[a] The work in the authors' laboratory was supported by Grants from the NIH, GM 30365 and GM 34396.

[b] Tel: (508) 856-2450; fax: (508) 856 6231; e-mail: carlos.hirschberg@ummed.edu.

pure, sealed, and of the same membrane topological orientation as *in vivo*. Transport of solutes into the lumen of these vesicles can be measured using filtration and centrifugation assays.[9,10]

Both assays have yielded comparable results and have allowed the following general characteristics of transport for the above nucleotides and nucleotide derivatives to be obtained: (1) Transport is organelle specific. Several nucleotides and nucleotide derivatives are transported solely, or at a much faster rate, into vesicles from either the Golgi apparatus or the endoplasmic reticulum. CMP-sialic acid,[11] GDP-fucose,[11] PAPS,[12] and UDP-galactose[13] are transported solely into vesicles from the Golgi apparatus and not into those from the endoplasmic reticulum. UDP-N-acetylgalactosamine,[13] UDP-N-acetylglucosamine,[14] UDP-glucuronic acid,[15] and UDP-xylose[15] are transported into vesicles from the Golgi apparatus at approximately twice the rate as into vesicles from the endoplasmic reticulum; ATP is transported into both vesicles at comparable rates,[16–18] whereas UDP-glucose is transported into vesicles from the endoplasmic reticulum at a considerably faster rate than into the Golgi apparatus.[19] GDP-mannose is transported into Golgi vesicles from yeast and protozoa but not into Golgi vesicles from mammals.[11,21,32] (2) The entire nucleotide or nucleotide derivative is transported. (3) Transport is saturable with apparent K_m values between 1 and 10 µM. (4) Transport is temperature dependent. (5) Transport is competitively inhibited by the corresponding nucleoside mono- and diphosphate and is not inhibited by either sugars or sulfate. (6) Transport does not require ATP as an energy source and is neither inhibited nor stimulated by ionophores.

TRANSPORTERS OF NUCLEOTIDE SUGARS AND ATP ARE ANTIPORTERS

Experiments *in vitro* have shown that following transport of nucleotide sugars, PAPS, and ATP into the lumen of Golgi vesicles, the solutes become concentrated within the lumen relative to their concentration in the medium.[9] The lack of either stimulation or inhibition by ATP and different ionophores in these reactions leads to the suggestion that the previous concentration effect may be coupled to exit (down a concentration gradient) of solutes within the vesicles.[20] Evidence for this hypothesis was obtained by incubating Golgi vesicles from rat liver with nucleotide sugars labeled in the nucleoside moiety with one radioisotope, followed by reincubation of the same vesicles with the same nucleotide sugar labeled in the sugar with a different radioisotope. It was found that exit of the first radiolabel, a nucleoside monophosphate, could only be effected upon addition of the corresponding nucleotide sugar. Thus, GMP could only exit vesicles that had been incubated with GDP-fucose but not with GDP-mannose, which does not enter mammalian Golgi vesicles.[20]

A second line of evidence supporting antiporters in the above reaction comes from experiments with Golgi vesicles preloaded with the putative antiporter. Thus, the rate of UDP-N-acetylglucosamine (UDP-GlcNAc) entry into Golgi vesicles was faster when these vesicles had been preincubated with UMP than with buffer alone.[10] Because the rate was dependent on pH with that at 7.5 (UMP is dianionic) being faster than at 5.45 (UMP is monoionic), it was inferred that the species exiting the vesicles was UMP^{-2}. Similar experiments were also done with proteoliposomes preincubated with either UMP or CMP and determining that the rate of entry of uridine and cytidine nucleotide sugars was faster compared to proteoliposomes preincubated in the presence of buffer.

Studies with *Saccharomyces cerevisiae* have also provided genetic evidence supporting the antiporter hypothesis. This yeast contains a luminal Golgi GDPase[21–23] whose hypothesized role is to convert GDP into GMP, the putative antiporter for

GDP-mannose entry into the Golgi lumen. GDP-mannose, following its entry into the Golgi lumen and transfer of mannose to mannans, yields, as the other reaction product, GDP, which in turn is a substrate for the GDPase. Experiments *in vivo* demonstrated that gene disruption of the GDA gene resulted in inhibition of Golgi mannosylation of proteins and lipids;[23] experiments *in vitro* with Golgi vesicles derived from the gene-disrupted strain and the wild-type demonstrated that the rate of GDP-mannose entry into those vesicles lacking their GDPase was 5-fold slower than into wild-type vesicles;[24,25] this demonstrated a direct connection between the lack of *in vivo* Golgi mannosylation of macromolecules and decreased entry of GDP-mannose into the Golgi lumen.

PHYSIOLOGIC RELEVANCE OF NUCLEOTIDE SUGAR TRANSPORT INTO THE GOLGI LUMEN: THE EXISTENCE OF MUTANTS

To date, mammalian,[26–29] yeast,[30] and *Leishmania*[31,32] mutants in nucleotide sugar transport into the Golgi lumen have been described. These mutants have a 95–100% deficiency of the corresponding sugar in their macromolecules. This phenotype can be specifically attributed to a defect in a specific transport activity in the Golgi membrane.

The first mutants characterized as being deficient in nucleotide sugar transport into the Golgi apparatus where Chinese hamster ovary (CHO) cell lines. CHO Lec2[26,27] and CHO 1021[28] are mutants that are resistant to wheat germ agglutinin and belong to the same complementation group. Their proteins and lipids contain 2–5% of wild-type levels of sialic acid, and the rate of CMP-sialic acid transport into Golgi vesicles was 2–5% of that of vesicles from wild-type cells.[33] This transport defect was specific for the above nucleotide sugar. CHO Lec8[26,27] and clone 13[28] are mutants that belong to the same complementation group and have a 95% deficiency of galactose and sialic acid in proteins and lipids. Golgi vesicles from mutant cells transport UDP-galactose at 2–5% of the rate of vesicles from wild-type cells, whereas vesicles from both cells transport other nucleotide sugars at comparable rates.[34] A MDCK cell line deficient in UDP-galactose transport into the Golgi lumen has also been described.[29]

A mutant *Kluyveromyces lactis* yeast deficient in transport of UDP-GlcNAc into the Golgi lumen has also been described.[30] The mutant can transport GDP-mannose at comparable rates as wild-type cells and lacks terminal *N*-acetylglucosamine in its mannan chains. A mutant *Leishmania donovani*[32] with a specific defect in transport of GDP-mannose into Golgi vesicles has recently been described. The mutant can transport UDP-galactose into the Golgi lumen at comparable rates with wild-type cells. The mutant that is avirulent, compared to the wild type that is virulent, is deficient in lipophosphoglycan, a complex glycolipid on its cell surface.

These studies demonstrate that transport of nucleotide sugars into the Golgi lumen is required for subsequent glycosylation of proteins and lipids and strongly suggests the existence of individual nucleotide sugar transporters in the Golgi membrane. The next section will show that these mutants have been crucial for cloning some of these transporters by phenotypic correction.

PRIMARY SEQUENCE OF NUCLEOTIDE SUGAR TRANSPORTERS

The primary amino acid sequence of Golgi membrane nucleotide sugar transporters from mammals,[35,36] yeast,[37] and *Leishmania*[31] has been determined to date. As can be seen in FIGURE 1, all these transporters appear to be very hydrophobic, multitransmembrane spanning proteins. So far, all transporters have been cloned by correction of mutant phenotypes. Expression of the murine CMP-sialic acid transporter cDNA in *S. cerevisiae* has directly demonstrated that the protein is the transporter *per se*.[38] The transporters for UDP-GlcNAc and CMP-sialic acid have a leucine zipper motif, suggesting that this region may be involved in oligomerization of the protein in the membrane. However, the Golgi transporters for GDP-mannose from *Leishmania*[31] and

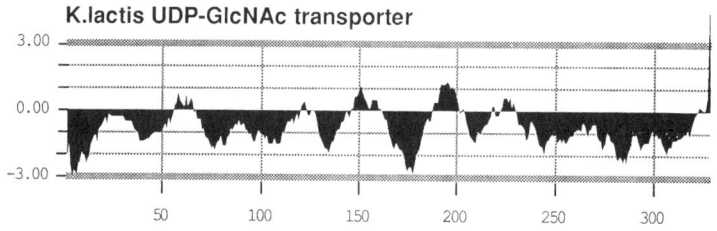

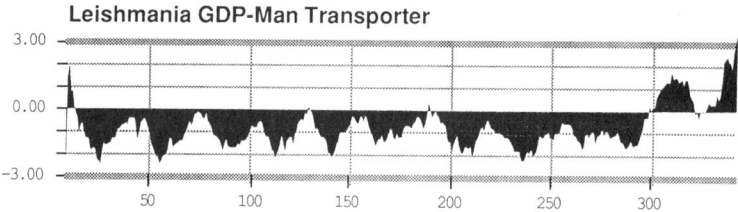

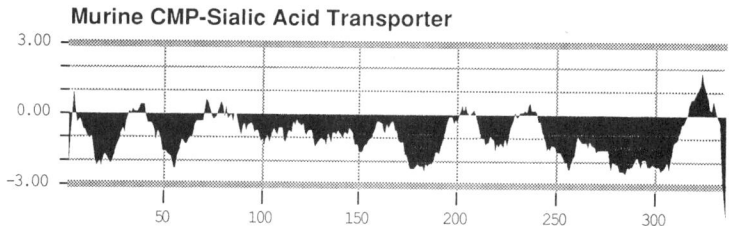

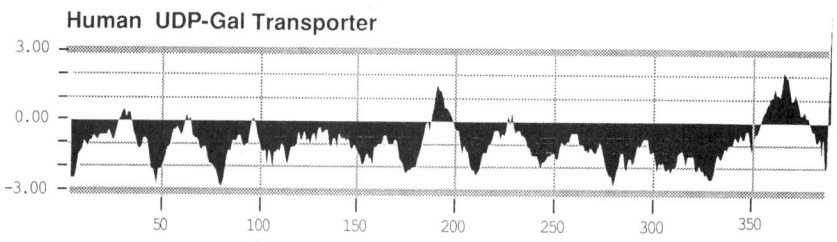

FIGURE 1. Kyte-Doolittle hydrophilicity plots of four Golgi membrane nucleotide sugar transporters; window size = 17.

human UDP-galactose[36] do not have a leucine zipper motif. Previously, radiation target inactivation studies had suggested that the PAPS transporter is a homodimer in the Golgi membrane *in situ.*[39]

The lack of identity or similarity, at the amino acid level, between the *K. lactis* transporter for UDP-GlcNAc and the human UDP-galactose transporter is surprising, particularly if one considers that all UDP-nucleotide sugars have UMP as a common antiporter. The 40% of identity between the transporter for UDP-galactose from humans and the murine CMP-sialic acid is puzzling, although the CMP-sialic acid transporter cannot transport UDP-galactose.[38]

An amino acid sequence will also be obtained from purified nucleotide sugar Golgi transporters from the Golgi apparatus. So far, the Golgi transporter for PAPS has been purified to homogeneity[39] whereas those for UDP-GalNAc, UDP-glucuronic acid, and ATP have been partially purified. Purification was accomplished through a combination of conventional and affinity-chromatographic procedures, using as an assay reconstitution of Triton X-100 solubilized proteins inserted in phosphatidylcholine liposomes.[40,41] A protein of 75 kD has been identified as the putative PAPS transporter.[39]

TRANSPORTERS OF NUCLEOTIDE SUGARS REGULATE GLYCOSYLATION OF MACROMOLECULES WITHIN THE GOLGI LUMEN

Two experimental lines support the hypothesis that transporters of nucleotide sugars regulate which macromolecules become glycosylated in the Golgi apparatus lumen. A mutant MDCK cell line has been described that is approximately 98% deficient in UDP-galactose transport into the Golgi lumen.[29] The cell line has marked reduced galactosylation of glycoproteins, glycosphingolipids, and keratan sulfate, a proteoglycan that contains galactose in its glycosaminoglycan polymer.[42] By contrast, chondroitin sulfate and heparan sulfate, proteoglycans that solely contain galactose in the linkage region between the polymer and the protein, are not reduced.[42] We favor the hypothesis that the deficient galactosylation of keratan sulfate is the result of a higher K_m for the galactosyltransferase involved in addition to galactose in the polymer, compared to those galactosyltransferases that add galactose to the linkage region.

The other evidence supporting a role for nucleotide sugar transport into the Golgi lumen being a regulator in macromolecular biosynthesis comes from experiments with *S. cerevisiae*. Strains where the Golgi GDPase was disrupted showed a virtual complete deficiency in Golgi mannosylation of *O*-linked mannoproteins, *N*-linked vacuolar proteins, and of mannosylation of phosphoceramides.[23] Surprisingly, invertase, a secreted glycoprotein, was found to have shorter *N*-linked mannan chains rather than a complete absence, as would have been expected. Although this selectivity may be the result of a series of possibilities, we favor the one that mannosyltransferases involved in *N*-linked mannan chain biosynthesis of secreted proteins have a lower K_m compared to the other mannosyltransferases. Nevertheless, the possibility of subcompartments for the above mannosylation reactions cannot be ruled out.

TRANSPORTERS OF NUCLEOTIDE SUGARS AND ATP IN THE ENDOPLASMIC RETICULUM

So far, transporters for UDP-glucose,[19,43] UDP-GlcNAc,[14] UDP-glucuronic acid,[15,44,45] UDP-xylose,[15] and ATP[17,18,46] have been identified in the endoplasmic reticulum. UDP-glucose appears to be necessary for reglucosylation of nascent polypeptide chains within the lumen as part of their quality control.[7,8,47] Transport of UDP-GlcNAc and addition of *O*-GlcNAc appears to occur in the lumen of the endoplasmic reticulum without a defined function as of yet.[48,49] Transport of UDP-glucuronic acid and UDP-xylose may be required for glucuronidation and xylosylation of bile acids in the lumen of the endoplasmic reticulum.[43–45] Transport of ATP appears to be necessary for the quality control of properly folded proteins within the endoplasmic reticulum.[5,8,47] So far, only the endoplasmic reticulum transporter for ATP has been successfully reconstituted.[18,46]

CONCLUSIONS AND FUTURE DIRECTIONS

Future studies of nucleotide sugar, ATP, and PAPS transporters in the Golgi apparatus and endoplasmic reticulum will most likely cover three areas: (a) structure of the transporters, (b) regulation of transport and possible diseases, and (c) targeting and subcellular distribution of transporters.

As more primary amino acid sequences of the above transporters become available, questions regarding binding domains for nucleotide sugars, nucleotide sulfate, ATP, and the corresponding antiporters will be important. Equally important will be establishment of their secondary, tertiary, and quaternary structures within the membrane.

Among studies on the regulation of transport of the above nucleotides and nucleotide derivatives, important questions will be understanding the regulation of the transporter proteins *per se,* as well as their mRNAs during different physiological conditions, during development; and the existence of possible diseases. Gene disruption studies as well as RNA antisense studies are expected to provide important new insights into the regulation of these transporters.

Determination of those structural features that result in some of these transporters being localized to specific organelles, although others are not, is an important open problem. Within the Golgi apparatus, the question of polarization of these transporters within this organelle as well as the possibility of complexes of these proteins with the corresponding transferases will need to be addressed, together with questions on membrane traffic and recycling.

In conclusion, the last years have resulted in major advances in understanding of these transporters; nevertheless, these studies are just the beginning in what we hope will be an exciting era of discovery about these novel groups of proteins.

ACKNOWLEDGMENT

We thank K. Welch and A. Stratton for excellent secretarial assistance.

REFERENCES

1. PALADE, G. 1975. Intracellular aspects of the process of protein synthesis. Science **189:** 347–358.
2. LINGAPPA, V.R., J.R. LINGAPPA, R. PRASSAD, K. EBNER & G. BLOBEL. 1978. Coupled cell-free synthesis, segregation and core glycosylation of a secretory protein. Proc. Natl. Acad. Sci. USA **75:** 2338–2342.
3. PFEFFER, S.R. & J.E. ROTHMAN. 1987. Biosynthetic protein transport and sorting by the endoplasmic reticulum and golgi. Annu. Rev. Biochem. **56:** 833–851.
4. KATZ, F.N., J.E. ROTHMAN, V.R. LINGAPPA, G. BLOBEL & H.F. LODISH. 1977. Membrane assembly *in vitro.* Synthesis, glycosylation and asymmetric insertion of a transmembrane protein. Proc. Natl. Acad. Sci. USA **74:** 3278–3282.

5. FLYNN, G.C., T.G. CHAPPELL & J.E. ROTHMAN. 1989. Peptide binding and release by proteins implicated as catalysts of protein assembly. Science **245:** 385–390.
6. MUNRO, S. & H.R.B. PELHAM. 1986. An Hsp 70-like protein in the ER: Identity with 78 kD glucose-regulated protein and immunoglobulin heavy chain binding protein. Cell **46:** 291–300.
7. SOUSA, M.C., M.A. FERRERO-GARCIA & A.J. PARODI. 1992. Recognition of the oligosaccharide and protein moieties of glycoproteins by the UDP-Glc:glycoprotein glucosyltransferase. Biochemistry **31:** 97–105.
8. HELENIUS, A. 1994. How N-linked oligosaccharides affect glycoprotein folding in the endoplasmic reticulum. Mol. Cell. Biol. **5:** 253–265.
9. HIRSCHBERG, C.B. & M.D. SNIDER. 1987. Topography of glycosylation in the rough endoplasmic reticulum and golgi apparatus. Annu. Rev. Biochem. **56:** 63–88.
10. WALDMAN, B.C. & G. RUDNICK. 1990. UDP-GlcNAc transport across the golgi membrane: Electroneutral exchange for dianionic UMP. Biochemistry **29:** 44–52.
11. SOMMERS, L.W. & C.B. HIRSCHBERG. 1982. Transport of sugar nucleotides into rat liver golgi: A new golgi marker activity. J. Biol. Chem. **257:** 10811–10817.
12. SCHWARZ, J.K., J.M. CAPASSO & C.B. HIRSCHBERG. 1984. Translocation of adenosine 3′-phosphate 5′-phosphosulfate into rat liver golgi vesicles. J. Biol. Chem. **259:** 3554–3559.
13. ABEIJON, C. & C.B. HIRSCHBERG. 1987. Subcellular site of synthesis of the N-acetygalactosamine (α1-0) serine (or threonine) linkage in rat liver. J. Biol. Chem. **262:** 4153–4159.
14. PEREZ, M. & C.B. HIRSCHBERG. 1985. Translocation of UDP-N-acetylglucosamine into vesicles derived from rat liver endoplasmic reticulum and golgi apparatus. J. Biol. Chem. **260:** 4671–4678.
15. NUWAYHID, N., J.H. GLASER, J.C. JOHNSON, H.E. CONRAD, S.C. HAUSER & C.B. HIRSCHBERG. 1986. Xylosylation and glucuronosylation reactions in rat liver golgi apparatus and endoplasmic reticulum. J. Biol. Chem. **261:** 12936–12941.
16. CAPASSO, J.M., T.W. KEENAN, C. ABEIJON & C.B. HIRSCHBERG. 1989. Mechanism of phosphorylation in the lumen of the golgi apparatus: Translocation of adenosine 5′ triphosphate into golgi vesicles from rat liver and mammary gland. J. Biol. Chem. **264:** 5233–5240.
17. CLAIRMONT, C.A., A. DEMAIO & C.B. HIRSCHBERG. 1992. Translocation of ATP into the lumen of the rough endoplasmic reticulum-derived vesicles and its binding to lumenal proteins including BiP (GRP 78) and GRP 94. J. Biol. Chem. **267:** 3983–3990.
18. GUILLEN, E. & C.B. HIRSCHBERG. 1995a. Transport of adenosine triphosphate into rat liver endoplasmic reticulum proteoliposomes. Biochemistry **34:** 5472–5476.
19. PEREZ, M. & C.B. HIRSCHBERG. 1986. Topography of glycosylation reactions in the rough endoplasmic reticulum membrane. J. Biol. Chem. **261:** 6822–6830.
20. CAPASSO, J.M. & C.B. HIRSCHBERG. 1984. Mechanisms of glycosylation and sulfation in the golgi apparatus: Evidence for nucleotide sugar/nucleoside monophosphate and nucleotide sulfate/nucleoside monophosphate antiports in the golgi apparatus membrane. Proc. Natl. Acad. Sci. USA **81:** 7051–7055.
21. ABEIJON, C., P. ORLEAN, P.W. ROBBINS & C.B. HIRSCHBERG. 1989. Topography of glycosylation in yeast: Characterization of GDP-mannose transport and lumenal guanosine diphosphatase activities in golgi-like vesicles. Proc. Natl. Acad. Sci. USA **86:** 6935–6939.
22. YANAGISAWA, K., D. RESNICK, C. ABEIJON, P.W. ROBBINS & C.B. HIRSCHBERG. 1990. A guanosine diphosphatase enriched in golgi vesicles of *Saccharomyces cerevisiae:* Purification and characterization. J. Biol. Chem. **265:** 19351–19355.
23. ABEIJON, C., K. YANAGISAWA, E. MANDON, A. HAUSLER, K. MOREMAN, C.B. HIRSCHBERG & P.W. ROBBINS. 1993. Guanosine diphosphatase is required for protein and sphingolipid glycosylation in the golgi lumen of *Saccharomyces cerevisiae.* J. Cell Biol. **122:** 307–323.
24. BERNINSONE, P., J.J. MIRET & C.B. HIRSCHBERG. 1994. The golgi guanosine diphosphatase is required for transport of GDP-mannose into the lumen of *Saccharomyces cerevisiae* golgi vesicles. J. Biol. Chem. **269:** 207–211.
25. BERNINSONE, P., Z.Y. LIN, E. KEMPNER & C.B. HIRSCHBERG. 1995. Regulation of yeast golgi glycosylation: Guanosine diphosphatase functions as a homodimer in the membranes. J. Biol. Chem. **270:** 14564–14567.

26. STANLEY, P. 1980. Altered glycolipids of CHO cells resistant to wheat germ agglutinin. Am. Chem. Soc. Symp. Series B. **128:** 213–221.
27. STANLEY, P. 1985. Membrane mutants of animal cells: Rapid identification of those with a primary defect in glycosylation. Mol. Cell. Biol. **5:** 923–929.
28. BRILES, E.B., E. LI & S. KORNFELD. 1977. Isolation of wheat germ agglutinin-resistant clones of Chinese hamster ovary cells deficient in membrane sialic acid and galactose. J. Biol. Chem. **252:** 1107–1116.
29. BRANDLI, A.W., G.C. HANSSON, E. RODRIGUEZ-BOULAN & K. SIMONS. 1988. A polarized epithelial cell mutant deficient in translocation of UDP-galactose into the golgi complex. J. Biol. Chem. **264:** 16283–16290.
30. ABEIJON, C., E.C. MANDON, P.W. ROBBINS & C.B. HIRSCHBERG. 1996. A mutant yeast deficient in golgi transport of uridine diphosphate N-acetylglucosamine. J. Biol. Chem. **271:** 8851–8854.
31. DESCOTEAUX, A., Y. LUO, S.J. TURCO & S.M. BEVERLEY. 1995. A specialized pathway affecting virulence glycoconjugate of *Leishmania*. Science **269:** 1859–1872.
32. MA, D., D.G. RUSSELL, S.M. BEVERLEY & S.J. TURCO. 1997. Golgi GDP-mannose uptake requires *Leishmania* LP62: A member of a eukaryotic family of putative nucleotide sugar transporters. J. Biol. Chem. **272:** 3799–3805.
33. DEUTSCHER, S.I., N. NUWAYHID, P. STANLEY, E.I.B. BRILES & C.B. HIRSCHBERG. 1984. Translocation across golgi vesicle membranes. A CHO glycosylation mutant deficient in CMP-sialic acid transport. Cell **39:** 295–299.
34. DEUTSCHER, S.L. & C.B. HIRSCHBERG. 1986. Mechanism of galactosylation in the golgi apparatus: A Chinese hamster ovary cell mutant deficient in translocation of UDP-galactose across golgi vesicle membranes. J. Biol. Chem. **261:** 96–100.
35. ECKHARDT, M., M. MUEHLENHOFF, A. BETHE & R. GERARDY-SCHAHN. 1976. Expression cloning of the golgi CMP-sialic acid transporter. Proc. Natl. Acad. Sci. USA **93:** 7572–7576.
36. MIURA, N., N. IISHIDA, M. HOSHINO, M. YAMAGUCHI, T. HARA, D. AYUSAWA & M. KAWAKITA. 1996. Human UDP-galactose translocator: Molecular cloning of a complementary DNA that complements the genetic defect of a mutant cell line defect in UDP-galactose translocator. J. Biochem. (Tokyo) **120:** 236–241.
37. ABEIJON, C., P.W. ROBBINS & C.B. HIRSCHBERG. 1996. Molecular cloning of the golgi apparatus uridine diphosphate N-acetylglucosamine transporter from *Kluyveromyces lactis*. Proc. Natl. Acad. Sci. USA **93:** 5963–5968.
38. BERNINSONE, P., M. ECKHARDT, R. GERARDY-SCHAHN & C.B. HIRSCHBERG. 1997. Functional expression of the murine golgi CMP-sialic acid transporter in *Saccharomyces cerevisiae*. J. Biol. Chem. **272:** 12616–12619.
39. MANDON, E.C., M.E. MILLA, E. KEMPNER & C.B. HIRSCHBERG. 1994. Purification of the golgi adenosine 3′ phosphate 5′-phosphosulfate transporter, a homodimer within the membrane. Proc. Natl. Acad. Sci. USA **91:** 10707–10711.
40. MILLA, M.E. & C.B. HIRSCHBERG. 1989. Reconstitution of golgi vesicle CMP-sialic acid and adenosine 3′ phosphate 5′ phosphosulfate transport into proteoliposomes. Proc. Natl. Acad. Sci. USA **86:** 1786–1790.
41. MILLA, M.E., C.A. CLAIRMONT & C.B. HIRSCHBERG. 1992. Reconstitution into proteoliposomes and partial purification of the golgi apparatus membrane UDP-galactose, UDP-xylose and UDP-glucuronic acid transport activities. J. Biol. Chem. **267:** 103–107.
42. TOMA, L., M.A.S. PINHAL, C.P. DIETRICH, H.B. NADER & C.B. HIRSCHBERG. 1996. Transport of UDP-galactose into the golgi lumen regulates the biosynthesis of proteoglycans. J. Biol. Chem. **271:** 3897–3901.
43. VANSTAPEL, F. & N. BLANKAERT. 1988. Carrier-mediated translocation of uridine diphosphate glucose into the lumen of the endoplasmic reticulum-derived vesicles from rat liver. J. Clin. Invest. **82:** 1113–1122.
44. HAUSER, S.C., J.C. ZIURYS & J.L. GOLAM. 1988. A membrane transporter mediates access of uridine 5′-diphosphoglucuronic acid from the cytosol into the endoplasmic reticulum of rat hepatocytes: Implications for glucuronidation reactions. Biochim. Biophys. Acta **967:** 149–157.
45. BERG, C.L., A. RADOMINSKA, R. LESTER & J.L. GOLLAN. 1995. Membrane translocation and

regulation of uridine diphosphate-glucuronic acid uptake in rat liver microsomal vesicles. Gastroenterology **108:** 183–192.
46. MAYINGER, P. & D.I. MEYER. 1993. An ATP transporter is required for protein translocation into the yeast endoplasmic reticulum. EMBO J. **12:** 659–666.
47. BRAAKMAN, I., J. HELENIUS & A. HELENIUS. 1992. Role of ATP and disulfide bonds during protein folding in the endoplasmic reticulum. Nature **356:** 260–262.
48. ABEIJON, C. & C.B. HIRSCHBERG. 1988. Intrinsic membrane glycoproteins with cytosol-oriented sugars in the endoplasmic reticulum. Proc. Natl. Acad. Sci. USA **85:** 1010–1014.
49. ABEIJON, C. & C.B. HIRSCHBERG. 1992. Topography of glycosylation reactions in the endoplasmic reticulum. Trends Biochem. Sci. **17:** 31–36.

Development of Salivary Gland Cell Lines for Studies of Signaling and Physiology[a]

STEPHEN P. SOLTOFF,[b,f] SHELLEY A. GRUBMAN,[c] AND DOUGLAS M. JEFFERSON[c,d,e]

[b]*Department of Medicine, Division of Signal Transduction, Beth Israel Deaconess Medical Center, Harvard Institutes of Medicine, 330 Brookline Avenue, Boston, Massachusetts 02215, USA*
[c]*Department of Pediatrics, New England Medical Center, Boston, Massachusetts 02111, USA*
[d]*Department of Physiology, Tufts University School of Medicine, Boston, Massachusetts 02111, USA*
[e]*Department of Medicine, New England Medical Center, Boston, Massachusetts 02111, USA*

ABSTRACT: We developed and characterized an immortalized rat parotid cell line to use in salivary gland studies. The cells were immortalized by retroviral transduction of SV40 large T antigen into isolated parotid cells. Using immunocytochemical techniques, we found that the immortalized epithelial cells were ductal, rather than acinar, in nature. Cells were grown under coculture conditions with lethally irradiated NIH3T3 cells. One cell line, which was designated RPG1/SV40 cells (for rat parotid gland 1/SV40 transformant), was selected for characterization. These cells formed a sheet epithelium with tight junctions and a measurable transepithelial resistance. RPG1/SV40 cells responded to muscarinic receptor (carbachol) and/or P_2 purinoceptor (ATP and UTP) stimuli with increases in the following: (1) intracellular free-calcium concentration ($[Ca^{2+}]i$); (2) the short-circuit current (I_{SC}) across the epithelium; (3) the tyrosine phosphorylation of PKCδ; and (4) MAP kinase activity. Thus, the cells appear to be useful for a wide range of studies involving physiology, biochemistry, and signal transduction approaches.

INTRODUCTION

Many physiological and biochemical aspects of fluid and protein secretion have been studied using freshly isolated dissociated cells from rodent salivary glands or by using *in vivo* techniques. In studies outlined in this paper, we present results from a rat salivary gland cell line that we developed for investigations into salivary gland function. Rat salivary glands have been used as a model system to study various aspects of stimulus-secretion coupling, including those related to fluid and electrolyte secretion as well as protein secretion (exocytosis). Parasympathetic and sympathetic innervation of parotid glands provides the main control of secretion. Fluid secretion is stimulated by neurotransmitters released from parasympathetic nerves. The activation of multiple receptors, including those for acetylcholine and substance P, increase the intracellular free calcium concentration ($[Ca^{2+}]i$), which alters membrane permeability by the activation of Ca^{2+}-sensitive ion channels.[1] Ca^{2+}-mobilizing secretagogues promote the hydrolysis

---

[a] This work was supported in part by NIDR DE10877, NIDR DE09596, and NIDDK P30DK34928.
[f] Tel: (617) 667-0949; fax: (617) 667-0957; e-mail: ssoltoff@bidmc.harvard.edu

of phosphatidylinositol-4,5-bisphosphate (PI-4,5-P_2) to diacylglycerol (DAG) and inositol 1,4,5-trisphosphate (IP_3), and this occurs through the activation of phospholipase C, which is linked to these receptors by a regulatory heterotrimeric GTP-binding protein.[2]

Salivary glands have been difficult to culture for more than a few days and quickly lose tissue specific function; this precludes some types of studies, particularly exocytosis.[3,4] Although we set out to develop a parotid cell line with acinar characteristics, including the maintenance of secretory granules so that we could study exocytosis, the cell line that we most fully characterized appears to be of ductal origin. To some degree it may not be possible that salivary gland cell lines mimic fully their parental origin, but this does not preclude the usefulness of such lines to continue studies relating to the salivary glands. Immortalized salivary cell lines provide a new and useful reagent for continued studies of salivary gland function.

In studies outlined in this paper, we describe the production of a salivary cell line and its characterization. In particular, we demonstrate that the immortalized parotid cells: (a) have multiple receptors found on parental cells and respond to receptor agonists with an elevation of $[Ca^{2+}]i$; (b) form tight junctions, which allows the measurement of short-circuit currents, an indication of net transcellular fluid and electrolyte transport across the sheet epithelium; and (c) respond to receptor agonists with the activation of muliple signaling proteins, including PKC and proteins involved in the mitogen-activated protein (MAP) kinase cascade.

More specific information regarding the characterization of this cell line will be published in a future manuscript. The information presented below outlines some of the approaches that we have taken to develop this line, to characterize its origin, and to use it to advance our understanding of signal transduction mechanisms and ion transport properties of salivary gland epithelial cells.

PRODUCTION OF IMMORTALIZED PAROTID CELL LINES

A suspension of rat parotid cells was made by treating freshly dissected parotid gland with trypsin and collagenase, as previously described.[5] This renders a collection of single cells and small groups of cells that are primarily acinar in nature, but that contain some ductal cells as well. The parotid cells were cocultured with lethally irradiated virus-producing NIH3T3 cells for 4–7 days (FIG. 1). Cells are grown in a Dulbecco modified Eagle medium (DMEM)/Ham's F12 (3:1, v/v) mixture, supplemented with the following: adenine, 1.8×10^{-4} M; insulin, 5 µg/mL; transferrin, 5 µg/mL; triiodothyronine, 2×10^{-9} M; hydrocortisone, 1.1×10^{-6} M; cholera toxin, 1×10^{-10} M; epidermal growth factor, 1.64×10^{-6} M; and 10% fetal calf serum (to maintain the NIH3T3 cells). After transformation, cholera toxin was replaced with epinephrine (5.5×10^{-6} M). We have successfully immortalized other epithelial cell lines by the transduction of SV40 large T antigen into cells using retroviruses,[6-8] and others have also used SV40 to immortalize different types of salivary cells.[9,10] The retroviral construct (FIG. 2) used in the present studies contains both SV40 large T antigen and a selectable marker for G418 (a neomycin analogue) resistance. The virus-infected parotid cells were cocultured with G418-resistant lethally irradiated NIH3T3 cells. Those parotid cells not expressing the viral construct were eliminated by G418 drug selection. Parotid cells that survived selection with G418 were passaged multiple times by coculture with lethally irradiated NIH3T3 cells. In other cells lines that we produced,[7] the coculture of epithelial cells and NIH3T3 cells was important in the maintenance of differentiated epithelial cell function, including tight junction formation and the ability to respond to appropriate agonists. The parotid cells had a typical epithelial cobblestone appearance and grew in

1. Cell isolation

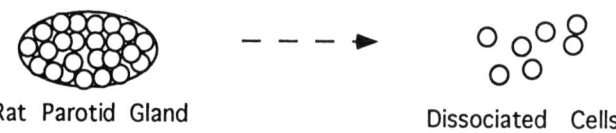

2. Plate with lethally irradiated retrovirus producer cells for 4-7 days

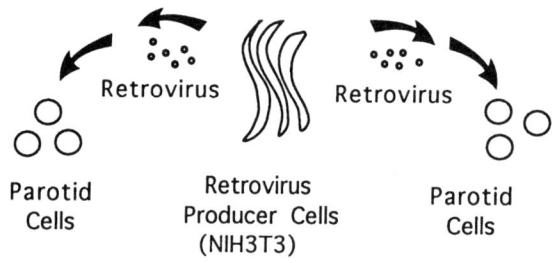

3. Co-culture of cells with lethally irradiated NIH3T3 cells

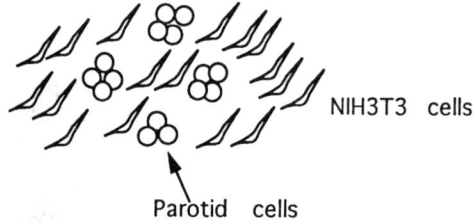

4. G418 antibiotic selection (10-12 days)

5. Characterization of G418-resistant cells
   Continued co-culture on lethally irradiated NIH3T3 cells

FIGURE 1. General immortalization protocol for development of rat parotid cell line. Other epithelial cell lines also have been immortalized using this protocol.

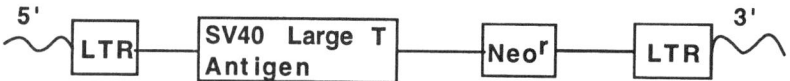

FIGURE 2. Oncogene construct used to immortalize parotid cells. LTR, long terminal repeat; Neo^r, 3'-phosphotransferase gene, which confers neomycin resistance.

colonies between the NIH3T3 cells (FIG. 3). Eventually, the epithelial cells became confluent, at which time they were split into new dishes containing lethally irradiated NIH3T3 cells. For all studies reported here, parotid cells were passaged once without coculture to derive a pure epithelial cell population.

CHARACTERIZATION OF AN IMMORTALIZED CELL LINE: RPG1/SV40 CELL

Immunocytochemical studies were performed to distinguish epithelial and nonepithelial cell types, and to determine the nature of the epithelial cells. Antibodies to muscle-specific proteins (alpha-actin, myosin) were used to screen for myoepithelial cells; a pan-cytokeratin antibody was used to identify epithelial cells; and antibodies to the various cytokeratins were used to screen for cells of epithelial origin, as well as to discern between cells of acinar and ductal origin. These antibodies were used to examine immortalized cells and also were used on fixed tissue sections of dissected rat parotid glands, which served as a reference to correlate staining with morphological cell type.

Resulting cell lines were screened for their responses to agonists of receptors known

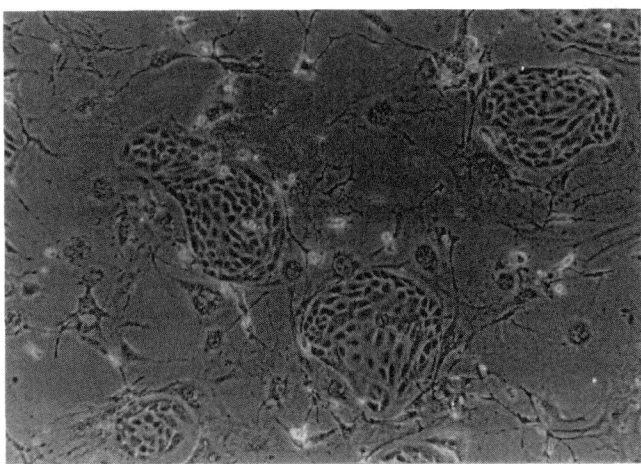

FIGURE 3. Low-power phase contrast micrograph of parotid cell colonies. The parotid cells maintain a cobblestone-like appearance, which is typical of epithlial cells in culture. Some of the cocultured NIH3T3 cells, which are elongated cells, can be seen between the colonies. Eventually the parotid cells will become fully confluent on the dish.

to be present on parotid cells. Typically, alterations in [Ca^{2+}]i (Fura-2 fluorescence) were measured to determine if particular [Ca^{2+}]i-mobilizing receptors were present. One cell line, which we called RPG1/SV40 (rat parotid gland 1/SV40 transformant), responded to several agonists (see below). It stained positively with a pan-cytokeratin antibody and thus was identified as a cell of epithelial origin. It also stained positively with several cytokeratins that were unique to ductal cells and that did not stain acinar cells in fixed tissue sections of the rat parotid gland. We chose this cell line to characterize more fully and to use in various studies outlined below.

RGP1/SV40 CELLS HAVE PLC-COUPLED MUSCARINIC RECEPTORS AND P_2 PURINOCEPTORS

Parotid cells have muscarinic and P_2 purinergic receptors (purinoceptors) that are linked through GTP-dependent proteins to phospholipase C. Carbachol and ATP, the respective agonists to these receptors, produced a rapid increase in the [Ca^{2+}]i of RPG1/SV40 cells. The response of the cells to ATP was mimicked by UTP, suggesting that these effects were mediated by a P_{2Y2} (formerly designated P_{2U}) purinoceptor, which recognizes both nucleotides.[11-13] By various criteria, including the maintenance of epithelial appearance and the ability to respond to these agonists with an increase in [Ca^{2+}]i, the cells maintained their phenotype for multiple passages.

RPG1/SV40 CELLS FORM TIGHT JUNCTIONS AND RESPOND TO AGONISTS WITH AN INCREASE IN SHORT-CIRCUIT CURRENT

RPG1/SV40 cells formed tight juctions between cells and grew as a sheet epithelium. The electrical resistance across a monolayer of RPG1/SV40 cells increased as a function of time in culture. Typically, the transepithelial resistance increased to ~500 Ohm cm^2. In these experiments, RPG1/SV40 cells from a confluent dish (no NIH3T3 cells remaining) were plated onto Millipore Millicell-HA inserts (12 mm diameter) that were coated with collagen. This allowed the short-circuit current (I_{SC}) across the epithelium to be measured. Carbachol and ATP produced large increases in the I_{SC}, which changed in parallel fashion to the alterations in [Ca^{2+}]i produced by these agents. Presumably, under these conditions the I_{SC} is a reflection of the net Cl^- secretory current across the RPG1/SV40 epithelium, and the increase in I_{SC} is due to the opening of Ca^{2+}-sensitive Cl^- channels. These studies suggest that net fluid and electrolyte secretion in RPG1/SV40 cells can be regulated by changes in [Ca^{2+}]i, as has been demonstrated in other salivary and nonsalivary epithelial cells.

PKCδ AND MAP KINASE ARE DOWNSTREAM EFFECTORS OF P_{2Y2} RECEPTORS IN RPG1/SV40 CELLS

We examined several other signaling proteins in this cell line. We found that PKCδ, a Ca^{2+}-insensitive PKC family member that is subgrouped as a "novel PKC" (nPKC), became phosphorylated on tyrosine residues in cells exposed to ATP or UTP for as brief as 10–15 seconds. PKCδ was also phosphorylated on tyrosine in rat parotid acinar cells exposed to carbachol or substance P.[14] Inasmuch as phorbol esters (which bind to the DAG binding site of PKCδ) could promote the same response in both parotid acinar cells and RPG1/SV40 cells, it appears that the production of DAG initiates the recruitment of PKCδ to the plasma membrane, where it becomes phosphorylated by an

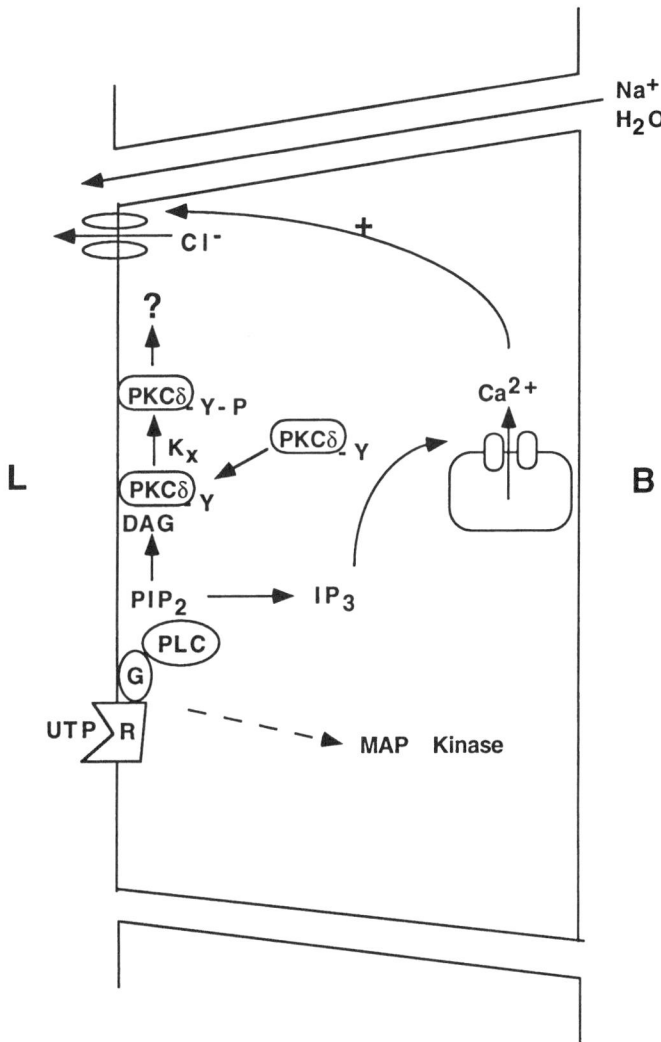

FIGURE 4. Summary of various effector molecules activated by UTP acting on RPG1/SV40 cells. UTP binds to its receptor (R), which is linked to phospholipase C (PLC) by a GTP-binding protein (G). PLC promotes the hydrolysis of phosphatidylinositol 4,5-bisphosphate (PIP_2) to inositol-1,4,5-trisphosphate (IP_3) and diacylglycerol (DAG). IP_3 promotes the elevation of $[Ca^{2+}]i$, including the release of Ca^{2+} from intracellular stores. $[Ca^{2+}]i$ elevation promotes an increase in the short-circuit current, a measurement of net transepithelial fluid and electrolyte secretion, presumably through the opening of Ca^{2+}-sensitive Cl^- channels. UTP also promotes the phosphorylation (-P) of PKCδ on tyrosine (Y) residues, due in part to the increased production of DAG at the membrane. The phosphorylation involves the action of an unknown kinase (K_x), which phosphorylates PKCδ that is recruited from the cytosol to the membrane. UTP also increases MAP kinase activity. L = luminal space; B = basolateral space.

as yet unknown kinase. PKCδ may be an important signaling molecule involved in the activation of fluid secretion or other parotid functions.

A second signaling system that was activated by UTP was MAP kinase. The MAP kinase family of proteins includes Erk (extracellular signal-regulated) kinases, which play a critical role in transducing signals from growth factor receptors and G protein–linked receptors to the nucleus.[15] After receptor activation, the Erk kinase signaling pathway involves a cascade of signaling proteins that include various serine/threonine kinases, which culminate with the activation of Erk kinases, which can translocate to the nucleus and affect differentiation, proliferation, or other cellular processes. Thus, UTP activates multiple signaling proteins and phosphorylation events upstream of MAP kinase, and probably downstream as well.

SUMMARY

We have developed and used a new parotid cell line, RPG1/SV40 cells, from rat parotid glands. By various criteria, the cells are parotid ductal epithelial cells. The cells are grown and maintained under coculture conditions with lethally irradiated NIH3T3 cells, and they maintain their phenotype for more than 20 passages. Previous experience suggests that coculture of immortalized epithelial cells helps to maintain their differentiated phenotype. The cells responded to agonists of muscarinic receptors and/or P_2 purinoceptors with increases in $[Ca^{2+}]i$, I_{sc}, PKCδ tyrosine phosphorylation, and MAP kinase activation. These responses are summarized in FIGURE 4. Thus, these cells are useful for a variety of signal transduction studies related to salivary gland research.

REFERENCES

1. TURNER, R. J. 1993. Ion transport related to fluid secretion in salivary glands. *In* The Biology of the Salivary Glands. edited by K. Dobrosielski-Vergona, Ed.: 105–127. CRC Press. Boca Raton, FL.
2. BAUM, B.J., I.S. AMBUDKAR & V.J. HORN. 1993. Neurotransmitter control of calcium mobilization. *In* Biology of the Salivary Glands. K. Dobrosielksi-Vergona, Ed.: 153–179. CRC Press. Boca Raton, FL.
3. KISER, C.S., F. RAHEMTULLA & B. MANSSON-RAHEMTULLA. 1990. Monolayer culture of rat parotid acinar cells without basement membrane stratess. In Vitro Cell. & Dev. Biol. **26:** 878–888.
4. OLIVER, C. 1980. Isolation and maintenance of differentiated exocrine gland acinar cells *in vitro*. In Vitro (Rockville) **16:** 297–305.
5. SOLTOFF, S. P., M.K. MCMILLIAN, L.C. CANTLEY, E.J. CRAGOE, JR. & B.R. TALAMO. 1989. Effects of muscarinic, alpha-adrenergic, and substance P agonists and ionomycin on ion transport mechanisms in the rat parotid acinar cell. The dependence of ion transport on intracellular calcium. J. Gen. Physiol. **93:** 285–319.
6. GRUBMAN, S. A., R.D. PERRONE, D.W. LEE, S.L. MURRAY, L.C. ROGERS, L.I. WOLKOFF, A.E. MULBERG, V. CHERINGTON & D.M. JEFFERSON. 1994. Regulation of intracellular pH by immortalized human intrahepatic biliary epithelial cell lines. Am. J. Physiol. **266:** G1060–G1070.
7. JEFFERSON, D.M., J.D. VALENTICH, F.C. MARINI, S.A. GRUBMAN, M.C. IANNUZZI, H.L. DORKIN, M. LI, K.W. KLINGER & M.J. WELSH. 1990. Expression of normal and cystic fibrosis phenotypes by continuous airway epithelial cell lines. Am. J. Physiol. **259:** L496–L505.
8. PERRONE, R.D., C. JOHNS, S.A. GRUBMAN, E. MOY, D.W. LEE, J. ALROY, G.R. SANT & D.M. JEFFERSON. 1996. Immortalized human bladder cell line exhibits amiloride-sensitive sodium absorption. Am. J. Physiol. **270:** F148–F153.
9. AZUMA, M., T. TAMATANI, Y. KASAI & M. SATO. 1993. Immortalization of normal human

salivary gland cells with duct-, myoepithelial, acinar-, or squamous phenotype by transfection with SV40 Ori⁻ mutant deoxyribonucleic acid. Lab. Invest. **69:** 24–42.
10. QUISSELL, D., K.A. BARZEN, D.C. GRUENERT, R.S. REDMAN, J.M. CAMDEN & J.T. TURNER. 1997. Development and characterization of SV40 immortalized rat submandibular acinar cells. In Vitro Cell. Dev. Biol. **33:** 164–173.
11. ABBRACCHIO, M. P. & G BURNSTOCK. 1994. Purinoceptors: are there families of P2X and P2Y receptors? Pharmacol. & Ther. **64:** 445–475.
12. LUSTIG, K.D., A.K. SHIAU, A.J. BRAKE & D. JULIUS. 1993. Expression cloning of an ATP receptor from mouse neuroblastoma cells. Proc. Natl. Acad. Sci. USA **90:** 5113–5117.
13. WOLKOFF, L.I., R.D. PERRONE, S.A. GRUBMAN, D.W. LEE, S.P. SOLTOFF, L.C. ROGERS, M. BEINBORN, S.L. FANG, S.H. CHENG & D.M. JEFFERSON. 1995. Purinoceptor P_{2U} identification and function in human intrahepatic biliary epithelial cell lines. Cell Calcium **17:** 375–383.
14. SOLTOFF, S. P. & A. TOKER. 1995. Carbachol, substance P, and phorbol ester promote the tyrosine phosphorylation of protein kinase Cδ in salivary gland epithelial cells. J. Biol. Chem. **270:** 13490–13495.
15. MALARKEY, K., C.M. BELHAM, A. PAUL, A. GRAHAM, A. MCLEES, P.H. SCOTT & R. PLEVIN. 1995. The regulation of tyrosine kinase signalling pathways by growth factor and G-protein-coupled receptors. Biochem. J. **309:** 361–375.

Transcriptional Regulation of Salivary Proline-rich Protein Gene Expression[a]

DAVID K. ANN[b] AND H. HELEN LIN

Department of Molecular Pharmacology and Toxicology, University of Southern California, Los Angeles, California 90033, USA

ABSTRACT: Mechanisms governing gene expression and regulation in eukaryotes are remarkably complex. The results from *in vivo* transgenic and *in vitro* transfection studies designed to identify *cis*-element(s) and *trans*-factor(s) associated with the salivary proline-rich proteins (PRPs) gene expression are utilized as a paradigm to discuss the regulation of salivary-specific gene expression. Particular attention is given to the molecular mechanism(s) underlying the salivary PRP *R15* gene regulation. In rodents, the PRPs are selectively expressed in the acinar cells of salivary glands, and are inducible by the β-agonist isoproterenol as well as by dietary tannins. The results from a series of experiments using chimeric reporter constructs containing different lengths of the *R15* distal enhancer region, their mutations, and various expressing constructs are analyzed and discussed. These data suggest that the inducible nuclear orphan receptor NGFI-B may participate in the regulation of salivary acinar cell-specific and inducible expression of the rat *R15* gene via three distinct distal NGFI-B sites. Taken together, a model for the induction of *R15* gene expression by isoproterenol is proposed. However, the exact molecular basis of this NGFI-B-mediated transactivation of cAMP-regulated *R15* expression remains to be established.

INTRODUCTION

It is becoming apparent that there is a significant degree of gene regulation at the levels of alternative splicing, polyadenylation, and mRNA stability. This review is mainly limited to a discussion of the modulation of initiation of transcription via binding of proteins (*trans*-factors) to DNA sequences (*cis*-elements) flanking the coding sequences of genes. Two basic models have been proposed to explain the effects that *trans*-factors have on transcription rates when bound to their cognate *cis*-elements.[1,2] The first model involves the alteration of DNA topology by assembling a three-dimensional multimeric complex. The roles of several proteins that appear to be involved in rearranging chromatin structure are explained by this model.[2] The second model involves protein–protein interactions between the bound *trans*-factors and members of the general transcriptional machinery.[1] These two models are not mutually exclusive, and both rely on the ability of *trans*-factor(s) to recognize a specific DNA sequence(s) in order to impart specificity to the response.

Multiple pathways that mediate salivary gene regulation and proliferation/differentiation have been proposed. One of the classical and best characterized pathways is the one mediated by the β-adrenergic receptor agonist, isoproterenol (Ipr). Chronic Ipr injections induce adaptive growth of both parotid and submandibular glands. This growth is the result of both cell enlargement and a moderate proliferative response of

---

[a] This work is supported in part by USPHS Grant RO1-DE10742 (to D.K.A.).
[b] Address for correspondence: David K. Ann, Department of Molecular Pharmacology and Toxicology, PSC-210B, 1985 Zonal Avenue, University of Southern California-HSC, Los Angeles, California 90033. Phone, 213/342-3146; fax, 213-342-1681; e-mail, ann@hsc.usc.edu

terminally differentiated acinar cells.[3-5] Characteristically, this increase in the size of salivary glands is associated with qualitative and quantitative changes in salivary-specific gene expression, including upregulation of the major secretory proteins, proline-rich proteins (PRPs), and downregulation of amylase[6] and parotid secretory protein (PSP).[7]

This review will mainly focus on the regulation of salivary-specific genes, in particular PRP R15 gene expression. We will present information on the identification and characterization of *cis*-element(s) in the distal enhancer region, which mediates the salivary cAMP-inducibility on *R15* gene. Additional evidence describing a novel parotid-specific cAMP-responsive element(s) and its putative trans-factor(s), NGFI-B, will also be discussed. Finally, we will briefly speculate on the role(s) of signal transduction pathway(s) and other Ipr-mediated mechanism(s) in regulating salivary PRP expression.

SALIVARY GLAND–SPECIFIC PROLINE-RICH PROTEIN GENES

The salivary PRPs are encoded by a multigene family, which in turn belongs to a superfamily including glutamine/glutamic acid-rich protein (GRPs).[8-10] The biochemistry, genetics, and molecular cloning of various PRP cDNAs and genes have been reviewed extensively (for details, see Refs. 11–14). In rodents, the salivary PRPs are exclusively synthesized and secreted by the acinar cells, and their expression is dramatically induced by the β-adrenergic stimulation or by ingesting dietary tannins.[6,15,16] The response to dietary tannins suggests that one of the functions of PRPs is to protect organisms from the toxic effects of tannins, common in the human diet.[16]

The expression of PRP in rodent parotid glands is developmentally regulated in parallel with the postnatal differentiation of salivary acinar cells.[17] Initially, PRP transcripts are barely detected in parotid glands of the postnatal day-14 rat by *in situ* hybridization and only in a few well-differentiated acinar cells.[18] Then there is a burst of PRP transcription which coincides with the appearance of high density of functional β-adrenergic receptor starting at postnatal day 21. But toward the end of weanling period, only low levels of PRP expression are detected in parotid acinar cells.[18] After postnatal day 28, the rodent PRP protein and mRNA levels drastically increase as a consequence of such experimental conditions as chronic daily Ipr injection and tannin-feeding that raise the intracellular cAMP levels, suggesting that the tissue-specific induction of PRP expression is regulated at the level of transcription.[6,15,19-22] These PRP genes, however, take longer to respond to Ipr treatment than do those primary response genes such as Fos and Jun and appear to be regulated through a mechanism different from that of the primary response or the immediate-early response.

MOLECULAR MECHANISM GOVERNING SALIVARY-SPECIFIC GENE EXPRESSION AND REGULATION

Chronic daily administration of Ipr leads to salivary gland hyperplasia and hypertrophy and also reprograms salivary-specific gene expression. These changes are in part mediated by the rise of intracellular cAMP levels via β-receptor activation. Classically, transcriptional activation in response to increased intracellular cAMP levels has been found to be regulated by the cAMP response element (CRE), which binds *trans*-factors such as the CRE-binding protein (CREB)/activating transcription factors (ATF) family. Sequence analyses of PRP genomic clones and *in vitro* transient transfection assays indicate the presence of <u>s</u>alivary-specific <u>c</u>AMP-<u>r</u>esponsive <u>e</u>lements

(SCREs) in the proximal 5′-flanking region of the PRP genes.[23–26] In addition, nuclear helix-loop-helix proteins, SCBPs, have been demonstrated to bind to the 5′-border of the SCRE and to activate reporter gene expression in the cotransfection assays.[27]

Recently, we have taken a transgenic approach to locate the regulatory regions that are essential for tissue-specific and inducible expression of the rat PRP gene, *R15*, *in vivo*. The expression profiles of 18 independent transgenic lines harboring fusion constructs containing 10-, 6-, or 1.7-kb contiguous *R15* 5′-flanking region, respectively, and the CAT reporter gene were analyzed.[28] Our data indicate that (i) the 6-kb *R15* 5′-flanking region is sufficient to reproduce the correct spatiotemporal transgene regulation *in vivo*; (ii) there are no noticeable differences among the expression profiles of independently established transgenic lines that harbor 10-kb and 6-kb of *R15* 5′-flanking region; and (iii) the *R15* 5′-DNA sequences up to −1.7 kb relative to transcription start site, which contain the previously identified *cis*-elements in the proximal promoter including the SCRE, fail to confer Ipr/tannins-inducibility to transgene expression in the salivary glands.[28]

Although several *trans*-factors are shown to be important for regulating the PRP proximal promoter activity,[27, 29] the results from transgenic mice studies suggest that the distal regulatory elements located between −6 and −1.7 kb of the *R15* 5′-flanking region are essential to recapitulate the correct spatial and inducible *R15* expression pattern *in vivo*. Thus, we have designated this 4.3-kb (−6 to −1.7) fragment as the *R15* *s*alivary-specific and *I*pr/*t*annins-dependent *r*egulatory region (SITR).[28] Recently, an upstream regulatory region located between −2.4 and −1.7 kb of the *R15* 5′-flanking region was further demonstrated to be indispensable for the parotid-specific and inducible reporter gene expression *in vivo* by transgenic approach.[30] Additionally, we have reported that the 1.7-kb of *R15* 5′-flanking region is able to direct acinar cell type-specific expression.[28]

INVOLVEMENT OF NUCLEAR ORPHAN RECEPTOR NGFI-B IN TRANSCRIPTIONAL ACTIVATION OF THE *R15* GENE BY cAMP

In an effort to define the regulatory network that coordinately controls tissue-specific and inducible gene expression, studies on the rat PRP *R15* gene expression are used as examples. The *R15* gene appears to be a remodeling gene, as it has two Ipr-inducible hypersensitive sites at approximately −9400 and −1900 nt, respectively.[28] With heterologous promoter constructs and transient transfection in parotid cells, we further delineated the minimal control region of the abovementioned *R15* SITR as extending from −1995 to −1812 nt relative to the transcription start site.[30] This SITR minimal control region also coincides with one of the previously identified Ipr-dependent hypersensitive sites.[28] However, sequencing analysis indicates that there is no consensus CRE site in this 184-bp (−1995 to −1812 nt) distal regulatory element. Instead, several hexameric elements that are either identical or homologous to an estrogen or retinoic acid receptor half site, AGGTCA (reviewed in Refs. 31 and 32), are located within this element.

Members of the nuclear orphan receptor superfamily, including NGFI-B, NURR1, and SF-1, are demonstrated to bind to their respective response element, which is homologous to the abovementioned AGGTCA half site, as monomers, and to activate specific gene expression.[31, 32] Recent publications show that NGFI-B and the related orphan nuclear receptor NURR1 can heterodimerize with the 9-*cis*-retinoic acid receptor RXR.[33,34] This heterodimerization allows the NGFI-B to activate gene transcription in a ligand-dependent manner via retinoic acid response elements (RARE), which are composed of direct repeats separated by 5 nucleotides (DR+5). The heterodimerization between NGFI-B and RXR is interesting because one of the putative NGFI-B binding sites in the *R15* distal enhancer shares similarity with the DR+5 RARE.[30] However, our preliminary data suggest that 9-*cis* retinoic acid has no effect on the regulation of endogenous PRP expression or on transfected reporter construct activity in salivary cells.

To address the functional role(s) of the AGGTCA hexamer sequences in regulating salivary PRP expression, we performed co-transfection experiments and mutagenesis studies. The results from these analyses suggest that NGFI-B or a closely related factor, NURR1, is involved as a major *trans*-regulator in the tissue-specific induction of PRP expression brought about by chronic Ipr-injection or tannin-feeding through cAMP as a second messenger.[30] This conclusion is based on several observations: (i) a pCMV-NGFI-B expression construct stimulates the activity of a TK promoter linked to the 184-bp enhancer fragment; (ii) expression of a dominant negative mutant pCMV-NGFI-B(Δ25-195) construct decreases NGFI-B transactivation to almost background level, even when transfected at one-eighth the amount of the co-transfected wild-type pCMV-NGFI-B construct; and (iii) mutations on the three NGFI-B sites completely abolish the NGFI-B-mediated transcriptional activation.[30] In addition, we tested the transactivation activity of NGFI-B mutant that carries mutation on two serine residues at position 340 and 350 of NGFI-B, which reside within the DNA-binding domain. Our data showed that when the serine residues of NGFI-B are replaced by two glutamates, the transactivation activity on heterologous TK promoter via the 184-bp distal enhancer is reduced to less than 20% of wild-type activity in Pa-4 cells (Fig. 1). It has been demonstrated that the phosphorylation of serine 350 of NGFI-B decreases its binding activity and nuclear localization.[35] This serine→glutamate mutation in the construct we used was thought to mimic the negative charges on the serine molecules introduced by phosphorylation. Substitution of both serine340 and serine350 to alanines, presumably mimicking the unphosphorylated status, resulted in a modest change of NGFI-B transactivation activity (FIG. 1). An independent line of evidence suggest-

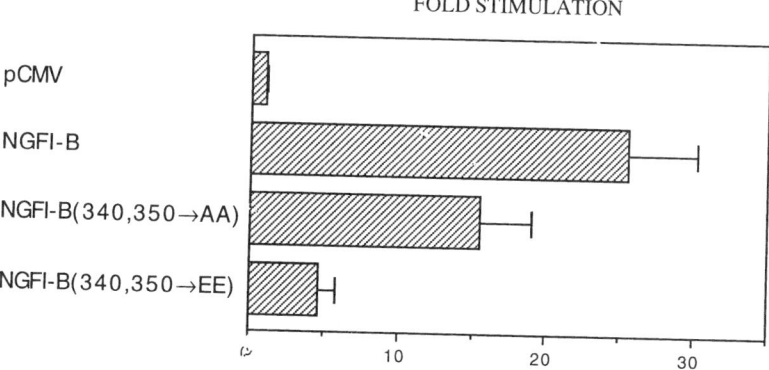

FIGURE 1. NGFI-B is involved in the transcriptional activation of R15 gene by cAMP. Transient transfection of Pa-4 cells with NGFI-B construct, its mutants and vector control pCMV together with reporter plasmid, R15-TK-CAT, is as described previously.[30] Twenty-four hours after the start of transfection, the cells were treated with 10 μM forskolin to activate protein kinase A pathway. Control plasmid pSV2-luciferase was co-transfected to normalize the transfection efficiency, and CAT assay was subsequently performed.[30] Fold stimulation of CAT activity is calculated by setting the CAT activity of the control pCMV vector at one.

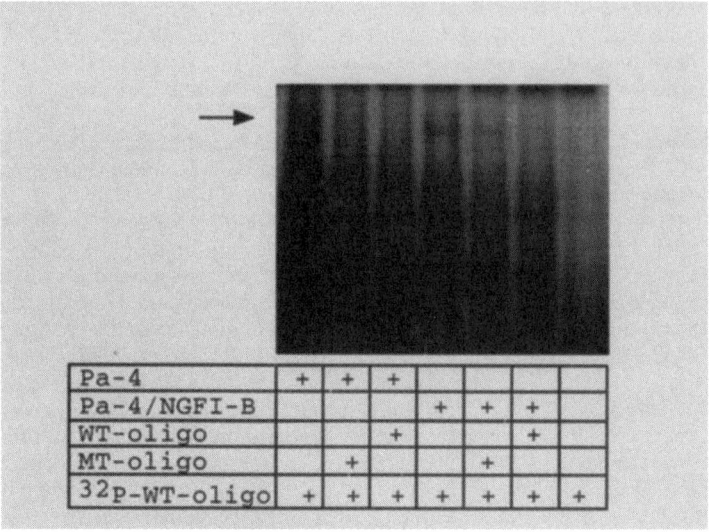

FIGURE 2. NGFI-B binds to distal enhancer of R15 gene. The gel mobility shift assay was performed as described previously.[23] Nuclear extracts were prepared from Pa-4 cells transfected with pCMV-NGFI-B (Pa-4/NGFI-B) and the parental Pa-4 cells. Labeled probe (10,000 cpm) was incubated with 2 μg of nuclear extract for 20 min at room temperature following a pre-incubation with either wild-type (WT-oligo) or mutant (MT-oligo) cold competitors at 100-fold excess. The *arrow* indicates the position of the retarded probe.

ing the transactivation activity of NGFI-B comes from a mobility shift analysis. As shown in FIGURE 2, NGFI-B binds to the labeled 184-bp enhancer fragment (lane 4) and this binding can be blocked by the addition of unlabelled wild-type oligo (lane 6), whereas oligo with mutated NGFI-B binding sequences showed minimal competition against the labeled probe (lane 5). However, this retarded band was not detected when nuclear extract of the parental Pa-4 cells was used. Taken together, we conclude that the transcriptional stimulation from the 184-bp (−1995 to −1812) distal fragment is highly dependent on the nuclear orphan receptor, NGFI-B.

CONCLUDING REMARKS

Modification, in particular phosphorylation/dephosphorylation, of transcription factors is a frequent event of transcriptional activation (reviewed in Ref. 36). Davis and Lau have shown that cAMP regulates NGFI-B activity in two ways.[37] First, cAMP can increase NGFI-B levels by transcriptional activation, and second, cAMP alters the phosphorylation state of NGFI-B to enhance its activity. In particular, cAMP increases the phosphorylation at the N-terminus and causes the hypophosphorylation of serine 350 of NGFI-B. On the basis of currently available information, a model for the induction of *R15* expression by Ipr is proposed. In this model, we speculate that the distal Ipr-dependent hypersensitive site is involved in establishing an open chromatin arrangement over the *R15* gene during the initial phase of Ipr treatment. This chromatin remodeling allows activated transcription factors, such as NGFI-B, and perhaps other *trans*-acting factors, such as CREB and SCBPs, to play a major role in the induction of *R15* expression.

Nevertheless, it is unclear how these modifications contribute to the salivary cell specificity of *R15* expression via the 184-bp minimal control region. Many of the necessary interactions are still poorly understood. While the data from *in vitro* experiments suggest that NGFI-B has an important influence on the expression of *R15* through the identified NGFI-B sites, it is possible that the induction of *R15* expression may also require the removal of negative repressor(s) through a modification process involving the protein kinase A pathway. Alternatively, the expression of *R15* could be controlled by tissue-specific protein–protein interactions involving adaptors/coactivators or heterodimerization. Thus, an additional factor or factors might be required for efficient salivary *R15* gene regulation by cAMP. Conceivably, the tissue-specific and inducible *R15* gene expression *in vivo* is regulated through complex mechanisms that depend on a multitude of *cis*-elements and *trans*-factors as well as modifications.

APOLOGIA

The authors apologize to all those whose work has not been directly referenced because of space constraints.

REFERENCES

1. TJIAN, R. & T. MANIATIS. 1994. Transcriptional activation: a complex puzzle with few easy pieces. Cell **77:** 5–8.
2. STARGELL, L.A. & K. STRUHL. 1996. Mechanisms of transcriptional activation in vivo: two steps forward. Trends Genet **12:** 311–315.
3. BROWN-GRANT, K. 1961. Enlargement of salivary gland in mice treated with isopropylnoadrenaline. Nature **191:** 1076–1078.
4. BARKA, T., R.M. GUBITS & H.M. VAN DER NOEN. 1986. Beta-adrenergic stimulation of c-fos gene expression in the mouse submandibular gland. Mol. Cell. Biol. **6:** 2984–2989.
5. SCHNEYER, C.A. 1962. Salivary gland changes after isoproterenol-introduced enlargement. Am. J. Physiol. **203:** 232–236.
6. ANN, D.K. *et al.* 1987. Induction of tissue-specific proline-rich protein multigene families in rat and mouse parotid glands by isoproterenol. Unusual strain differences of proline-rich protein mRNAs. J. Biol. Chem. **262:** 899–904.
7. POULSEN, K. *et al.* 1986. Coordination of murine parotid secretory protein and salivary amylase expression. EMBO J. **5:** 1891–1896.
8. HEINRICH, G. & J.F. HABENER. 1987. Genes encoding proteins with homologous contiguous repeat sequences are highly expressed in the serous cells of the rat submandibular gland. J. Biol. Chem. **262:** 5262–5270.
9. MIRELS, L. *et al.* 1987. Molecular characterization of glutamic acid/glutamine-rich secretory proteins from rat submandibular glands. J. Biol. Chem. **262:** 7289–7297.
10. ROSINSKI CHUPIN, I. *et al.* 1993. Localization of mRNAs of two androgen-dependent proteins, SMR1 and SMR2, by in situ hybridization reveals sexual differences in acinar cells of rat submandibular gland. J. Histochem. Cytochem. **41:** 1645–1649.
11. BENNICK, A. 1982. Salivary proline-rich proteins. Mol. Cell. Biochem. **45:** 83–99.
12. BENNICK, A. 1987. Structural and genetic aspects of proline-rich proteins. J. Dent. Res. **66:** 457–461.
13. CARLSON, D.M. 1993. Salivary proline-rich proteins: biochemistry, molecular biology, and regulation of expression. Crit. Rev. Oral Biol. Med. **4:** 495–502.
14. ANN, D.K. & H.H. LIN. 1993. Macaque salivary proline-rich protein: structure, evolution, and expression. Crit. Rev. Oral Biol. Med. **4:** 545–551.
15. MEHANSHO, H. *et al.* 1983. Modulation of proline-rich protein biosynthesis in rat parotid glands by sorghums with high tannin levels. Proc. Natl. Acad. Sci. USA **80:** 3948–3952.

16. MEHANSHO, H. et al. 1987. Induction of proline-rich proteins in hamster salivary glands by isoproterenol treatment and an unusual growth inhibition by tannins. J. Biol. Chem. **262:** 12344–12350.
17. REDMAN, R.S. 1987. Development of the salivary glands. *In* The Salivary System. L. M. Sreebny, Ed.: 1–20. CRC Press, Inc. Boca Raton, FL.
18. LAZOWSKI, K.W. et al. 1992. Reciprocal expression of c-jun, proline-rich protein and amylase genes during rat parotid salivary gland development. Differentiation **51:** 225–232.
19. MUENZER, J. et al. 1979. Purification of proline-rich proteins from parotid glands of isoproerenol-treated rats. J. Biol. Chem. **254:** 5623–5628.
20. WRIGHT, P.S. & D.M. CARLSON. 1988. Regulation of proline-rich protein and alpha-amylase genes in parotid-hepatoma hybrid cells. FASEB J. **2:** 3104–3107.
21. WRIGHT, P.S., C. LENNEY & D.M. CARLSON. 1990. Regulation of proline-rich protein gene expression by cyclic AMP in primary cultures of hamster parotid glands. J. Mol. Endocrinol. **4:** 81–87.
22. LAYFIELD, R. et al. 1992. cDNA clones for mouse parotid proline-rich proteins. mRNA regulation by isoprenaline and the nucleotide sequence of proline-rich protein cDNA MP5. Eur. J. Biochem. **204:** 591–597.
23. LIN, H.H. & D.K. ANN. 1992. Identification of cis- and trans-acting factors regulating the expression of rat salivary-specific RP4 gene. Gene Expr. **2:** 365–377.
24. LIN, H.H. & D.K. ANN. 1991. Molecular characterization of rat multigene family encoding proline-rich proteins. Genomics **10:** 102–113.
25. LIN, H.H., E.E. KOUSVELARI & D.K. ANN. 1991. Sequence and expression of the MnP4 gene encoding basic proline-rich protein in macaque salivary glands. Gene **104:** 219–226.
26. ANN, D.K. & D.M. CARLSON. 1985. The structure and organization of a proline-rich protein gene of a mouse multigene family. J. Biol. Chem. **260:** 15863–15872.
27. LIN, H.H., W.Y. LI & D.K. ANN. 1993. The helix-loop-helix proteins (salivary-specific cAMP response element-binding proteins) can modulate cAMP-inducible RP4 gene expression in salivary cells. J. Biol. Chem. **268:** 10214–10220.
28. TU, Z. J. et al. 1993. Isoproterenol/tannin-dependent R15 expression in transgenic mice is mediated by an upstream parotid control region. Gene Expr. **3:** 289–305.
29. ROBERTS, S.G., R. LAYFIELD & C.J. MCDONALD. 1991. The mouse proline-rich protein MP6 promoter binds isoprenaline-inducible parotid nuclear proteins via a highly conserved NFκB/rel-like site. Nucleic Acids Res. **19:** 5205–5211.
30. LIN, H.H., Z.J. TU & D.K. ANN. 1996. Involvement of nuclear orphan receptor NGFI-B in transcriptional activation of salivary-specific R15 gene by cAMP. J. Biol. Chem. **271:** 27637–27644.
31. KASTNER, P., M. MARK & P. CHAMBON. 1995. Nonsteroid nuclear receptors: what are genetic studies telling us about their role in real life? Cell **83:** 859–869.
32. MANGELSDORF, D.J. & R.M. EVANS. 1995. The RXR heterodimers and orphan receptors. Cell **83:** 841–850.
33. PERLMANN, T. & L. JANSSON. 1995. A novel pathway for vitamin A signaling mediated by RXR heterodimerization with NGFI-B and NURR1. Genes & Dev. **9:** 769–782.
34. FORMAN, B.M. et al. 1995. Unique response pathways are established by allosteric interactions among nuclear hormone receptors. Cell **81:** 541–550.
35. HIRATA, Y. et al. 1993. The phosphorylation and DNA binding of the DNA-binding domain of the orphan nuclear receptor NGFI-B. J. Biol. Chem. **268:** 24808–24812.
36. KARIN, M. 1990. The AP-1 complex and its role in transcriptional control by protein kinase C. Mol. Aspects Cell. Regul. **6:** 143–161.
37. DAVIS, I.J. & L.F. LAU. 1994. Endocrine and neurogenic regulation of the orphan nuclear receptors Nur77 and Nurr-1 in the adrenal glands. Mol. Cell Biol. **14:** 3469–3483.

Protein Secretion by Rat Parotid Acinar Cells

Pathways and Regulation

J. DAVID CASTLE[a]

Department of Cell Biology, University of Virginia Health Sciences Center, Charlottesville, Virginia 22908, USA

> ABSTRACT: Protein secretion from rat parotid acinar cells occurs in both the absence and presence of secretory agonists. Release takes place by four pathways that are distinguished by combined examination of their timing following biosynthetic labeling, their relative composition of salivary proteins, and their sensitivity to secretagogue stimulation. Following pulse-labeling with a radioactive amino acid, two unstimulated export pathways are detected—a constitutive-like pathway that is coupled to maturation of secretory granules and the later unstimulated exocytosis of secretory granules. In both cases, protein release is insensitive to secretory antagonists. Two regulated secretory pathways are also detected. The major regulated pathway comprises stimulated exocytosis of secretory granules and requires application of β-adrenergic agonists (≥ 1 μM). A newly discovered minor regulated pathway resembles the constitutive-like pathway in secretory composition but requires low-dose stimulation by either β-adrenergic or cholinergic agonists. The latter pathway may provide a significant component of basal secretion by the parotid gland during periods between meals.

Parotid glands are one of the three sets of major salivary glands and are notable for their contribution to the protein, and fluid and electrolyte composition of saliva. Within these glands, the primary secretory unit for all of these components is the acinar cell. Acinar cells maintain an extensive internal membrane system that functions in salivary protein export and a battery of plasma membrane-associated ion pumps and ion and water channels that function in transport of fluid and electrolytes. These two major secretory functions are differentially regulated by the neural and, to a lesser extent, hormonal stimuli that control salivary output. In the rat parotid gland, which is the focus of this report, individual acinar cells are innervated by both sympathetic and parasympathetic nerve terminals. The rate of protein secretion is controlled mainly by noradrenalin that is released from sympathetic terminals and acts through β-adrenergic receptors located on the basolateral surface of the acinar cell. Elevated cyclic AMP serves as an intracellular signal to couple β receptor stimulation to protein secretion. By contrast, the rates of fluid and electrolyte secretion are controlled by acetylcholine released from parasympathetic terminals and acting through muscarinic cholinergic receptors and to a lesser extent by noradrenalin acting through α-adrenergic receptors. Both of these signaling pathways regulate Ca^{2+} activity in the acinar cell cytoplasm, which in turn controls transepithelial ion flux and passive water flow (reviewed in ref. 1). The molecular mechanisms that constitute these signaling pathways are of great interest at present, and recent progress suggests that events in salivary acinar cells are analogous to those that have been more extensively studied in other secretory cell types.[2–5] The present report focuses on salivary protein secretion by parotid acinar cells. The main emphasis is on distinguishing multiple pathways that are used for protein se-

---

[a] Tel: (804) 924-1786; fax: (804) 982-3912; e-mail: jdc4r@virginia.edu

cretion and on examining how they each might contribute to salivary output both in the presence and absence of stimulation.

The parotid acinar cell is more or less pyramid shaped, and organelles making up its secretory pathway are highly polarized within the cytoplasm. The extensive endoplasmic reticulum (ER), where salivary proteins are initially sequestered during synthesis, occupies most of the cytoplasm surrounding the nucleus at the base of the pyramid. A prominent Golgi complex, where salivary proteins undergo posttranslational modification followed by packaging for export in the *trans*-Golgi network (TGN), is located in the center of the cell above the ER. Membrane-bounded secretory granules that are the products of the packaging operation accumulate in the cytoplasm between the Golgi complex and the apex of the pyramid. They serve as an intracellular store for salivary proteins prior to undergoing exocytosis at the apical cell surface. The functional specialization of acinar cells is so extensive that more than 80–90% of the total protein synthesized at any given time is destined to follow the secretory pathway from ER to Golgi and then into forming secretory granules. As a consequence of this situation, it is possible to monitor protein transport experimentally using biosynthetic labeling. Accordingly, brief (pulsed) labeling of acinar cell proteins with radioactive amino acid and tracking of the labeled protein during subsequent chase incubation by radioautography shows that passage from ER to Golgi to granule forming is mostly complete by 60 minutes.[6]

Analogous biosynthetic labeling is also very useful for monitoring the process of secretion by parotid acinar cells. Historically, this approach was used to demonstrate that most proteins being synthesized by rat parotid tissue/ acinar cells *in vitro* are ultimately released as salivary components,[7] that secretion is mainly regulated by β-adrenergic agonists,[8] and that older secretion granules undergo exocytosis before younger ones do in response to stimulation.[9] More recent studies from my laboratory have also used this approach to identify and characterize secretory pathways that operate in the absence of agonist stimulation[6,10] and to identify a new pathway that is stimulated selectively by low doses of agonists.[11]

FIGURE 1a depicts a typical profile of protein secretion that occurs when parotid tissue is pulse labeled with [^{35}S]methionine *in vitro* and then chase incubated in the absence of secretory stimulation. At regular time intervals during incubation, the medium is removed and replaced, and a fixed proportion of the medium at each time point is examined for its radioactive protein content. During the final time interval, isoproterenol (40 µM) is added to elicit massive granule exocytosis for comparison to the preceding unstimulated output. The profile shows that proteins are secreted in two kinetically distinct phases. The early phase first appears at about 30 minutes postpulse and peaks at about 80 to 90 minutes, substantially after newly synthesized proteins have reached immature granules.[6] Then it declines until it becomes obscured by the appearance of a second broader phase. The latter peaks more than 10 hours postpulse and then slowly declines thereafter; it has seldom been followed to completion before applying secretory stimulation in our experiments. SDS-PAGE and fluorography of the radiolabeled proteins released during each phase of unstimulated secretion and also following stimulation is illustrated in FIGURE 1b. Comparison of the profiles indicates that the same polypeptides are released in each case. However, whereas the relative composition of labeled polypeptides in the late phase is almost the same as that in stimulated secretion, the relative composition in the early phase differs significantly. We interpreted these findings to indicate that there are two pathways of unstimulated secretion that operate in parotid acinar cells.[6] The late phase was considered to correspond to unstimulated exocytosis of secretory granules, whereas the early phase was thought to resemble a constitutive secretory pathway. Notably, this early phase pathway differed from the usual constitutive secretory pathways that have been characterized in other cell types in at least three significant ways. First, it transported the same secretory proteins as

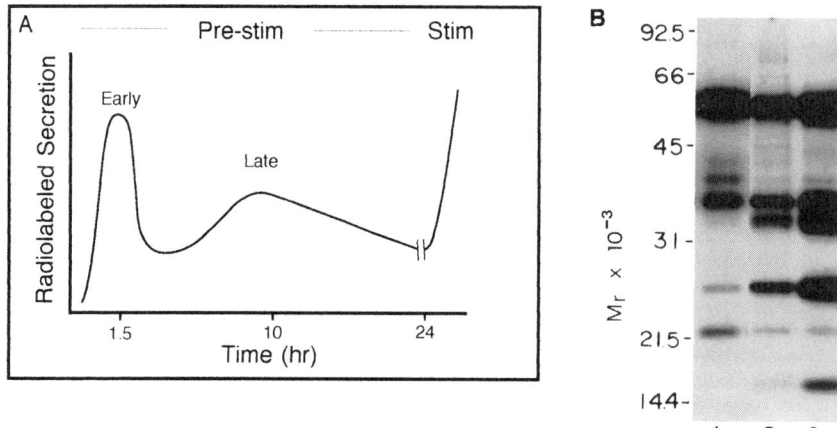

FIGURE 1. A: Output of biosynthetically labeled protein by parotid tissue during chase incubation following *in vitro* pulse labeling with [^{35}S]methionine. In the period before stimulation (< 24 h), radiolabeled proteins are released in two kinetically distinct phases labeled early and late. Both phases are unaffected by addition of antagonists propranolol, phentolamine, and atropine. During the final period of incubation, 40 μM isoproterenol is added and stimulates secretion of stored salivary proteins. **B:** Profiles of radiolabeled salivary proteins secreted during the early phase (1), late phase (2), and period of stimulation (3). Note that the same major proteins appear in all phases but in different relative amounts. The compositions in 2 and 3 resemble the content of stored granules, whereas that in 1 does not.

found in the regulated secretory pathway (secretion granules) rather than different proteins. Second, according to our radioautographic results,[6] it largely occurred after proteins had reached immature granules rather than before (as would occur by direct transport to the cell surface from the TGN). Third, once started, the pathway has a longer duration (half-time) than the duration of the usual constitutive secretory pathway (reviewed in ref. 12). For these reasons, early phase secretion in parotid acinar cells has been considered to occur by a constitutive-like pathway, a name given by Kuliawat and Arvan,[13] as a distinction from the constitutive pathway.

To account for the post-Golgi onset and distinct composition of early phase secretion, the constitutive-like pathway has been postulated to arise by vesicular budding from immature granules. Accordingly, vesicular content of the constitutive-like pathway is mainly thought to reflect "negative selection" during the parallel process of condensing secretory proteins within the maturing granule (FIG. 2a). That is, proteins that aggregate least efficiently within the condensing granule core are relatively enriched in constitutive-like secretion. Indirect support for this hypothesis is provided by experiments in which the membrane-permeant weak base, ammonium chloride, is used to perturb the condensation process.[10] Under these conditions, the magnitude of constitutive-like secretion increases and its composition changes to more nearly reflect the relative composition stored in granules (FIGS. 3 and 4 in ref. 10). Both effects are predicted by the coupling of constitutive-like secretion to granule maturation (FIG. 2b). Incidently, the altered secretory profile observed using ammonium chloride also implies that the protein composition within the constitutive-like pathway is condition dependent and argues against the possibility that it might derive from separate cells than those that make storage granules.

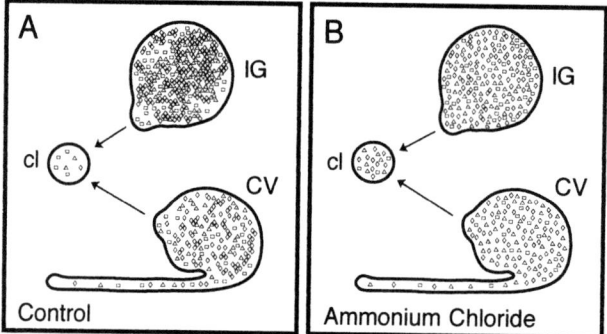

FIGURE 2. A: Cartoon depicting the coupled processes of condensation of stored proteins within maturing granules and generation of vesicles that serve as carriers of constitutive-like secretion. The closed triangle and diamond (▲, ♦) identify proteins that are condensed and stored efficiently in the granule core, whereas the closed square (■) represents proteins that are less efficiently condensed and stored and thus are enriched in constitutive-like secretion. **B:** Addition of the weak base, ammonium chloride, perturbs maturation; it decreases condensation and consequently increases the amount of secretion in the constitutive-like pathway and abrogates the distinct composition of proteins that follow this route. cl, constitutive-like pathway; IG, immature granules; CV=condensing vacuole.

Once the vesicular carriers that are thought to comprise the constitutive-like secretory pathway have budded from immature granules, their itinerary enroute to the cell surface is unclear. Although direct delivery to the surface may occur, the extended half-time that has been derived for the transport process[6,13,14] is compatible with less direct transit. Indeed, compelling evidence suggests that vesicles budding from immature secretory granules may be a major route of delivery of lysosomal hydrolase precursors to the endocytic/prelysosomal pathway in regulated secretory cells.[15] Thus part or all of the constitutive-like secretory pathway may involve such a detour.

The discovery that parotid acinar cells possess two different unstimulated secretory pathways in addition to stimulated granule exocytosis increases the number of known export pathways for the major salivary proteins to three. Recently, we have been examining the secretory output of rat parotid tissue in response to stimulation by low doses of secretory agonists that may relate to the low levels of secretory stimulation occurring during nonfeeding periods in animals. Surprisingly, we have identified what we believe to be a fourth secretory pathway that is activated selectively by low doses of agonists.[11] Discovery of this pathway was aided by using *in vitro* biosynthetic labeling. Evidently, this strategy facilitates detection of secretion of small amounts of radiolabeled

FIGURE 3. a and b: Secretion of parotid salivary proteins during successive 40-min intervals of chase incubation following a 5-min pulse labeling with Tran[^{35}S]label. Pilocarpine (0.1 μM) was added from 240–280 min in b, whereas isoproterenol (40 μM) was added from 400–4440 min in both a and b. Note the peak of constitutive-like secretion of labeled proteins at 80 min in both a and b. The relative radioactive composition of proteins secreted in response to pilocarpine in b is identical to that in constitutive-like secretion and differs from that secreted in response to isoproterenol in both a and b. **c:** Secretion of amylase enzyme activity during the successive intervals of chase incubation in a (closed circles) and b (open circles). Note that unstimulated output re-

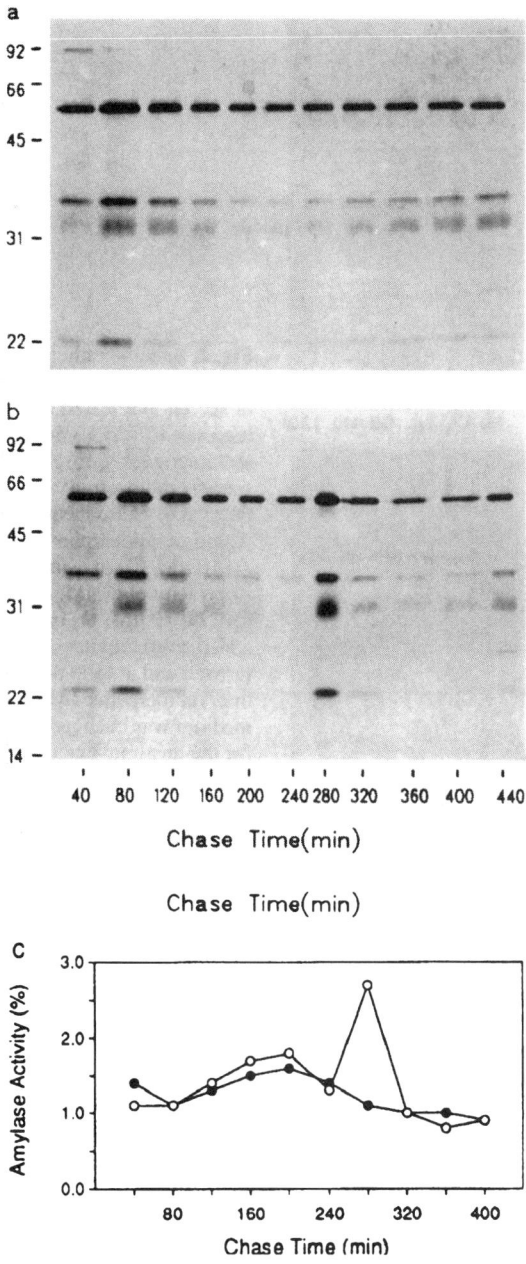

mains between 1.0–1.6% of total in the absence of stimulation and that pilocarpine increases output by ~1% of total during the 240–280 min interval in b. The enzyme activity released in response to isoproterenol (400–440 min) is not shown but is > 30% in each case. (J.D. Castle & A.M. Castle.[11] With the permission from the *Journal of Cell Science.*)

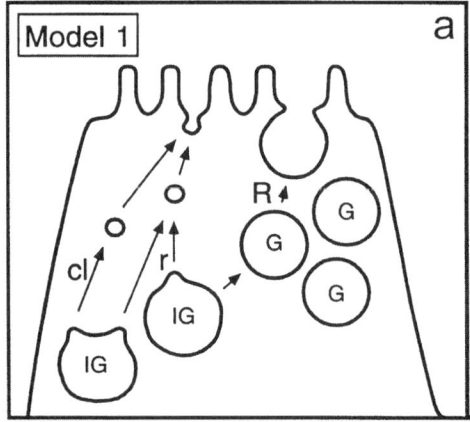
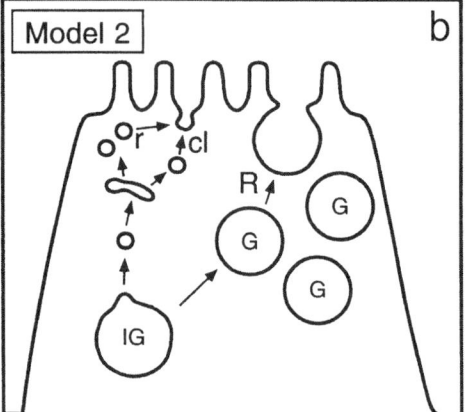
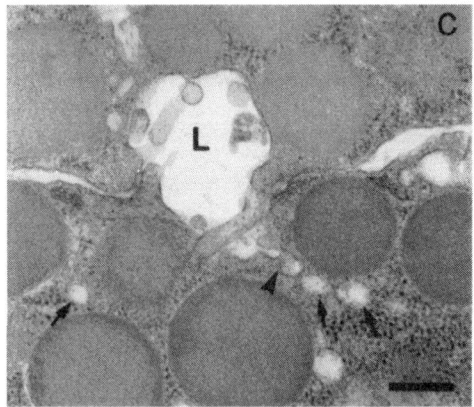

protein concomitant with the release of potentially larger amounts of unlabeled salivary protein (*e.g.,* by ongoing unstimulated exocytosis of secretory granules). An example of secretion by this newly regulated pathway is shown using SDS/PAGE and fluorography in FIGURE 3, a and b. In this illustration, secretion during each time interval of chase incubation has been assayed for amylase enzyme activity, and the same amount of enzyme has been loaded in each lane of the gel. Thus the intensity of the amylase band (58 K) directly reflects specific radioactivity. Enzyme activity secreted as a percent of total is also plotted in the bottom panel (FIG. 3c). Panels a and b of FIGURE 3 both show a peak of unstimulated release of labeled protein by the constitutive-like pathway between 40 and 120 minutes, while the rate of secretion of enzyme activity remains nearly constant. During the interval 240–280 minutes in FIGURE 3b, the tissue was treated with 0.1 µM pilocarpine. Although the agonist causes a small increase in amylase secretion (FIG. 3c), the specific radioactivity of protein secreted in this time interval is clearly elevated. Strikingly, the composition of radiolabeled proteins that are released in response to agonist is the same as released by the constitutive-like pathway and thus is unlike what is discharged by granule exocytosis (FIG. 1b). Because the output of secretion caused by low doses of secretory agonist is rather small, we refer to this new secretory pathway as the minor regulated pathway.

We have conducted a variety of experiments to establish that the minor regulated pathway has the following characteristics. (1) From the pattern observed in FIGURE 3, it is clear that the minor regulated pathway preferentially releases secretory proteins that are newly synthesized relative to the large quantity of unlabeled proteins that are already packaged in secretion granules at the time of stimulation. (2) The pathway is stimulated by low doses of isoproterenol (5–100 nM) that are below those required to elicit granule exocytosis. (3) The pathway is also stimulated by cholinergic agonists (pilocarpine (as in FIG. 5) and carbachol, 20 nM (not shown)) at doses that are well below those that induce cytoplasmic vacuolation.[8,16] (4) Densitometric measurements show that the radiochemical composition released in response to either isoproterenol or pilocarpine is identical to that found in constitutive-like secretion and distinct from that released when granule exocytosis is stimulated by 40 µM isoproterenol (FIG. 3 in ref. 11). (5) When the time intervals of stimulation are shortened, it can be seen that the response to agonist addition is quite rapid; with 0.1 µM of either isoproterenol or pilocarpine, the specific radioactivity of secreted amylase peaks in ≤ 10 minutes. At lower doses of agonist, the peak is reached more slowly (see FIG. 2 in ref. 11). (6) If agonist addition is continued in successive time intervals, it takes about 90 minutes for the specific radioactivity of amylase to decrease to the level observed in the control. What is

---

FIGURE 4. a, b: Two models of the minor regulated secretory pathway in rat parotid acinar cells. In model 1, the minor regulated pathway (r) and constitutive-like pathway (cl) both derive directly from immature granules (IG). R is the major regulated pathway corresponding to stimulated granule exocytosis. To account for stimulation of the minor regulated pathway at late chase times, r is shown to continue further along the granule maturation pathway and may even involve mature granules (G). The formation of the vesicular carriers for r is regulated by low doses of muscarinic and β-adrenergic agonists. In model 2, vesicular carriers originating from immature granules intersect an apical endosome where the cl and r pathways split; cl proceeds continually to the cell surface, whereas r requires agonist stimulation. Thus r is a storage population and is refilled from the apical endosome following discharge. **c:** Electron micrograph showing electron-lucent vesicles (arrows) in pilocarpine-treated tissue (5 min, 0.1 µM) that may represent the carriers of the minor regulated pathway. Note that the carriers are frequently in close aposition to secretion granules and that one appears to be in the act of fusing with the apical surface (arrowhead) bordering the lumen (L). Bar corresponds to 1 µm. Panels a and b are reprinted from Castle and Castle,[11] with permission of the *Journal of Cell Science.*

more, persistent stimulation can release as much as 10% of newly synthesized amylase when initiated just after the peak of constitutive-like secretion. Thus the pathway is likely to be activated in a substantial fraction of acinar cells. (7) When stimulation is applied either immediately following the peak of constitutive-like secretion or much later during chase incubation (up to 6 h tested so far), the increment in radioactive amylase secretion is the same (FIG. 4a in ref. 11). This finding suggests that the minor regulated pathway does not correspond to stimulation of the constitutive-like pathway but instead reflects stimulation from a storage pool of secretory products. (8) Although the minor regulated and constitutive-like pathways are distinct, they appear to draw on the same pool of secretory proteins, at least in part. Indeed, we have observed that during time intervals following those in which low-dose agonist stimulation was applied, the specific radioactivity of unstimulated secretion (presumably during the tail end of constitutive-like secretion) was decreased to about half the level observed in the control (FIGS. 1b and 4b in ref. 11).

Although our findings regarding the new minor regulated pathway so far are indirect, we have developed two possible models for its origin that are consistent with the characteristics above (FIG. 4 a and b). In model one, the minor regulated pathway is hypothesized to originate by agonist-dependent vesicular budding from granules. Thus it initially parallels the constitutive-like pathway in immature granules but also is suggested to be stimulable much later in the granule maturation process. In model two, the constitutive-like and minor regulated pathways are hypothesized to have a common origin by a single budding process from immature granules. However, the vesicles are directed to another intracellular compartment, possibly the apical endosome that has been characterized in epithelial cells.[17,18] At this site, the pathways divide, such that constitutive-like carriers proceed continually to the cell surface without regulation, while the minor regulated vesicles form a reserve that only proceeds to the cell surface for exocytosis when low doses of secretory agonists are applied.

To date we have not yet identified a marker for the minor regulated pathway. As well, further studies will be required to distinguish whether one of the two models (or even another) is more appropriate. Despite these limitations, we have tentatively identified a morphological correlate for the minor regulated pathway by electron microscopy. Electron micrographs of parotid tissue stimulated 5 min *in vitro* with 0.1 µM pilocarpine show small electron-luscent vesicles in close proximity to secretory granules in the apical cytoplasm, and there is suggestive evidence that these vesicles are capable of exocytosis at the apical surface (FIG. 4c).

The presence of two regulated secretory pathways in parotid acinar cells that are distinguished by their sensitivity to secretagogue stimulation is reminiscent of the situation in neurons where synaptic vesicles are selectively discharged by low frequency signaling and large dense core vesicles are released only at higher frequencies.[19] Indeed this may be a general feature of neuroendocrine and possibly other regulated secretory cells (reviewed in ref. 20). Notably, the parotid minor regulated pathway is distinct from these potential relatives, in that it secretes proteins rather than classical neurotransmitters. A number of interesting possibilities come to mind for the role of the minor regulated pathway in the parotid secretory process. First is the intriguing possibility that the minor regulated pathway represents a significant component of so-called basal salivary secretion. Between periods of food intake, low-level neural stimulation is presumed to maintain salivary output. Depending on the magnitude of this output, relative to that occurring by stimulus-independent exocytosis of granules, the minor regulated pathway may be a prominent component of basal secretion. If so, its potential dysfunction in relation to various dry mouth disorders would be of great interest. Second, maybe the minor regulated pathway, along with the constitutive-like pathway, secretes some unique salivary components. Because unique polypeptides are not apparent in the electrophoretic profiles for these pathways, such components would probably be rather scarce. Third, the minor regulated pathway may contribute in a previously unrealized way to fluid and electrolyte secretion or as a general primer that is needed for large-scale secretion. This pathway is distinguished from the the major regulated pathway by its broad-spectrum activation by cholinergic and adrenergic stimuli. Together with the relatively rapid kinetics that we have observed, these features suggest that the minor regulated pathway may provide an essential first response to stimulation. Finally and potentially related to the latter possibility, the minor regulated pathway may function in regulated recycling of cell-surface components in much the same way that vesicles in adipocytes and renal collecting tubules, respectively, relocate glucose transporters and water channels to the cell surface in response to insulin and vasopressin. Indeed, there is growing evidence that recycling to the apical cell surface from subplasmalemmal endosomes may be regulated in epithelial cells,[17,18,21] and this capability may have been put to a specific purpose in the acinar cell.

ACKNOWLEDGMENTS

The author is grateful to Drs. Anna Castle, Peter Arvan, and Mark von Zastrow for their many valuable contributions in developing this area of research and to Amy Huang for her help in preparing the illustrations.

REFERENCES

1. BAUM, B.J. 1987. Regulation of salivary secretion. *In* The Salivary System. L.M. Sreebny, Ed.: 123–134. CRC Press. Boca Raton, Fl.
2. FUJITA-YOSHIGAKI, J., Y. DOHKE, M. HARA-YOKOYAMA, Y. KAMATA, S. KOZAKI, S. FURUYAMA & H. SUGIYA. 1996. Vesicle-associated membrane protein 2 is essential for cAMP-regulated exocytosis in rat parotid acinar cells. J. Biol. Chem. **271:** 13130–13134.
3. GAISANO, H.Y. L. SHEU, J.K. FOSKETT & W.S. TRIMBLE. 1994. Tetanus toxin light chain cleaves a vesicle-associated membrane protein (VAMP) isoform 2 in rat pancreatic zymogen granules and inhibits enzyme secretion. J. Biol. Chem. **269:** 17062–17077.
4. GAISANO, H.Y., M. GHAI, P.N. MALKUS, L. SHEU, A. BOUQUILLON, M.K. BENNETT & W.S. TRIMBLE. 1996. Distinct cellular locations of the syntaxin family of proteins in rat pancreatic acinar cells. Mol. Biol. Cell **7:** 2019–2027.
5. GLENN, D.E. & R.D. BURGOYNE. 1996. Botulinum neurotoxin light chains inhibit both Ca2+-induced and GTP analogue-induced catecholamine release from permeabilized adrenal chromaffin cells. FEBS Lett. **386:** 137–140.
6. ZASTROW, M.V. & J.D. CASTLE. 1987. Protein sorting among two distinct export pathways occurs from the content of maturing exocrine storage granules. J. Cell Biol. **105:** 2675–2684.
7. WALLACH, D., N. KIRSCHNER & M. SCHRAMM. 1975. Non-parallel transport of membrane proteins and content proteins during assembly of the secretory granule in rat parotid gland. Biochim. Biophys. Acta **375:** 87–105.
8. BATZRI, S., Z. SELINGER & M. SCHRAMM. 1971. Potassium ion release and enzyme secretion: adrenergic regulation by a- and p-receptors. Science **174:** 1029–1031.
9. SHARONI, Y., S. EIMERI & M. SCHRAMM. 1976. Secretion of old versus new exportable protein in rat parotid slices. J. Cell Biol. **71:** 107–122.
10. ZASTROW, M.V., A.M. CASTLE & J.D. CASTLE. 1989. Ammonium chloride alters secretory protein sorting within the maturing exocrine storage compartment. J. Biol. Chem. **264:** 6566–6571.
11. CASTLE, J.D. & A.M. CASTLE. 1996. Two regulated secretory pathways for newly synthesized salivary proteins are distinguished by doses of secretagogues. J. Cell Sci. **109:** 2591–2599.
12. ARVAN, P. & D. CASTLE. 1992. Protein sorting and secretion granule formation in regulated secretory cells. Trends Cell Biol. **2:** 327–331.
13. KULIAWAT, R. & P. ARVAN. 1992. Protein targeting via the constitutive-like secretory path-

way in isolated pancreatic islets: passive sorting in the immature granule compartment. J. Cell Biol. **118:** 521–529.
14. ARVAN, P. & J.D. CASTLE. 1987. Phasic release of newly synthesized secretory proteins in the unstimulated rat exocrine pancreas. J. Cell Biol. **104:** 243–252.
15. KULIAWAT, R. & P. ARVAN. 1994. Distinct molecular mechanisms for protein sorting within immature secretory granules of pancreatic p-cells. J. Cell Biol. **126:** 77–86.
16. LESLIE, B.A. & J.W. PUTNEY. 1983. Ionic mechanisms in secretagogue-induced morphological changes in rat parotid gland. J. Cell Biol. **97:** 1119–1130.
17. BAROSO, M. & E.S. SZTUL. 1994. Basolateral to apical transcytosis in polarized cells is indirect and involves BFA and trimeric G protein sensitive passage through the apical endosome. J. Cell Biol. **124:** 83–100.
18. CARDONE, M.H., B.L. SMITH, W. SONG, D. MOCHLY-ROSEN & K.E. MOSTOV. 1994. Phorbol myristate acetate-mediated stimulation of transcytosis and apical recycling in MDCK cells. J. Cell Biol. **124:** 717–727.
19. LUNDBERG, J.M. & T. HOKFELT. 1983. Coexistence of peptides and classical neurotransmitters. Trends Neurosci. **6:** 325–333.
20. DECAMILLI, P. & F. NAVONE. 1987. Regulated secretory pathways of neurons and their relation to the regulated secretory pathway of endocrine cells. Ann. N.Y. Acad. Sci. **493:** 461–479.
21. BROWN, D. & I. SABOLIC. 1993. Endosomal pathways for water channel and proton pump recycling in kidney epithelial cells. J. Cell Sci. Suppl. **17:** 49–59.

Salivary Abnormalities in Prader-Willi Syndrome

P. SUZANNE HART[a]

Department of Pediatrics/Section on Medical Genetics, Bowman Gray School of Medicine, Medical Center Boulevard, Winston-Salem, North Carolina 27157, USA

ABSTRACT: Prader-Willi syndrome (PWS) is characterized by psychomotor and growth retardation, infantile hypotonia, characteristic facies, small hands and feet, dental abnormalities, and early onset of childhood hyperphagia with consequent obesity. PWS is associated with abnormalities of chromosome 15. Approximately 75% of patients have a deletion of 15q11q13 on the paternal homologue, whereas 20–25% have inherited both chromosome 15s from the mother and none from the father, a condition known as maternal uniparental disomy (UPD). Thus, it is a lack of paternal alleles in the 15q11q13 region that results in PWS. Thick, sticky saliva is a consistent finding in patients with PWS. We have characterized salivary flow and composition in individuals with PWS. Salivary flow in patients with PWS is approximately 20% of that in controls. In addition, the salivary ions and proteins are present in increased amounts, possibly reflecting a concentration effect relative to decreased water in the saliva. Both deletion and uniparental disomy patients exhibit these findings, suggesting that the gene(s) involved are subject to imprinting.

INTRODUCTION

Prader-Willi syndrome (PWS) was first described by Prader *et al.* in 1956.[1] It is estimated to occur in 1 in 10,000–25,000 newborns, making it the most common dysmorphic form of obesity.[2,3] Individuals with Prader-Willi syndrome exhibit infantile hypotonia, mild to moderate mental retardation, hypogonadism, short stature, hyperphagia leading to obesity, thick saliva, and a characteristic facial appearance that includes a narrow forehead, almond-shaped eyes, and a down-turned mouth with a thin upper lip.

Early diagnosis of PWS remains difficult. Although symptoms change dramatically with age,[3] infants and young children display fewer features than older children and adults.[4] Expression of the most important diagnostic criteria are age related and include hyperphagia, obesity, mental retardation, and hypogonadism.[5] Recently a set of diagnostic criteria for PWS has been developed.[4] There are major criteria weighted at one point each and minor criteria weighted at one half point each. For individuals three years of age or younger, five points are required to make the diagnosis, 4 of which must come from the major category. For individuals older than three years, a total of eight points are required, of which five must come from the major criteria. Over 95% of patients reported in the literature are of Northern European ancestry. It is thought that PWS is probably underdiagnosed in young children and in many ethnic groups, including African-Americans.[3,6]

Abnormalities of chromosome 15 have been identified in approximately 99% of individuals with PWS and are believed to account for PWS. Approximately 75% of PWS patients exhibit a deletion of bands q11-q13 of chromosome 15.[7-9] In all cases, the

---

[a] Tel: (910) 716-2213; fax: 910-716-2554; e-mail: pshart@bgsm.edu

deletion occurs on the paternal homologue.[8] The majority of patients who do not have a deletion have UPD, that is, both of their chromosome 15s have been inherited from their mother and none from the father.[10,11] Thus, it is a lack of paternal contribution of loci in the 15q11q13 region that results in PWS. Interestingly, Angelman's syndrome (AS), a clinically distinct disorder, can result from maternal deletions of 15q11q13 and paternal uniparental disomy of chromosome 15.[12-14] These parent-of-origin effects on inheritance indicate that development of PWS and AS are consequences of genomic imprinting, that is, genes within this region are expressed differently, depending upon the sex of the parent of origin.[15,16] Analysis of patients with microdeletions has demonstrated that the PWS and AS regions are actually distinct, although most patients have large deletions that span the PWS and AS critical regions.[17]

Dental abnormalities reported to occur in association with PWS include delayed tooth eruption, hypoplastic enamel, abnormal saliva, periodontal disease, supernumerary teeth, and rampant caries. Thick, viscous saliva has been implicated as a diagnostic clue of PWS in infancy[18] and is one of the minor criteria for assigning a diagnosis of PWS.[4] Unstimulated (0.243 ± 0.72 g/2 min, n=4) and stimulated (data not given) whole salivary flow rates in PWS patients have been reported to be less than 20% of that for controls (unstimulated flow rate of 1.139 ± 0.221 g/2 min).[19] Despite the recognition that abnormal saliva is a consistent finding in PWS, little is known about the nature and mechanism of altered saliva in this patient population. We now report the composition of saliva from individuals with PWS.

MATERIAL AND METHODS

Saliva Collection

All samples were collected at parent support groups in New York, Maryland, and North Carolina; and genetics clinics in New York, North Carolina, and Connecticut. Whole unstimulated saliva was collected by having the subject swallow and then pool saliva in their mouth for 2 minutes. The saliva was then suctioned from the mouth into a preweighed collection tube by a vacuum pump. For young children or severely retarded individuals, a French feeding tube connected to a collection tube was inserted into the mouth. Total collection time was 5–10 min, depending on patient cooperation. Flow rates were expressed as milligrams per minute. If the patient was able, stimulated saliva was collected by having the subject chew on a small piece of paraffin. A detailed history was taken and included past and current medications, as well as the time of the last teeth brushing and the dentifrice used. Information regarding the influence of medications on saliva was determined from a search of the literature.

Salivary Composition in PWS

Calcium, fluoride, sodium, phosphate, chloride, and total protein concentrations were measured as described below. Saliva samples were analyzed for total available fluoride using the method described by Whitford and Reynolds.[20] One hundred microliter saliva samples were placed in the Taves apparatus. The fluoride content was measured by specific ion electrode (Orion, Model 94-08A, Orion Research Inc. Cambridge, MA) and comparison made to standards diffused at the same time. The remaining solution in the Taves dish, now devoid of fluoride, was analyzed for calcium, phosphate, sodium, and chloride. Calcium was analyzed by atomic absorption in the presence of potassium chloride (KCl) to avoid ionization in the nitrous oxide/acetylene flame that is used to avoid interference by other ions, including phosphate. Sodium was also measured by atomic absorption using KCl.[21] Phosphate was assayed spectrophotometrically by the molybdate method.[22] Chloride was measured using an ion-specific electrode (Orion, Model 94-17BN). In this way, the acid-diffusible fluoride, calcium, phosphate, chloride, and sodium in the original saliva sample were measured very efficiently with only one sample preparation of 100 microliters. A Beckman DU640 spectrophotometer was used for the assay of phosphate. A Perkin-Elmer 1100B atomic absorption unit was used for determinations of calcium and sodium. Total protein concentration was analyzed by the Bradford assay.[23] Comparison was made to a standard curve of the concentration (μg/mL) of albumin as a function of the net absorbance at 595 nanometers.

RESULTS

To date, saliva has been collected from 22 white (1–53 years of age) and 3 black (ages 1, 27, and 48 years) individuals with PWS. As shown in TABLE 1, the underlying molecular defect was deletion (17/25), uniparental disomy (3/25), and unknown (5/25). Saliva collections were attempted on another 15 subjects, but, due to the combination of low flow and viscosity, collections were unsuccessful. The average flow rate for unstimulated saliva was 0.16 ± 0.05 g/min for the 25 PWS individuals compared to 0.54 g/min for controls (TABLE 1). Stimulated salivary flow was 0.38 ± 0.11 g/min for the PWS individuals compared to 2.38 g/min for controls. Flow rates were similar for all ages, and for deletion and nondeletion individuals with PWS. Both unstimulated and stimulated flow rates were found to differ significantly between PWS individuals and controls ($p < 0.05$).

As shown in TABLE 1, all measured components were increased in saliva from PWS subjects. Both deletion and nondeletion patients had similiar concentrations of ions and protein in their saliva. Although the Bradford method underestimates the amount of protein in saliva,[24] the same method was used for both patients and controls, ensuring the detection of relative quantitative changes. Using a t-test, all components were found to differ significantly from controls ($p < 0.05$). Thus, individuals with PWS have decreased salivary flow and their saliva is altered in composition. In addition, these data indicate that the alterations in the ions and total protein composition may actually reflect a concentration effect as opposed to increased secretion of these components.

DISCUSSION

The salivary flow rates of this study are consistent with those of Bray *et al.*[19] who measured flow rates in four individuals with PWS. In addition, there were no significant differences between deletion and nondeletion patients, confirming that the clinical observation of thick saliva is an important diagnostic clue for the majority of PWS individuals.

Decreased salivary flow rates in individuals with PWS occur in two major ways: (1) PWS individuals secrete saliva of normal composition, but at a lower rate; or (2) PWS individuals secrete saliva of altered composition, also at a lower rate. Compositional analysis was performed on the saliva samples in order to distinguish between these two hypotheses. As noted above, all of the components studied were found to be present in increased concentrations in saliva from individuals with PWS, supporting the second hypothesis. Thus, individuals with PWS have decreased salivary flow, and their

TABLE 1. Summary of Salivary Compositional Analysis

Case	Age (yr)	Molecular Diagnosis	Unstimulated Flow Rate (g/min)	Stimulated Flow Rate (g/min)	F[c] (µM)	Ca (mM)	P[d] (mM)	Cl (mM)	Na (mM)	Protein (mg/mL)
1	53	Unknown[a]	0.20	0.45	6.95	2.66	7.89	30.2	12.8	1.4
2	21	Disomy	0.18	0.42	6.37	2.89	9.20	27.4	11.6	2.4
3	1	Deletion	0.22	—	6.50	2.75	8.37	29.7	13.0	2.5
4	48	Deletion	0.12	0.28	6.50	2.25	7.50	27.1	12.0	2.0
5	7	Deletion	0.24	0.53	5.90	2.59	10.0	29.0	12.4	2.6
6	36	Deletion	0.13	0.30	6.90	3.59	9.42	28.4	11.4	2.2
7	8	Deletion	0.08	0.20	6.02	3.25	11.4	30.6	11.1	2.8
8	8	Deletion	0.18	0.40	5.75	2.45	10.4	31.6	12.9	2.5
9	27	Deletion	0.16	0.35	6.43	2.55	9.98	29.2	13.1	2.6
10	24	Deletion	0.08	0.20	6.25	2.76	10.3	30.8	12.1	2.2
11	22	Deletion	0.24	0.54	6.38	3.64	12.1	29.4	12.7	2.4
12	22	Deletion	0.12	0.28	6.82	2.79	9.48	30.9	11.6	2.6
13	18	Deletion	0.26	0.60	5.87	2.86	8.23	27.6	13.4	2.3
14	12	Unknown[a]	0.12	0.28	6.72	3.78	11.0	30.1	12.1	3.1
15	2	Disomy	0.14	—	5.80	2.68	10.4	31.8	11.6	2.6
16	3	Deletion	0.10	—	6.05	2.34	10.1	29.0	11.6	2.2
17	11	Deletion	0.22	0.48	6.47	3.67	13.2	28.2	13.8	2.0
18	9	Disomy	0.17	0.38	6.25	2.31	9.47	30.0	11.7	1.9
19	1	Unknown[a]	0.15	—	5.95	2.68	10.3	27.6	12.4	2.3
20	5	Deletion	0.14	0.32	5.26	2.70	11.4	30.1	13.1	2.5
21	6	Unknown[a]	0.20	0.46	6.19	3.36	8.27	27.2	12.4	2.0
22	7	Unknown[a]	0.19	0.40	6.43	3.14	10.7	29.1	12.9	2.4
23	1	Deletion	0.10	—	5.98	2.76	12.1	30.5	12.1	3.0
24	13	Deletion	0.14	0.30	6.00	3.30	11.3	30.9	12.8	2.8
25	8	Deletion	0.18	0.37	7.24	3.66	13.6	29.3	13.0	2.0
All PWS Mean (SE)	—	—	0.16[b] (0.01)	0.38[b] (0.02)	6.16[b] (0.09)	2.94[b] (0.09)	10.2[b] (0.31)	29.8[b] (0.28)	12.4[b] (0.14)	2.4[b] (0.06)
Controls Mean (SE)	—	—	0.54 (0.12)	2.38 (0.57)	3.74 (0.70)	1.30 (0.03)	6.50 (0.08)	24.0 (0.59)	8.03 (0.21)	1.9 (0.09)

[a] Normal cytogenetic and FISH analysis; no DNA studies conducted.
[b] Mean values of PWS individuals were significantly different from those of control subjects (p < 0.05).
[c] Fluoride.
[d] Phosphate.

saliva is altered in composition. In addition, these data indicate that the alterations in the ions and total protein composition may actually reflect a concentration effect as opposed to increased secretion of these components.

Based on clinical observations and the salivary data on PWS subjects, it appears that a gene or genes important in salivary secretion maps to the 15q11q13 region. A prime candidate would be a member of the water channel genes known as aquaporins.[25] Six distinct human aquaporins have been identified to date.[25-31] Except for *AQP2*, mutations in human aquaporins have not yet been associated with a disease phenotype. Although the molecular pathways by which salivary glands secrete water are not yet known, *AQP5* gene expression has been identified in rat and human salivary glands.[30,31] As human *AQP5* was mapped to 12q13,[30] abnormalities of *AQP5* would not be expected to account for the salivary dysfunction noted in PWS.

Although it is not currently known what gene or genes in the 15q11q13 region are important in salivary secretion, it appears that the expression of such sequences is subject to imprinting, as has been demonstrated for many other genes in this region.[32-36] The finding that individuals with PWS, regardless of the underlying molecular mechanism (deletion, uniparental disomy), secrete saliva that is altered in composition suggests that expression is solely from the paternal allele. If imprinting were not involved, individuals with maternal uniparental disomy would be expected to have normal salivary flow and composition, as they have two maternal alleles. More studies are needed to determine the sequences in 15q11q13 important in salivary secretion and whether or not these sequences are truly subject to imprinting.

REFERENCES

1. PRADER, A, A. LABHART & H. WILLI. 1956. Ein syndrom von adipositas, Kleinwuchs, Kryptorchismus, und Oligophrenie nach myotonieartigem Zustand in Neugeborenenalter. Schweiz. Med. Wochenschr. **86:** 1260–1261.
2. ZELLWEGER, H. & R.T. SOPER. 1979. The Prader-Willi syndrome. Med. Hyg. **37:** 3338–3345.
3. CASSIDY, S.B. 1984. Prader-Willi syndrome. Curr. Probl. Pediatr. **14:** 1–55.
4. HOLM, V.A., S.B. CASSIDY, M.G. BUTLER, J.M. HENCHETT, L.R. GREENSWAG, B.Y. WHITMAN & F. GREENBERG. 1993. Prader-Willi syndrome: Consensus diagnostic criteria. Pediatrics **91:** 398–402.
5. CHITAYAT, D., E.B. DAVIS, B.C. MCGILLIVRAY, M.R. HAYDEN & J.G. HALL. 1989. Perinatal and first year follow-up of patients with Prader-Willi syndrome: normal size of hands and feet. Clin. Genet. **35:** 161–166.
6. HUDGINS, L & S.B. CASSIDY. 1991. Hand and foot length in Prader-Willi syndrome. Am. J. Med. Genet. **41:** 5–9.
7. DONLON, T.A. 1988. Similar molecular deletions of chromosome 15q11.2 are encountered in both the Prader-Willi and Angelman syndromes. Hum. Genet. **80:** 285–290.
8. NICHOLLS, R.D., J.H. KNOLL, K. GLATT, J.H. HERSH, T.D. BREWSTER, J.M. GRAHAM JR., D. WURSTER-HILL, R. WHARTON & SA LATT 1989. Restriction fragment length polymorphisms within proximal 15q and their use in molecular cytogenetics and the Prader-Willi syndrome. Am. J. Med. Genet. **33:** 66–77.
9. GREGORY, C.A., A.J. KIRKILIONIS, C.R. GREENBERG, A.E. CHUDLEY & J.L. HAMERTON. 1990. Detection of molecular rearrangements in Prader-Willi syndrome patients by using genomic probes recognizing four loci within the PWCR. Am. J. Med. Genet. **35:** 536–545.
10. NICHOLLS, R.D., J.H. KNOLL, M.G. BUTLER, S. KARAM & M. LALANDE. 1989. Genetic imprinting suggested by maternal uniparental heterodisomy in nondeletion Prader-Willi syndrome. Nature **342:** 281–285.
11. MASCARI, M.J., W. GOTTLIEB, P.K. ROGAN, M.G. BUTLER, J. ARMOUR, A. JEFFREYS, D. WALLER, R.L. LADDA & R.D. NICHOLLS. 1992. The frequency of uniparental disomy in Prader-Willi syndrome: implications for molecular diangosis. N. Engl. J. Med. **326:** 1599–1607.

12. PEMBREY, M., S.J. FENNELL, J. VANDENBERGHE, M. FITCHETT, D. SUMMERS, L. BUTLER, C. CLARKE, M. GRIFFITH, E. THOMPSON, M. SUPER & M. BARAITSER. 1989. The association of Angelman's syndrome with deletions within 15q11-q13. J. Med. Genet. **26:** 73–77.
13. HAMABE, J., Y. KUROKI, K. IMAIZUMI, T. SUGIMOTO, Y. FUKUSHIMA, A. YAMAGUCHI, N. IZUMIKAWA & N. NIIKAWA. 1991. DNA deletion and its parental origin in Angelman syndrome patients. Am. J. Med. Genet. **41:** 64–68.
14. NICHOLLS, R.D., G.S. PAI, W. GOTTLIEB & E.S. CANTU. 1992. Paternal uniparental disomy in Angelman syndrome. Ann. Neurol. **32:** 512–518.
15. HALL, J.G. 1990. Genomic imprinting: Review and relevance to human disease. Am. J. Hum. Genet. **46:** 857–873.
16. NICHOLLS, R.D. 1993. Genomic imprinting and uniparental disomy in Angelman and Prader-Willi syndromes: A review. Am. J. Med. Genet. **46:** 16–25.
17. MAGENIS, R.E., S. TOTH-FEJAL, L.J. ALLEN, M. BLACK, M.G. BROWN, S. BUDDEN, R. COHEN, J.M. FREIDMAN, D. KALOUSEK, J. ZONANA, D. LACY, S. LA FRANCHI, M. LAHR, J. MACFARLANE & C.P.S. WILLIAMS. 1990. Comparison of the 15q deletions in Prader-Willi and Angelman syndromes: specific regions, extent of deletions, parental origin, and clinical consequences. Am. J. Med. Genet. **35:** 333–349.
18. STEPHENSON, J.B.P. 1992. Neonatal presentation of Prader-Willi syndrome. Am. J. Dis. Child. **146:** 151–152.
19. BRAY, G.A., W.T. DAHMS, R.S. SWERDLOFF, R.H. FISER, R.L. ATKINSON & R.E. CARREL. 1983. The Prader-Willi syndrome: A study of 40 patients and a review of the literature. Medicine **62:** 59–80.
20. WHITFIELD, G.M. & K.E. REYNOLDS. 1979. Plasma and developing enamel fluoride concentrations during chronic acid-base disturbances. J. Dent. Res. **58:** 2058–2065.
21. DAWES, C. 1969. The effect of flow rate and duration of stimulation on the concentrations of proteins and the main electrolytes in human parotid saliva. Arch. Oral Biol. **14:** 277–294.
22. CHEN, P.S., T.Y. TORIBARA & H. WARNER. 1956. Micro-determination of phosphorous. Anal. Chem. **28:** 1756–1758.
23. BRADFORD, M.M. 1976. A rapid and sensitive method for the quantitation of microgram quantities of protein utilizing the principle of protein-dye binding. Anal. Biochem. **72:** 248.
24. NAKAMURA, M. & J. SLOTS. 1983. Salivary enzymes: origin and relationship to periodontal disease. J. Periodontal Res. **18:** 559–569.
25. AGRE, P., G. PRESTON, B. SMITH, J.S. JUNG, S. RAINA, C. MOON, W.B. GUGGINO & S. NIELSEN. 1993. Aquaporin CHIP: the archetypal molecular water channel. Am. J. Physiol. **265:** F463–F476.
26. DEEN, P.M.T., D.O. WEGHUIS, A. GEURTS VAN KESSEL, B. WIERINGA & C.H. VAN OS. 1994. The human gene for water channel aquaporin 1 (AQP1) is localized on chromosome 7p15→p14. Cytogenet. Cell. Genet. **65:** 243–246.
27. SAITO, F., S. SASAKI, A.B. CHEPELINSKY, K. FUSHIMI, F. MARUMO & T. IKEUCHI. 1995. Human AWP2 and MIP genes, two members of the MIP family, map within chromosome band 12q13 on the basis of two-color FISH. Cytogenet. Cell Genet. **68:** 45–48.
28. YANG, B., T. MA & A.S. VERKMAN. 1995. cDNA cloning, gene organization, and chromosomal localization of a human mercurial insensitive water channel. J. Biol. Chem. **270:** 22,907–22,913.
29. MULDERS, S.M., G.M. PRESTON, P.M.T. DEEN, W.B. GUGGINO, C.H. VAN OS & P. AGRE. 1995. Water channel properties of major intrinsic protein of lens. J. Biol. Chem. **270:** 9010–9016.
30. LEE, M.D., K.Y. BHAKTA, S. RAINA, R. YONESCU, C.A. GRIFFIN, N.G. COPELAND, D.J. GILBERT, N.A. JENKINS, G.M. PRESTON & P. AGRE. 1996. The human *Aquaporin-5* gene. J. Biol. Chem. **271:** 8599–8604.
31. RAINA, S., G.M. PRESTON, W.B. GUGGINO & P. AGRE. 1995. Molecular cloning and characterization of an aquaporin cDNA from salivary, lacrimal, and respiratory tissues. J. Biol. Chem. **270:** 1908–1912.
32. OZCELIK, T., S. LEFF, W. ROBINSON, T. DONLON, M. LALANDE, E. SANJINES, A. SCHINZEL & U. FRANCKE. 1992. Small nuclear ribonucleoprotein polypeptide N (SNRPN), an expressed gene in the Prader-Willi syndrome critical region. Nat. Genet. **24:** 265–269.

33. GLENN, C.C., K.A. PORTER, M.T.C. JONG, R.D. NICHOLLS & D.J. DRISCOLL. 1993. Functional imprinting and epigenetic modification of the human *SNRPN* gene. Hum. Mol. Gen. **2:** 2001–2005.
34. MITSUYOSHI, N., J.S. SUTCLIFFE, B. DURTSCHI, A. MUTIRANGURA, D.S. LEDBETTER & A.L. BEAUDET. 1994. Imprinting analysis of three genes in the Prader-Willi/Angleman region: SNRPN E6-associated protein and PAR-2 (D15s225E). Hum. Mol. Genet. **3:** 309–315.
35. NAKAO, M. 1994. Imprinting analysis of three genes in the Prader-Willi/Angleman region: *SNRPN, E6*-associated protein and *PAR-2 (D15S225E)*. Hum. Mol. Genet. **10:** 1877–1882.
36. WEVRICK, R., J.A. KERNS & U. FRANCKE. 1994. Identification of a novel paternally expressed gene in the Prader-Willi syndrome region. Hum. Mol. Genet. **3:** 1877–1882.

Acquired Salivary Dysfunction
Drugs and Radiation

PHILIP C. FOX[a]

Clinical Investigations Section, Gene Therapy and Therapeutics Branch, National Institute of Dental Research, National Institutes of Health, Building 10, Room 1N-113, 10 Center Drive MSC 1190, Bethesda, Maryland 20892-1190, USA

ABSTRACT: When considering the effects of drugs on salivary glands, a distinction should be drawn between the complaint of oral dryness (xerostomia), a symptom, and measurable secretory hypofunction, a sign. In general, the symptom of xerostomia is often not accompanied by objective reductions in salivary output, and xerostomia is not a reliable indicator of secretory hypofunction. Whereas therapeutic pharmaceutical side effects represent the most prominent cause of xerostomia, with over 500 drugs associated with this symptom, only a small number of drugs have been demonstrated to reduce salivary output substantially. There are examples in which drugs with a high prevalence of xerostomia complaints do not affect secretory function. The mechanisms responsible for this discrepancy between subjective and objective findings have not been fully identified. It is hypothesized that alterations in systemic or mucosal hydration may play a role. Of the drugs with true salivary hypofunctional actions, most have direct anticholinergic properties. In almost all cases, the salivary effects of pharmaceuticals are not permanent, and function returns to pretreatment levels when the medication is stopped.

By contrast, the effects of irradiation on the salivary glands are permanent when exposures exceed 50 Gy. About 40,000 individuals per year receive irradiation that involves the salivary glands (by external beam or internal sources—radon implants and ^{131}I) for treatment of cancers of the head and neck region. Although these radiation effects have been recognized as a significant clinical problem for more than 80 years, the specific mechanisms responsible for radiation-induced salivary gland dysfunction are still not understood. With the exception of studies documenting the secretory functional deficits following head and neck irradiation, limited studies have been done in humans. The majority of experimental work has been done in rodents. A variety of mechanisms, including mitotic and interphase cell death, direct DNA damage or effects of secondary metabolites, damage to progenitor cells, or altered gene expression, have all been proposed to explain the salivary epithelial cell death observed. Recent experimental studies with models of radiation-induced salivary damage in rats and a human salivary cell line suggest that the small percentage of surviving epithelial cells are capable of performing functions such as signal transduction and ion transport normally. Apoptotic cell death following irradiation has not been a prominent feature in these model systems.

The effects of head and neck radiation on the salivary glands and oral cavity continue to present multiple significant clinical problems both during and after radiotherapy. In recent years, there has been some progress in minimizing these effects through more careful shielding and pretreatment planning. Additionally, there are preliminary results from a clinical trial suggesting that the use of a secretagogue, pilocarpine HCl, given during the course of radiotherapy, may reduce the secretory hypofunctional effects. A multicenter trial is now underway to test this hypothesis. There is still a real need to develop more effective treatments for this condition.

The most common causes of acquired salivary gland dysfunctions in humans are systemic diseases, radiation therapy, and pharmaceutical side effects.[1] Although precise

[a]Tel: (301) 496-4278; fax: (301) 402-1228; e-mail: pfox@yoda.nidr.nih.gov

epidemiologic data are unavailable, millions of individuals in the United States have medical conditions or use therapies that may significantly affect salivary function. This in turn may lead to substantial compromise in oral functions, systemic health, and general quality of life. Xerostomia, the symptom of oral dryness that is most often associated with salivary gland hypofunction, has been reported to be present in up to 25% of institutionalized elders.[2] This symptom may have a prevalence of up to 10% in the general population and often is a signal of systemic disease.[3] Although salivary gland dysfunction has garnered increased research attention in recent years, it is still a problem that is incompletely understood and inadequately treated. The paper will review current knowledge of two of the major causes of salivary dysfunction, drugs and radiation.

DRUGS

The first consideration when examining the effects of pharmaceuticals on the salivary glands is to draw a distinction between the symptom of dry mouth (xerostomia) and measurable salivary hypofunction. Xerostomia is a reported side effect of over 500 medications.[4] It is among the more common listed side effects of pharmaceuticals generally and can be associated with any class of medication. However, xerostomia is not a reliable indicator of objectively determined salivary gland hypofunction.[5] Although xerostomia is found in most instances of salivary gland dysfunction, it also is associated with nonsalivary causes and can be present in spite of apparently completely normal salivary gland function. Indeed, only a relatively small number of drugs that report xerostomia as a prominent side effect have been shown to reduce salivary gland output in controlled trials.[6]

An example of the lack of correlation between symptoms of dry mouth and diminished salivary flow is a study by Atkinson *et al.*[7] Healthy volunteers were given a physiologic dose of furosemide, a potent diuretic that is known to induce xerostomia, in a double-masked, placebo-controlled, crossover trial. The mechanism of action of furosemide is through inhibition of the action of the Na/K/2Cl cotransporter in the kidney.[8] This cotransporter has been identified in the salivary glands, also, and is felt to be a major force in saliva production and secretion.[9] Following oral dosing with furosemide, a marked diuresis resulted, significantly greater than following placebo, as expected. Subjects also were queried hourly concerning symptoms of oral dryness. All subjects when given furosemide complained of xerostomia at several time points during the four-hour postdose observation period. By contrast, only a single subject at a single time point noted oral dryness following placebo. Unstimulated parotid and submandibular saliva were collected at baseline and hourly. In spite of the marked differences in the symptoms, there were no significant differences between the treatment groups in salivary flow at any time point. Additionally, there were not significant differences in salivary total protein concentration or in total output, hourly output, or average concentrations of salivary Na^+, K^+, or Cl^-. The mechanism for xerostomia was not determined but may be related to changes in tissue hydration or alterations in extracellular volume. This study emphasizes that we do not understand fully the factors that are responsible for subjective oral comfort and the sensations of oral mucosal wetness or dryness. It also highlights the lack of reliable correlation between the symptom of xerostomia and diminished salivary gland volume output.

There are a number of drugs that do lead to measurable salivary gland hypofunction.[7] Most have direct anticholinergic properties. Antihistaminics, tricyclic antidepressants, certain antihypertensives, hypnotics, and sedatives are drug groups associated with salivary gland functional alterations. It is important to recognize the potential for salivary gland dysfunction with these treatments and others, as preventive measures can be taken to provide symptomatic relief of the xerostomia and to limit the consequences of reduced salivation. Often, substitution of a different agent with similar therapeutic properties can alleviate the problem. In almost all cases, the salivary effects are not permanent, and function will return to pretreatment levels after stopping treatment with the offending agent.

RADIATION

By contrast, the effects of irradiation on the salivary glands are usually irreversible when exposures exceed ~ 50 Gy.[10] Irradiation to the head and neck region, which includes the salivary glands in the field of treatment, leads to rapid decreases in saliva output. Most head and neck cancer radiation treatment is delivered in fractionated doses, five days per week, for six to eight weeks. Within one week of radiotherapy (~ 10 Gy, delivered dose), salivary function declines by as much as 60%.[11] At the completion of a full course of radiotherapy, which averages about 70 Gy, salivary function is essentially absent. At these dose levels, there is very little improvement in function, even at late time points after treatment.[12] Although there is general belief that there is differential radiosensitivity of the major salivary glands, at the doses delivered in most modern therapeutic protocols, all glands in the field are markedly affected to about the same degree.

In the United States, about 40,000 individuals per year receive irradiation that involves the salivary glands. Most have had external beam radiotherapy for head and neck tumors. However, it should be remembered that individuals who receive internal sources of irradiation, such as treatment with ^{131}I for thyroid cancers[13] or radon "seed" implants in the head and neck, also may suffer significant salivary gland damage and dysfunction. All patients who have received therapeutic head and neck radiotherapy require careful preirradiation screening for potential oral complications, and vigorous posttreatment oral care.[14] Complications of radiotherapy, including stomatitis, oral infection, severe dental decay, and osteoradionecrosis, may have a significant impact on the efficacy of therapy, quality of life, and survival of the individual.[15]

Although radiation-induced effects on salivary function have been recognized for more than 80 years, the specific mechanisms responsible are still not understood completely. In humans, with the exception of numerous studies that have documented the secretory functional deficits following head and neck irradiation, there are very limited data. Histologically, it is believed that there is loss of salivary epithelial cells, predominantly acinar cells, with fibrosis of the remaining tissue.[16] There is also believed to be change in the vasculature locally. There are no comprehensive tissue studies of the salivary glands following different irradiation doses in humans. Many studies have been done in animal model systems, primarily rodents. In rat studies, significant alterations in the vasculature[17] and neural innervation[18] were not seen early after irradiation, at times when salivary output has been demonstrated to be markedly reduced.

Based on animal studies, a variety of mechanisms, including mitotic and interphase cell death, direct DNA damage or effects on DNA by secondary metabolites, damage to progenitor cells, or altered gene expression, have been proposed to explain the cell death and functional alterations found in the salivary glands. There is not agreement or definitive data on the mechanism of damage. Indeed, many studies presenting contradictory results are available.

In the rat model, it appears that even with significant reduction in salivary flow, salivary cells *in vitro* can perform a variety of cell functions adequately.[19] Recent studies with rats and using a human salivary cell line suggest that the small percentage of epithelial cells surviving after irradiation are capable of performing functions normally, such as signal transduction and ion transport.[20] They also were capable of normal growth and differentiation after a lag phase. Apoptotic cell death following irradiation has not been a prominent feature in these model systems (unpublished data). Further study of the mechanisms of irradiation-induced salivary gland dysfunction are essential, particularly in humans, in order to devise more effective means of prevention and repair of damaged glands.

The effects of head and neck radiotherapy on the salivary glands and oral cavity continue to present significant clinical problems, both during and after treatment. A number of approaches have been taken to reduce salivary damage caused by irradiation (radioprotection) and to improve salivary function following radiotherapy.

The effects of radiotherapy on salivary gland function can be lessened by positioning of the patient during treatment to minimize exposure of the glands. Shielding can also be helpful if it will not compromise the treatment fields. Careful attention to fields and beam direction using three-dimensional treatment planning and conformational dose delivery has resulted in significant sparing of salivary gland function in specific instances.[21]

A number of agents have been proposed as salivary radioprotectants during head and neck therapy.[22] These have met with limited success, and there is persistent concern that such agents may confer protection to tumor as well as nonaffected "bystander" tissues. A somewhat different approach has been taken in a pilot clinical trial using the secretogogue, pilocarpine HCL.[23] Pilocarpine (5 mg orally q.i.d.) was given beginning one day prior to the start of head and neck radiotherapy and was continued throughout the treatment period, for a total of 13 weeks. An identical-appearing placebo was used for a control in a double-masked design. The pilocarpine-treated group had a smaller decline in salivary function following radiotherapy compared to the placebo group. The mechanisms of action of the secretagogue as a salivary functional protectant are not known. Because the most pronounced protective effects were seen in the parotid glands, which were partially shielded from the irradiation, the pilocarpine may be acting primarily to maintain the nonirradiated salivary tissue at the borders of the radiation field. This result needs to be tested in larger protocols to confirm the findings and explore the mechanisms of the protection observed. At present, a multicenter trial is planned to examine the effects of pilocarpine given during the treatment phase in reducing salivary gland hypofunction caused by radiotherapy.

Pilocarpine has been shown also to be effective in treating postirradiation xerostomia and salivary gland hypofunction. Several large trials[24,25] in patients who had marked salivary gland dysfunction following radiotherapy have confirmed that 5–10 mg pilocarpine orally given t.i.d. or q.i.d. can reduce symptoms of oral dryness, improve oral functioning, and increase salivary output. Side effects of the medication were common, but generally mild. Pilocarpine is approved in the United States for treatment of postradiation xerostomia and is the only agent recognized for this indication. Most postradiation patients have little remaining salivary gland function. However, even modest improvements in output seem to lead to marked symptomatic improvement in many patients.[24] Longer-term studies will be necessary to determine if secretogogue stimulation in these patients results in increased function over time and a reduction in oral complications.

Newer approaches are suggested by a recent study using gene transfer techniques.[26] An adenovirus vector was used to transduce the gene for aquaporin 1, a water channel, into irradiated salivary glands of rats. Several months after exposure to irradiation, rats had significant reductions in salivary output compared to control nonirradiated animals. The adenovirus vector was administered to submandibular glands by retrograde ductal instillation. Expression of the aquaporin gene in the irradiated glands of these rats resulted in a two- to threefold increase in salivary secretion, approaching the levels of the nonirradiated controls. This is a novel approach to correction of radiation damage in salivary glands and may be applicable to treatment of other causes of irreversible salivary gland damage. Although further extensive testing is necessary, this work presents the first example of an exciting new therapeutic modality for radiation-induced salivary gland dysfunction.

REFERENCES

1. MANDEL, I.D. 1980. Sialochemistry in diseases and clinical situations affecting the salivary glands. Crit. Rev. Clin. Lab. Sci. **12**: 321–366.
2. HANDELMAN, S.L., J.M. BARIC, R.H. SAUNDERS et al. 1989. Hyposalivatory drug use, whole salivary flow, and dryness in older, long-term care residents. Spec. Care Dent. **4**: 12–18.
3. SREEBNY, L.M. & A. VALDINI. 1987. Xerostomia: a neglected symptom. Arch. Intern. Med. **147**: 1333–1337.
4. SREEBNY, L.M. & S.S. SCHWARTZ. 1986. A reference guide to drugs and dry mouth. Gerodontol. **5**: 75–99.
5. FOX, P.C., K.A. BUSCH & B.J. BAUM. 1987. Subjective reports of xerostomia and objective measures of salivary gland performance. J. Am. Dent. Assoc. **115**: 581–584.
6. ATKINSON, J.C. & P.C. FOX. 1992. Salivary gland dysfunction. Clin. Ger. Med. **8**: 499–511.
7. ATKINSON, J.C., J.B. SHIROKY, A. MACYNSKI & P.C. FOX. 1989. Effects of furosemide on the oral cavity. Gerodontol. **8**: 23–26.
8. KOWNIG, B., S. RICAPITO & R. KINNE. 1983. Chloride transport in the thick ascending limb of Henle's loop: potassium dependence and stochiometry of the NaCl cotransport system in plasma membrane vesicles. Pfluegers Arch. **399**: 173–179.
9. TURNER, R.J. 1993. Mechanisms of fluid secretion by salivary glands. Ann. N.Y. Acad. Sci. **694**: 24–35.
10. FRANZEN, L., U. FUNEGARD, T. ERICSON et al. 1992. Parotid gland function during and following radiotherapy of malignancies in the head and neck. A consecutive study of salivary flow and patient discomfort. Eur. J. Cancer **28**: 457–462.
11. MOSSMAN, K.L. 1983. Quantitative radiation dose-response relationships for normal tissues in man. II. Response of the salivary glands during radiotherapy. Radiat. Res. **95**: 392–398.
12. VALDEZ, I.H., J.C. ATKINSON, J.A. SHIP et al. 1993. Major salivary gland function in patients with radiation-induced xerostomia: flow rates and sialochemistry. Int. J. Radiat. Oncol. Biol. Phys. **25**: 41–47.
13. CREUTZIG, H. 1985. Sialadenitis following iodine-131 therapy for thyroid carcinoma. J. Nucl. Med. **26**: 817–818.
14. CONSENSUS DEVELOPMENT PANEL. 1990. Consensus statement: oral complications of cancer therapies. NCI Monogr. **9**: 3–8.
15. VALDEZ, I.H. 1991. Radiation-induced salivary dysfunction: clinical course and significance. Spec. Care Dent. **11**: 252–255.
16. KASHIMA, H.K., W.R. KIRKHAM & J.R. ANDREWS. 1965. Postradiation sialadenitis. A study of the clinical features, histopathologic changes and serum enzyme variations following irradiation of human salivary glands. Am. J. Roentgenol. Radium Ther. Nucl. Med. **94**: 271–291.
17. HIRAMATSU, Y., R.M. NAGLER, P.C. FOX & B.J. BAUM. 1994. Rat salivary gland blood flow and blood-to-tissue partition coefficients following x-irradiation. Arch. Oral Biol. **39**: 77–80.
18. KOHN, W.G., E. GROSSMAN, P.C. FOX et al. 1992. Effect of ionizing radiation on sympathetic nerve function in rat parotid glands. J. Oral Pathol. & Med. **21**: 134–137.
19. BODNER, L., B.L. KUYATT, A.R. HAND & B.J. BAUM. 1984. Rat parotid cell function *in vitro* following X irradiation *in vivo*. Radiat. Res. **97**: 386–395.
20. O'CONNELL, A.C. 1997. Radiation-induced xerostomia in cancer patients: current treatments and future therapies. Genetic modification of surviving cells [abstract]. J. Dent. Res. **76**: 251.

21. SHIP, J.A., A. EISBRUCH, E. D'HONDT et al. 1997. Parotid sparing study in head and neck cancer patients receiving bilateral radiation therapy: one-year results. J. Dent. Res. **76:** 807–813.
22. SODICOFF, M. & A.D. CONGER. 1983. Radioprotection of the rat parotid gland by WR-2721 and isoproterenol and its modification by propanolol. Radiat. Res. **94:** 97–104.
23. VALDEZ, I.H., A. WOLFF, J.C. ATKINSON et al. 1993. Use of pilocarpine during head and neck radiation therapy to reduce xerostomia and salivary dysfunction. Cancer **71:** 1848–1851.
24. JOHNSON, J.T., G.A. FERRETTI, W.J. NETHERY et al. 1993. Oral pilocarpine for post irradiation xerostomia symptoms and saliva production in patients with head and neck cancer: a multi-center, double-blind, placebo controlled study. N. Engl. J. Med. **329:** 390–395.
25. LEVEQUE, F.G., M. MONTGOMERY, D. POTTER et al. 1993. A multicenter, randomized, double-blind, placebo-controlled, dose-titration study of oral pilocarpine for treatment of radiation-induced xerostomia in head and neck cancer patients. J. Clin. Oncol. **11:** 1124–1131.
26. DELPORTE, C, B.C. O'CONNELL, X. HE et al. 1997. Increased fluid secretion after adenoviral-mediated transfer of the aquaporin-1 cDNA to irradiated rat salivary glands. Proc. Natl. Acad. Sci. USA **94:** 3268–3273.

Antigen Processing and Autoimmunity

Evaluation of mRNA Abundance and Function of HLA-linked Genes[a]

YINENG FU, GANG YAN, LIJIA SHI, AND DENISE FAUSTMAN[b]

Immunobiology Laboratory, Massachusetts General Hospital, Harvard Medical School, Boston, Massachusetts 02129, USA

ABSTRACT: Quantitative defects in the density of conformationally correct human lymphocyte antigen (HLA) class I complexes on the surface of lymphocytes are apparent in patients with diverse HLA-linked autoimmune diseases, including Type I diabetes and Sjögren's syndrome. First, HLA class I expression was investigated in individuals with two rare and genetically divergent polyglandular autoimmune diseases. Polyglandular failure patients whose disease showed HLA linkage, but not those whose disease was not HLA linked, exhibited decreased HLA class I expression on the surface of their lymphocytes as well as a reduced abundance of transcripts of the HLA-linked genes *Tap1* and *Tap2*, both of which encode proteins that contribute to HLA class I processing. Second, lymphocytes from patients with insulin-dependent diabetes mellitus (IDDM), Sjögren's syndrome, Graves' disease, and Hashimoto's disease showed varying degrees of decreased abundance of mRNAs that encode *Tap1*, *Tap2*, *Lmp2*, or *Lmp7* (the latter two proteins also contribute to HLA class I processing). Third, in twins discordant for IDDM, reduced transcript abundance was preferential to diabetic subjects. Fourth, functional assays of isolated diabetic proteasomes, the peptide cutting complex containing LMP2 and LMP7 proteins, revealed altered peptidase activity. These data suggest that defective transcription of HLA class I–processing genes could contribute to the quantitative defect in cell-surface expression in autoimmune lymphocytes of HLA-controlled disease.

INTRODUCTION

Major histocompatibility (MHC) class I molecules on the surface of antigen-presenting cells play an important role in the interaction of these cells with T lymphocytes. Thus, the exterior-facing peptide-binding groove of MHC class I molecules can present viral protein fragments to CD8+ cytotoxic T cells.[1,2] However, small peptides derived from endogenous intracellular proteins have also been identified in the peptide-binding groove of MHC class I molecules, suggesting a steric role for such self-peptides in MHC class I stability in the absence of viral infection.

We have previously shown that defective surface expression of class I molecules attributable to impaired complex formation with self-peptides appears to be an antigen-presenting cell defect characteristic of lymphocytes of humans with Type I diabetes and mutant NOD mice with Sjögren's syndrome and Type I diabetes. Furthermore, this defect in antigen presentation predicts future disease expression in high-risk first-degree relatives of such patients.[3] We proposed that the binding of self-peptides in the groove

---

[a] This work was supported, in part, by NIH Grant #RO1-DE11151-02 and Cure Diabetes Now.

[b] Address for correspondence: Denise Faustman, M.D., Ph.D., Massachusetts General Hospital-East, Immunobiology Laboratory, Building 149, 13th Street, CNY-3601, Charlestown, MA 02129. Tel: (617) 726-4084; fax: (617) 726-4095; e-mail: faustman@warren.med.harvard.edu

of human lymphocyte antigen (HLA) class I molecules is critical for T-cell education and for preventing certain types of autoreactivity. Quantitative defects in the expression of conformationally normal complexes of HLA class I molecules and self-peptides have been identified in a variety of other HLA class II-linked autoimmune diseases, including lupus erythematosus, Sjögren's syndrome, rheumatoid arthritis, Graves' diseases, Hashimoto's thyroiditis, and multiple sclerosis.[4,5] These blinded studies also detected asymptomatic "control" individuals with the class I assembly defect, and follow-up confirmed the presence of autoimmunity with autoantibodies to various target organs in these subjects.

Further evidence for a role of MHC class I and self-peptides on antigen-presenting cells in T-cell education has been obtained with genetic mouse models of altered class I expression. Disruption by homologous recombination of genes critical for class I assembly, including those encoding TAP, LMP, or β_2-microglobulin proteins, was associated with faulty T-cell education, altered T-cell numbers, altered host T-cell reactivity, and reactivity to self-proteins *in vitro* and, in some instances, *in vivo*.[3,6–10] In murine models, severe class I interruption appears to culminate in few peripheral CD8$^+$ T cells. In a recent rare human pedigree without TAP, the two young children's CD8$^+$ T-cell numbers were adequate and demonstrated cytotoxic activity.[11] Thus, differences in the surface density of conformationally correct complexes of class I and self-peptide appeared to affect T-cell education and can affect T-cell numbers, depending on the species. Transgenic low class I murine models and the rare human deficiency in TAP represents dramatic defects in reduced surface class I expression of at least 80% ablation. The defects in HLA class I assembly in autoimmune human antigen-presenting cells are of a magnitude of a 20–40% reduction in conformationally correct class I surface protein. T-cell avidity and T-cell selection may be determined by the affinity and density of complexes of class I and self-peptides.[12] T-cell avidity is thought to be critical for both positive and negative T-cell selection.[13]

Several genes that control class I assembly have been recently identified and are located in the HLA class II genomic region. In an exciting explosion of the literature over the past five years, both *Tap1* and *Tap2* are identified as HLA class II–linked genes that encode proteins that form an obligatory heterodimer essential for transporting small self-peptides from the cytoplasm into the endoplasmic reticulum (ER), the site of class I assembly.[14–20] HLA-class II linked *Lmp2* and *Lmp7* encode components of the proteasome, a large macromolecular complex that degrades endogenous cytoplasmic proteins into small fragments suitable for TAP-mediated translocation into the ER.[21–26]

Most human autoimmune diseases show statistically significant associations with the HLA class II genomic region, although precise HLA-linked mutations have not been identified. Furthermore, HLA class II genes that show an increased frequency in patients with autoimmune diseases are commonly present in normal individuals, and functional studies have not revealed specific class II malfunctions of specific alleles in autoimmune patients. It is possible that multiple HLA genes, acting in concert, contribute to the disease process, in which instance statistical analysis will generally average the linkage of the various genes and potentially identify only the polymorphic genes located most centrally. It is also possible that genes such as those encoding TAP or LMP proteins are, in part, responsible for autoimmunity and that the statistical class II linkage of disease actually reflects that location of multiple genes in the class II genomic region. Moreover, point mutations in an HLA gene associated with autoimmunity may never be found, because cassettes of linked genes function in unison to cause faulty class I expression and interrupted T-cell education. Genetic screening of DNA misses quantitative errors in gene expression that are observable only at the level of mRNA or protein abundance. Finally, it has been recognized for a long time and confirmed that the HLA region appears as the single most significant contributor to autoimmunity, yet the mechanism of disease conferment is elusive.

Quantitative defects in the expression of class I and self-peptides on the surface of antigen-presenting cells have been detected in the NOD mouse, a naturally occurring model of type I diabetes, by flow cytometric analysis with conformationally specific antibodies to class I molecules.[3,27] Although there have been varying reports concerning density of class I in the NOD, ranging from only observing B cells; not observing at all; only observing at the H-2K, but not H-2D locus; as well as its association to cell size, the most consistent and dramatic observation is with a conformationally specific antibody named M1/42.[28–30] NOD mice also show a decreased abundance of *Tap1* mRNA with near normal amounts of *Tap2* mRNA.[3] This quantitative defect in class I assembly presumably results, at least in part, from the decreased availability of *Tap1* mRNA. This decrease in *Tap1* mRNA abundance directly correlated with disease expression and predicts future hyperglycemia in young animals, although this data is associative.[31]

Although quantitative differences in *Tap* have not been functionally correlated with measurable changes in activity, alterations in *Lmp* gene transcription causes well-described functional changes in the ability of the proteasome to prepare peptides compatible with the *Tap* transporters and the class I–binding groove. The adequate transcription of MHC-linked *Lmp2* and *Lmp7* ensures a proteasome generating peptides compatible with transport into the ER and occupancy of the binding cleft of the MHC class I molecules. Adequate levels of *Lmp2* and *Lmp7* gene transcription increases the proteasome's generation of hydrophobic and basic substrates and reduces the hydrolysis of acid substrates. When *Lmp2* and *Lmp7* transcript abundance is reduced, the proteasome prepares peptides of low hydrophobic and basic activity and elevated acid cutting.[32–35] These peptides are less optimally suited for *Tap* transport and class I assembly.

NOD mice have been shown to be "cured" of various forms of immunostimulation, including viral infection and injection with complete Freund's adjuvant.[32,33,36–42] Two such cures, infection with mouse hepatitis virus and treatment with complete Freund's adjuvant, increase *Tap1* mRNA abundance, restore surface expression of peptide-filled MHC class I molecules, and eliminate measurable $CD8^+$ T-cell reactivity to class I self-antigen targets.[43] This murine data in an autoimmune model suggests similar human data of transcription abundance, and errors of class I processing genes should be sought.

It is not uncommon to identify multiple autoimmune diseases in the same individual or same family, the target organs often varying. Certain forms of polyglandular autoimmune diseases demonstrate risk mapping to the HLA region or to autosomal genes.[44–48] Multiple autoimmune diseases in the clinical setting of the early onset of candidiasis represents a rare subset of polyglandular failure with autosomal recessive inheritance.[49–51] These patients have been referred to as autoimmune polyglandular disease type I (APDI), autoimmune polyendocrinopathy-candidiasis-ectodermal dystrophy (APECED), or polyglandular deficiency with mucocutaneous candidiasis patients.[52] The recent assignment of the recessive disease locus to chromosome 21 confirms the lack of HLA-mediated risk (chromosome 6) with candidiasis and autoimmunity, and this contrasts dramatically from HLA-linked autoreactivity.[49,51] The underlying pathology at the site of end-organ damage may be unique in the recessive autosomal disease due to the reported lack of characteristic lymphoid infiltrates even in the setting of autoantibodies.[53]

In order to examine the possible HLA contribution to the antigen-presenting cell defects of altered class I assembly, we initially examined the abundance of mRNAs encoding *Tap1* and *Tap2* in lymphocytes by comparing individuals with these two rare autoimmune polyglandular diseases: HLA-linked multiple endocrine gland failure without mucocutaneous candidiasis, and HLA nonlinked polyglandular failure with mucocutaneous candidiasis.[44–47,49–54] These two rare diseases allowed the control of quantitative errors in HLA genes to be accessed. We also investigated whether errors in the assembly of class I molecule and self-peptide complexes would be quantitatively related to the abundance of transcripts encoding *Tap1*, *Tap2*, *Lmp2*, or *Lmp7* in diverse and common HLA-linked autoimmune diseases. These studies were done in large numbers of fresh peripheral blood lymphocytes (PBL) and transformed B-cell lines with stable phenotypes derived from individuals with established HLA class II–linked autoimmune diseases, such as Type I diabetes, Graves' disease, Hashimoto's thyroiditis, and Sjögren's syndrome. Examination of discordant diabetic twin pairs also allowed an assessment of the relation between expression of postgenomic HLA class II–linked gene expression and disease outcome. A possible functional consequence of altered transcript abundance was evaluated by a quantitative assay of *Lmp2*- and *Lmp7*-controlled proteasome activity, a step known in mutant cell lines to change peptide selection in the exterior facing groove of the class I protein, a structure essential for T-cell education.

MATERIAL AND METHODS

Patients

Patients with Type I diabetes (n = 59), Graves' disease (n = 1), Sjögren's syndrome (n = 5), Hashimoto's thyroiditis (n = 1), or Type II diabetes (n = 5) were identified in the outpatient clinics of the Massachusetts General Hospital. Only patients with histories and physical examinations consistent with their diagnosis were included in the study. Patients with Graves' disease, Sjögren's syndrome, and Hashimoto's disease showed serological evidence of their specific autoimmune disease. Patients with type I diabetes developed diabetes before age 20, were ketose prone, and were treated continuously with insulin. Normal volunteers and individuals with Type II diabetes had no family history of any of the diseases studied; all Type II diabetic patients developed diabetes after age 45 and had no history of urinary ketones. All control subjects were age matched (patient age ± 5 years).

Patients with polyglandular disease were clinically subdivided into two major classifications on the basis of early age of onset of polyglandular failure with mucocutaneous candidiasis versus the later age of onset (>30 years) of polyglandular failure without mucocutaneous symptoms (TABLE 1). Three patients with multiple endocrine deficiency without mucocutaneous candidiasis were studied: Patient 1 was a 35-year-old man who developed the disease at age 30; at the time of the examination, he had hypoadrenalism and hypothyroidism, as well as autoantibodies to salivary gland tissue and gastric parietal cells. Patient 2 was a 45-year-old woman who showed disease onset at age 32; she had multiorgan failure characterized by hypoadrenalism, hypoparathyroidism, premature ovarian failure, Sjögren's syndrome, anemia, and vitiligo. Patient 3 was a 52-year-old woman with premature ovarian failure, hypoadrenalism, Type I diabetes, Sjögren's syndrome, and celiac disease, with disease onset at 12 years of age. All three patients had a negative history of mucocutaneous candidiasis. Three patients with multiple endocrine deficiency and mucocutaneous candidiasis were also studied: Patient 4 was a 47-year-old woman with onset of mucocutaneous candidiasis at age 18. She also developed hypoadrenalism, hypothyroidism, and hypoparathyroidism; had a poorly characterized chronic anemia; and ceased menses at age 40. Patient 5 was a 20-year-old woman with mucocutaneous candidiasis, type I diabetes, premature ovarian failure, and hypothyroidism. Patient 6 was an 18-year-old woman with chronic muco-

TABLE 1. Comparison of the Clinical Features of the Major Syndromes Characterized by Multiple Endocrine Gland Failure[54a]

	Multiple Endocrine Deficiency Syndrome (Schmidt's Syndrome)	Polyglandular Deficiency with Mucocutaneous Candidiasis
Mucocutaneous candidiasis	Never observed	Present in all cases
Inheritance	Susceptibility related to HLA haplotype	Autosomal recessive; no apparent HLA association
Hypoadrenalism	Common	Common
Hypothyroidism	Common	Less common
Hypoparathyroidism	Less common	Common
Gonadal failure	Less common	Rare
Diabetes mellitus	Less common	Rare
Pituitary insufficiency	Rare	Rare
Autoantibodies to endocrine tissues and gastric parietal cells	Often present	Often present
Sex distribution	Strong female predominance	Female preponderance about 4:1
Time of onset	Usually evident during adult life	Typically evident during childhood but preceded by chronic mucocutaneous moniliasis
Other associated "autoimmune" diseases and characteristics	Pernicious anemia; - hyperthyroidism; celiac disease; alopecia vitiligo; myasthenia gravis; isolated red cell aplasia	Pernicious anemia; malabsorption; alopecia; vitiligo; IGA deficiency; hypergammaglobulinemia; chronic active hepatitis; proliferative glomerulonephritis

cutaneous candidiasis since age 7 and who subsequently developed hypoadrenalism, hypoparathyroidism, and Sjögren's syndrome.

All patients in these studies were maintained on their medication due to the life-saving nature of insulin. Because Type I and Type II polyglandular failure patients take similar medications and because these two groups had contrasting mRNA and flow cytometry data, we believe this study was adequately controlled. Further, the possible influence of medications was removed completely by analyzing immortalized and culture B-cell lines from the same patients.

Analysis of HLA Class I and Self-peptide Density on the Surface of Lymphocytes

PBL were isolated as previously described from 20 to 30 mL of blood freshly collected into heparinized tubes.[4] All patients were studied on at least two occasions separated by over six months. The mouse anti-human class I monoclonal antibody W6/32 (American Type Culture Collection, Rockville, MD) was used for the analysis of human MHC class I determinants because it detects a conformationally dependent form as well as the proteins encoded by diverse HLA alleles. The antibody was incubated with 1×10^6 cells in a volume of 0.2 mL excess of the 50% saturation point, thus eliminating the irrelevant Fc receptor binding and low-affinity binding to the class I heterodimer (class I and β_2-microglobulin without peptide apparent at higher concentrations). For indirect immunofluorescence, W6/32 was used with fluorescein isothiocyanate (FITC)–conjugated goat antibodies to mouse immunoglobulin (Ig) G2a (Tago, Burlingame, CA). Flow cytometer techniques are described in detail.[4]

Production of Epstein-Barr Virus (EBV)–transformed B-cell Lines

Infectious EBV culture supernatants were produced by growing the B95-8 cell line (American Type Culture Collection, Rockville, MD), an EBV-transformed marmoset lymphocyte cell line that releases high titers of transforming EBV particles in medium containing 10% fetal bovine serum. Fresh B cells were isolated from PBL by rosetting with sheep red blood cells and then cultured in medium containing 10% viral supernatant. All EBV cell lines were established in our laboratory with the exception of 12 lines derived from Type I diabetic patients that were obtained from the Human Biological Research Interchange (Philadelphia, PA).

Northern Blot Analysis

Peripheral blood (30 mL) was collected into green top tubes. The PBL pellet was placed on ice before mRNA isolation with a Fast Track kit (Invitrogen, San Diego, CA). One microgram of mRNA per lane was fractionated by electrophoresis on a 1% agarose gel, transferred to Gene Screen plus nylon membranes (Dupont, Delaware, MD), and cross-linked to the filters with an ultraviolet-activated cross-linker. The membranes were incubated at 45 °C for 4 to 12 h in a solution containing 50% formamide, 5 SSPE, 2 Denhardt's reagent, 0.1% SDS, and salmon sperm DNA (10 μg/mL). ^{32}P-Labeled cDNA probes were added directly to the prehybridization buffer, and hybridization was performed at 45 °C overnight. Membranes were washed three times in 1 SSC (standard saline citrate) and 0.1% SDS at room temperature for 20 min each time, and then at 56 °C for 15 min in 0.2 SSC and 0.1% SDS, and were finally exposed overnight at −80 °C to Fuji X-ray film.

Probes

Six probes were used in this study. The TAP1 probe originated from Dr. John Trowsdale at the Imperial Cancer Research Center. For transformation, the vector was grown in MC 1061/p3 cells. The TAP1 insert was removed from the vector via enzymatic cuts with Xba-I or Xho-I. The TAP2 probe originated from Dr. John Trowsdale and represented a 2.5 kb cDNA insert in bluescript. The vector conferred amp resistance and was grown in XL-blue cells. The insert was removed from the plasmid using Xba-I or Xho-I restriction enzymes. LMP7 was similarly a generous gift from Dr. John Trowsdale and represented a 1.3 kb insert in CDM8 with tetra-amp resistance. The plasmic was grown in MC 1061/p3 cells and enzymatically removed from the vector using Xha-I and Xba-I. LMP2 was a gift from Dr. John Trowsdale and represented an 800 bp insert in CDM8 with tetra/amp resistance. Similarly this probe was enzymatically removed with Xho-I or Xba-I enzymatic cuts and expanded on MC 1061/p3 cells. The HLA class I probe was purchased from ATCC (Rockville, MD). This probe was from HLA-B7 and represented a 1.4 kb insert on BR 322 with tetra resistance and was enzymatically removed from the vector with PST-I. The human actin probe was used for a control of absolute mRNA levels. This probe is a 1 kb insert in pGEM4 with amp resistance and removed with BAMH1 and Hind III.

Assay of Proteasome Activity

Proteasome activity was assayed as described with three substrates: a hydrophobic substrate (Suc-LLVY-MCA), a basic substrate (Boc-LRR-MCA), and an acidic substrate (Cbz-LLE-βNA).[55] All activity was accessed on B-cell lines. The proteasome preparations were adjusted to equivalent protein concentrations from the B-cell homogenates and then incubated with the fluorogenic peptide substrate at 37 ° C for 1 hour. The reaction was terminated by adding SDS to a final concentration of 10%, and the fluorescence intensity was measured with excitation and emission wavelengths of 380 and 440 nM for the hyperphobic substrate and 340 and 425 nM for the basic substrate.

Statistical Analysis

Data are presented as means ± SD and were analyzed by a t-test. A p value of < 0.05 was considered statistically significant. For data presented as a percentage change of a patient compared to a matched control, the following formula was used: (patient-control)/control.

Northern Blots

For Northern blots, the intensity of the mRNA signals was quantified using a Microtek Scanner. The scanned blots were then analyzed with an NIH Imager 1.41 program. All scanning was done on two occasions by two separate scientists. All mRNA levels were expressed as relative levels normalized for total mRNA load per gel lane. The relative intensity of mRNA was calculated using the following equation.

$$\text{Relative Intensity} = \frac{\text{Scanned Intensity of Specific Band}}{\text{Scanned Intensity of Specific Band.}}$$

RESULTS

Analysis of HLA Class I Presentation of Self-Peptides as well as TAP1 and TAP2 mRNA Abundance in Polyglandular Failure Patients with and without HLA-linked Disease

Although polyglandular autoimmune disease is clinically rare, genetically distinct subgroups of affected individuals can be identified. Polyglandular autoimmune failure patients with mucocutaneous candidiasis show non-HLA-linked genetic inheritance of disease, whereas those patients without mucocutaneous candidiasis demonstrate HLA-linked susceptibility. TABLE 1 highlights the characteristics of polyglandular autoimmune disease with and without mucocutaneous candidiasis.

Cell-surface expression of HLA class I molecules was analyzed on three occasions over a three-year time span. The mouse monoclonal antibody directed to human class

TABLE 2. Mean Fluorescence Intensity of Cell-surface HLA Class I Expression in Patients with Polyglandular Failure[a]

		Mean Fluorescence Intensity		
	N	T Cells	B Cells	Monocyte-Macrophages
Patients without mucocutaneous candidiasis	3	8 ± 3.9^b	16 ± 4.1^c	24 ± 1.7^d
Patients with mucocutaneous candidiasis	3	16 ± 2.8	27 ± 1.9	37 ± 1.0
Controls	9	18 ± 3.1	22 ± 3.2	36 ± 2.1

[a] Phenotyping was performed on at least three occasions spanning a 3-year period. Different age-matched controls were used for comparisons with patients at different time points. Data are means ± SD.

[b] $p = 0.001$ vs. respective control values. All p values for patients with mucocutaneous candidiasis compared to controls exceeded 0.25.

[c] $p = 0.04$ vs. respective control values.

[d] $p = 0.02$ vs. respective control values.

I, W6/32, detects peptide-filled conformationally correct forms of HLA class I molecules with high affinity but binds poorly to conformationally altered forms of class I molecules and was used to determine density. The density of conformationally correct class I molecules on the surface of T cells, B cells, and monocytes-macrophages from all three polyglandular failure patients without mucocutaneous candidiasis was significantly lower than that on the surface of the corresponding cell types from age-matched controls (FIG. 1, TABLE 2). Each patient showed the same trend compared to random

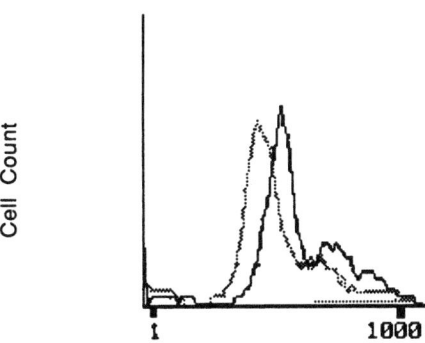

FIGURE 1. Histogram of HLA class I expression in patients with polyglandular failure without mucocutaneous candidiasis analyzed with the W6/32 fluorescence-conjugated antibody. The dashed line represents the patient and the solid line the control. The histogram shown represents a T- and B-cell lymphocyte gate on forward light scatter and two-color fluorescence with W6/32-FITC combined with B1-PE.

controls at each time point of study; consistently the class I presentation defect was detectable in the T cells, B cells, and monocytes-macrophages of the polyglandular autoimmune patients without candidiasis. One of the three patients with autoimmune polyglandular failure had disease onset at age 12 compared to the other two patients with disease onset at age 30 and 32 years. No difference in the magnitude of the class I defect and age of disease onset could be discerned. In contrast to these HLA-linked patients, HLA class I density was phenotypically normal in polyglandular failure patients with candidiasis relative to the same control population. The mean density of HLA class I on T cells was 16 ± 2.8 versus 18 ± 3.1 (p=.67); on B cells the mean density was 27 ± 1.9 versus 22 ± 3.2 (p=.87) and 37 ± 1.0 versus 36 ± 2.1 (p=.77) for patients with mucocutaneous candidiasis compared to random controls. Therefore, patients with multiple endocrine organ destruction selectively have the antigen-presenting cell defect detectable with faulty class I conformation when the disease is controlled, in part, by the HLA region.

Measurement of the basal abundance of transcripts that encode *Tap1* or *Tap2* in EBV cell lines derived from patient B cells avoids interference of systemic infections, drug treatment, or endogenous serum or hormone factors. EBV cell lines derived from each of the three polyglandular failure patients with autoimmunity linked to the HLA region (patients 1 to 3) showed decreased amounts of both *Tap1* and *Tap2* mRNAs compared with EBV cell lines derived from age-matched controls (FIG. 2). By contrast, *Tap1* and *Tap2* mRNA abundance in EBV cell lines of patients with non-HLA

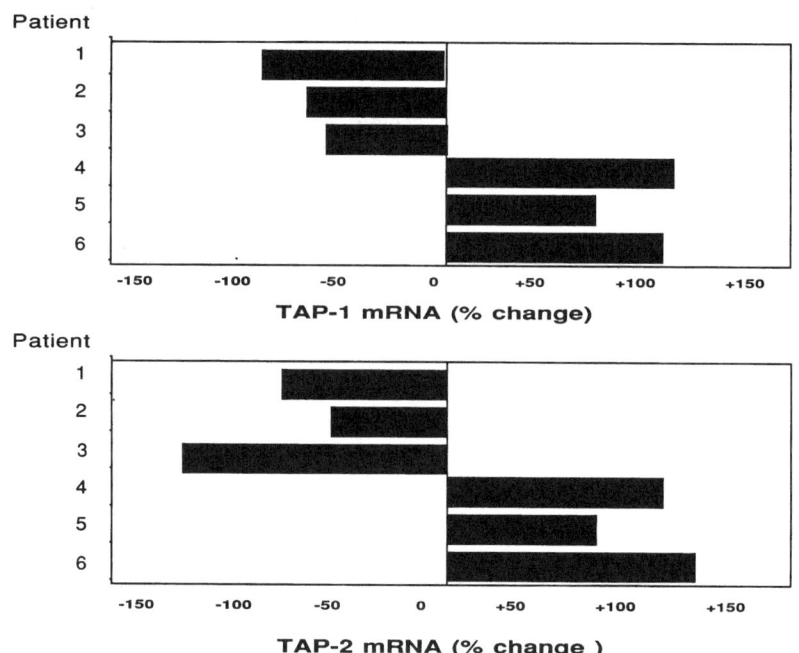

FIGURE 2. Abundance of TAP1 and TAP2 mRNAs in EBV cell lines derived from patients with polyendocrine failure without (patients 1 to 3) or with (patients 4 to 6) HLA linkage. Data are expressed as percentage change relative to EBV cell lines derived from age-matched controls. The percentage change was calculated as (patient-control)/control with normalization to actin.

linked autoreactivity (patients 4 to 6) was increased. The data presented represents a Northern blot of mRNA simultaneously prepared on one occasion for six EBV cell lines on the same membrane. The experiment was repeated on two additional occasions with similar trends. These observations with a limited number of patients with two genetically distinct autoimmune diseases indicate a selective contribution of HLA-linked genes to the class I assembly defect in HLA-linked autoimmunity.

Analysis of Patients with Type I Diabetes

Because Type I diabetes is a relatively common disease compared to both forms of polyglandular failure and demonstrates HLA-associated risk, we expanded our studies of transcript abundance of class I processing genes to this patient group. The abundance of transcripts encoding four proteins (TAP1, TAP2, LMP2, and LMP7) essential for normal class I presentation was determined in PBL from 27 patients with Type I diabetes, a common autoimmune disease with genetic risk factors associated with the HLA class II region. The abundance of TAP1, TAP2, and LMP2 (but not LMP7) mRNAs in pooled data from random subjects was significantly lower in PBL from Type I diabetic patients than in those from age-matched paired controls (FIG. 3).

PBL consist of T cells, B cells, and monocytes-macrophages, and the relative basal amounts of transcripts of the class I assembly genes vary slightly between these cell types. Thus, although the ratios of PBL subsets in individuals with Type I diabetes ap-

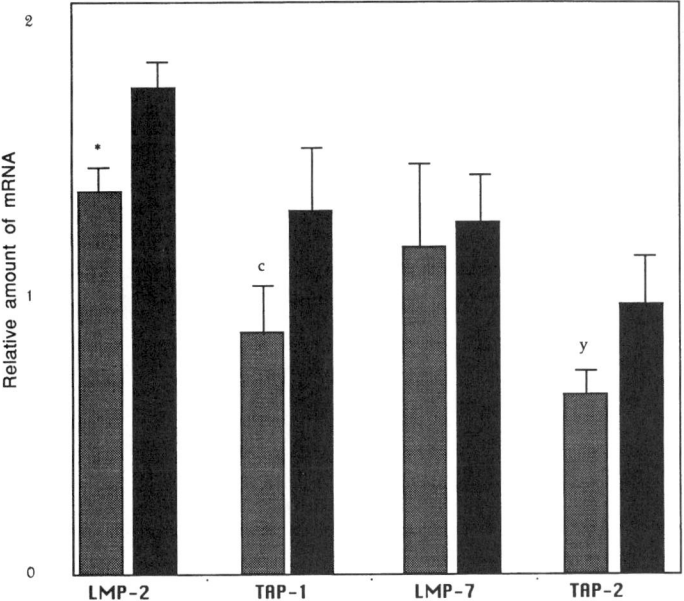

FIGURE 3. Relative abundance of transcripts encoding TAP1, TAP2, LMP2, and LMP7 in peripheral blood lymphocytes from individuals with Type I diabetes (gray boxes) and age-matched controls (black boxes). Data are means ± SD (n=27) and are expressed relative to control actin levels. *p = 0.005, cP = 0.007, yP = 0.02, vs. respective control values.

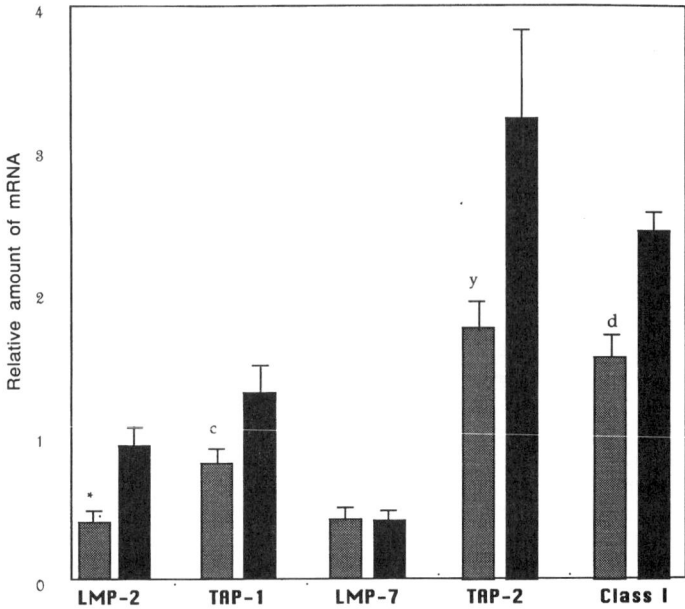

FIGURE 4. Relative abundance of transcripts encoding TAP1, TAP2, LMP2, LMP7, and HLA class I in EBV cell lines from diabetic patients (gray boxes) and age-matched controls (black boxes). Data are means ± SD (n=32) and are expressed relative to actin levels. *p = 0.02, cp = 0.05, yp = 0.004, dp = 0.007 vs. respective control values.

pear similar to those in controls, we also measured the abundance of *Tap1, Tap2, Lmp2,* and *Lmp7* mRNAs in EBV cell lines derived from patients and control subjects to normal levels for cellular subset distributions. Similar to the results with PBL, EBV cell lines from 32 random Type I diabetic patients showed significantly reduced amounts of transcripts encoding *Tap1, Tap2,* and *Lmp2* (but not *Lmp7*) (FIG. 4). The abundance of HLA class I mRNA was also significantly reduced in cell lines from Type I diabetic patients (FIG. 4), consistent with our previous observation that such cell lines show reduced surface expression of conformationally normal class I molecules.[3]

Individual diabetic patients expressed transcript abundance patterns for class I assembly genes distinct from that of the pooled data (TABLE 3). Patient 1, characterized by reduced abundance of *Tap1, Tap2,* and *Lmp2* mRNAs, but normal or increased amounts of *Lmp7* mRNA, was present in 41% of random diabetic patients either evaluated as PBL or as immortalized EBV cell lines. By contrast, 37% of Type I diabetic patients showed reduced amounts of all four mRNAs (pattern 2). Expression patterns 3 to 5 were less common. The frequencies of these expression patterns were identical for PBL and EBV cell lines from the same patient. Numerous patient samples, either fresh PBL or EBV cell lines, were analyzed on more than one occasion and yielded consistently altered levels of class I assembly gene expression. HLA class II genotyping was performed, and no consistent class II allele tracked with a specific pattern of altered transcription.

To control for hyperglycemia-induced changes in transcription of class I–process-

TABLE 3. HLA Class I Processing Genes: Patterns of mRNA Expression for IDDM Patients[a]

Patterns	Percent of Patients	Lmp2	Tap1	Lmp7	Tap2
1	41%	↓	↓	↑/–	↓
2	37%	↓	↓	↓	↓
3	11%	↓	↓	↓	↑/–
4	7%	↑	↓	↓	↓
5	4%	↑	↓	↓	↑

[a] Data represented corresponds to relative mRNA levels of IDDM patients compared to paired control samples.

ing genes, we analyzed transcript abundance in PBL from five Type II diabetic patients. The relative abundance of *Tap1, Tap2, Lmp2,* and *Lmp7* mRNAs did not differ significantly between patients and controls (data not shown). Therefore, the decreased abundance of transcripts of HLA class I–processing genes in autoimmune diabetes was not secondary to hyperglycemia-induced changes in gene transcription. This possibility was eliminated with the use of immortalized Type I diabetic cell lines and the similar evaluation of class I assembly gene expression of Type II diabetic PBL.

Analysis of Type I Diabetic Twins with Discordant Disease Penetrance

For most autoimmune diseases, identical twins show a disease concordance of less than 50 percent. Similarly, such animal models of autoimmunity as the diabetic NOD mouse exhibit variable disease expression among genetically identical animals. We have previously shown that reduced cell-surface expression of conformationally correct HLA class I molecules on defective antigen-presenting cells segregates with diabetes and is predictive of disease expression in human twins discordant for diabetes.[3] We have now measured the abundance of *Tap1, Tap2, Lmp2,* and HLA class I mRNAs in EBV cell lines from eleven sets of twins discordant for diabetes. The data clearly show that diabetic twins consistently showed a reduced abundance of *Tap1, Tap2, Lmp2,* and HLA class I transcripts compared with their normal twins or compared to random controls (TABLE 4, A and C). The data in the TABLE is presented as individual twin sets to highlight the trends. Most nondiabetic twins of discordant pairs showed increased amounts of *Tap2* and HLA class I mRNAs relative to random controls (TABLE 4B) and always elevated transcription products of LMP2, TAP1, TAP2, LMP7, and HLA class I compared to diabetic twins (TABLE 4A). Finally, all diabetic twins showed decreased amounts of *Tap1, Tap2, Lmp2,* and HLA class I mRNAs relative to control individuals, with the exception of diabetic twins from sets 10 and 11, who showed increased amounts of only *Tap2* mRNA (TABLE 4C). The data in TABLE 4 represents mRNA abundance of LMP2, TAP1, LMP7, TAP2, and HLA class I from the same cell line harvested the same day. This experiment was repeated with fresh mRNA production on three separate occasions.

Altered transcript abundance of *Lmp2* and *Lmp7* correlates with altered proteasome cutting activity. The effects of the altered abundance of LMP proteins can be assessed

TABLE 4. Abundance of TAP-1 and TAP-2 mRNAs in EBV Cell Lines from Discordant Diabetic Twin Sets Relative to Each Other and Age-matched Controls[a]

	A. Comparison of mRNA levels between identical twins				
Twins	LMP-2	TAP-1	LMP-7	TAP-2	HLA-Class I
1		−75%		−63%	−58%
2		−40%		−74%	−99%
3		−52%	−25%	−19%	
4	−49%	−42%		−45%	−59%
5	−40%	−64%			−71%
	B. Comparison of mRNA levels of nondiabetic twins to control individuals				
Twins	LMP-2	TAP-1	LMP-7	TAP-2	HLA Class I
1		+19%		+63%	+45%
2		−56%		+52%	+74%
3		−2%		−2%	+50%
4	+.3%	−13%		+33%	+74%
5	−48%	+5%			+78%
6		−44%		+12%	−30%
7		+129%		+241%	−77%
8		−15%		−6%	+38%
9		−47%		+70%	−37%
	C. Comparison of mRNA levels of diabetic twins to control individuals				
Twins	LMP-2	TAP-1	LMP-7	TAP-2	HLA CLASS I
1		−70%		−41%	−40%
2		−74%		−60%	−92%
3					
4	−49%	−50%		−27%	−30%
5	−50%	−54%		—	−66%
10		−11%		+23%	−19%
11		−21%		+34%	−20%

[a] All data are represented as the percent change. A. (Diabetic-nondiabetic twin)/nondiabetic twin. B. (Nondiabetic twin-control)/control. C. (Diabetic twin-control)/control.

by measuring proteasome activity.[32,35] The incorporation of MHC-linked *Lmp2* and *Lmp7* into the proteasome promotes the production of basic and hydrophobic peptides, peptides compatible with human TAP protein transport and optimal class I groove assembly. As Table 5 clearly shows, the diabetic twin B cell–isolated proteasomes have reduced hydrophobic and basic cutting activity and elevated acid substrate cutting. The discordant nondiabetic twin proteasomes exhibited proteasome cutting activity that was intermediary. These differences in proteasome activity are consistent with the observed reduced abundance of *Lmp2* or *Lmp7* transcripts.

Analysis of Patients with Other Autoimmune Diseases

In addition to HLA-linked polyglandular autoimmunity and Type I diabetes, several other autoimmune diseases demonstrate HLA linkage and are associated with antigen presentation defects attributable to faulty class I assembly. Examination of PBL from small numbers of patients with Sjögren's syndrome, Hashimoto's disease, or

TABLE 5. Proteasome Activity in B Cells from Diabetic Twins, Nondiabetic Twins, and Controls[a]

	Hydrophobic		Basic		Acid	
Diabetic	1273 ± 61		2086 ± 63		923 ± 33	
		.009		.005		.013
Normal Twin	1395 ± 114		2325 ± 89		768 ± 34	
		.000		.000 (.06)		.000
		.0001		.000		.000
Control	1906 ± 52		3126 ± 104		886 ± 32	

[a] All data are represented as means ± standard error. Data are expressed as fluorescence intensity units for at least 5 separate experiments. The p values were obtained from a paired t-test.

TABLE 6. Abundance of TAP-1 and TAP-2 mRNAs in PBL from Patients with Graves' Disease, Hashimoto's Disease, or Sjögren's Syndrome Expressed as Percentage Change Relative to PBL from Age-matched Controls

			mRNA (% change)	
	Patients	N	TAP-1	TAP-2
	Graves' disease	1	−54	−36
	Hashimoto's disease	1	−19	−47
	Sjögren's syndrome	5	−32	−44

Graves' disease also revealed a decreased abundance of *Tap1* and *Tap2* mRNAs (TABLE 6). This data is consistent with the possible similar genetic role of the HLA region in various autoimmune diseases with risk.

DISCUSSION

Our results suggest that autoimmune diseases with HLA linkage are characterized, in part, by quantitative defects in the amount of transcription products of such class I-processing genes as *Tap1, Tap2, Lmp2,* and/or *Lmp7.* These defects may be responsible, in part, for the previously observed impairment in the cell-surface expression of class I protein complexed with self-peptide and be related to the abnormal antigen presentation in such conditions. Patients with Type I diabetes, Sjögren's syndrome, polyglandular failure without mucocutaneous candidiasis, Graves' disease, and Hashimoto's disease all showed a reduced abundance of transcripts of most class I assembly genes. The observation that, regardless of the target organ attacked, similar decreases in the abundance of transcripts of HLA-linked class I–processing genes were apparent suggests that the class I assembly defects in individuals with clinically diverse autoimmune diseases are determined, in part, with a *cis-* or *trans-*contribution from within the HLA region and may prove a necessary milieu for inappropriate autoreactivity. This conclusion is further supported by the observation that multiple endocrine organ failure patients with non-HLA-linked disease lack defects in both class I assembly and the transcription of HLA class I–processing genes. Non-HLA-linked autoimmune disease may be caused by self-destructive mechanisms independent of defective antigen processing or class I assembly malfunction. These data correlate with recent evidence that polyglandular autoimmune patients with candidiasis can have an unusual histology picture devoid of lymphoid infiltrates in the setting of humoral autoreactivity.[53] Inasmuch as antigen processing is a critical step for T-cell education, this may be an error specific for this disease category.

Examination of lymphocytes from Type I diabetic patients, in detail, revealed subsets of patients with different but stable errors in quantitative expression of *Tap1, Tap2, Lmp2,* and *Lmp7*. Most patients showed reduced amounts of *Tap1, Tap2,* and *Lmp2* mRNAs but increased or normal amounts of *Lmp7* mRNA. The next most prevalent pattern was a reduced abundance of all four mRNAs of the HLA-linked antigen-processing genes. These consistent but subtle quantitative errors in the expression of class I–processing genes were observed in both PBL and EBV-transformed B-cell lines from the same patients on numerous occasions.

Identical twins show a marked discordance (>50%) in the penetrance of autoimmune disease. We have shown previously that only the affected twin in pairs discordant for Type I diabetes, exclusively, show the defect in antigen presentation and class I assembly.[3] We have now shown that the abundance of *Tap1, Tap2,* and *Lmp2* mRNAs tend to be only reduced in the diabetic twin of discordant pairs. The nondiabetic twin tended to overexpress class I–processing genes. It should also be noted that, although monozygotic twins are genetically identical, their immune systems are divergent, with unique B- and T-cell gene rearrangements driven by random occurrences.

The observed defects in transcription abundance of class I–processing genes in individuals with autoimmune disease represents an average of 20 to 50% reduction in transcript abundance. The magnitude of these defects is thus similar to that of the decrease in surface class I expression, which suggests that transcription of class I assembly genes could be rate limiting in maintaining the surface density of conformationally correct class I proteins. On a functional level, the altered proteasome activity of the diabetic twin was confirmed by the demonstration of preferential acid substrate cutting instead of hydrophobic and basic substrate cutting. Such a proteasome cutting pattern in diabetic antigen-processing cells is consistent with the proteasome producing a repertoire of peptides in the human, less optimally compatible with TAP and the class I–binding groove. The altered proteasome cutting activity correlates with the mRNA expression patterns. The current study does not provide data demonstrating that the reduced relative levels of class I processing transcripts are secondary to reduced production or increased degradation. Future studies will be directed towards this issue. Additionally, mRNA is cumbersome and labor intensive to measure, making it unfeasible for mass population screening. The purpose of this paper and data instead is to start to dissect the pathophysiology in diverse humans with autoimmunity at the functional level of altered antigen processing. Defects in surface class I expression and mRNA of this magnitude may be sufficient to affect T-cell education. Certainly they are consistent with alterations of peptide production for class I assembly. It is known that class I surface density decreases by 10 to 40% in mice in which the genes encoding *Lmp7* or *Tap1* have been ablated and that show abnormalities in T-cell selection characterized by altered T-cell subsets.[56]

The prominent role of antigen processing, maintenance of class I density, and T-cell education has been established in both humans and mouse models. Although the first human description of defective antigen-processing linked to autoimmunity and *in vitro* autoreactivity was challenging to the common beliefs at the time, more recent murine transgenic models have similarly been linked to the role of antigen processing, class I assembly, and autoreactivity.[3,31] For instance, total ablation of *Tap* genes culminates in altered T-cell selection and *in vitro* and sometimes *in vivo* autoreactivity, similar in many ways to diabetic models.[6-8] In the human, statistical linkage data attempting to identify the possible HLA disease gene controlling this defect is yielding data in favor of, as well as against, the *Tap* and *Lmp* genes, and therefore the true candidate (or type of defects where quantitative or qualitative, or both) will require further studies. In this study, quantitative differences in the assembly of conformationally normal class I and self-peptide complexes correlate with the expression of diverse forms of only HLA-linked autoreactivity, suggesting this genetic region could contribute candidate gene or genes. Further studies are required to elucidate the cause of the decreased expression of HLA class I–processing genes in individuals with HLA class II–linked autoimmune diseases, and to determine the mechanism of target specificity of these common afflictions.

ACKNOWLEDGMENTS

We thank Dr. John Trowsdale for cDNA probes, the Human Biological Data Interchange for diabetic cell lines, and Lynne Murphy for secretarial services.

REFERENCES

1. MARRACK, P. & J. KAPPLER. 1987. The T cell receptor. Science **238**: 1073–1079.
2. TSOMIDES, T.J. & H.N. EISEN. 1991. Antigenic structures recognized by cytotoxic T-lymphocytes. J. Biol. Chem. **266**: 3357–3360.
3. FAUSTMAN, D. *et al.* 1991. Linkage of faulty major histocompatibility complex class I to autoimmune diabetes. Science **254**: 1756–1761.
4. FU, Y. *et al.* 1993. Defective major histocompatibility complex class I expression on lymphoid cells in autoimmunity. J. Clin. Invest. **91**: 2301–2307.
5. LI, F. *et al.* 1995. Reduced expression of peptide-loaded HLA class I molecules on multiple sclerosis lymphocytes. Ann. Neurol. **38**: 147–154.
6. GLAS, R. *et al.* 1994. The CD8$^+$ T cell repertoire in β_2-microglobulin-deficient mice is biased towards reactivity against self-major histocompatibility complex class I. J. Exp. Med. **179**: 661–672.
7. ALDRICH, C.J. *et al.* 1994. Positive selection of self- and alloreactive CD8$^+$ T cells in TAP-1 mutant mice. Proc. Natl. Acad. Sci. USA **91**: 6525–6528.
8. APASOV, S. & M. SITOVSKY. 1993. Highly lytic CD8+, $\alpha\beta$ T-cell receptor cytotoxic T cells with major histocompatibility complex (MHC) class I antigen-directed cytotoxicity in β_2-microglobulin, MHC class I-deficient mice. Proc. Natl. Acad. Sci. USA **90**: 2837–2841.
9. LAMOUSE-SMITH, E. *et al.* 1993. β_2-M -/- knockout mice contain low levels of CD8+ cytotoxic T lymphocytes that mediate specific tumor rejection. J. Immunol. **151**: 6281–6290.
10. APASOV, S.G. & M.V. SITOVSKY. 1994. Development and antigen specificity of CD8+ cytotoxic T lymphocytes in β_2-microglobulin-negative, MHC class I-deficient mice in response to immunization with tumor cells. J. Immunol. **152**: 2087–2097.
11. DE LA SALLE, H. *et al.* 1994. Homozygous human Tap peptide transporter mutation in HLA class I deficiency. Science **265**: 237–241.
12. ASHTON-RICKARDT, P.G. *et al.* 1994. Evidence for a differential avidity model of T cell selection in the thymus. Cell **76**: 651–663.
13. HOGQUIST, K.A. *et al.* 1994. T cell receptor antagonist peptides induce positive selection. Cell **76**: 17–27.
14. DEVERSON, E.V. *et al.* 1990. MHC class II region encoding proteins related to the multidrug resistance family of transmembrane transporters. Nature **348**: 738–741.
15. TROWSDALE, J. *et al.* 1990. Sequences encoded in the class II region of the MHC related to the 'ABC' superfamily of transporters. Nature **348**: 741–744.
16. SPIES, T. *et al.* 1990. A gene in the human major histocompatibility complex class II region controlling the class I antigen presentation pathway. Nature **348**: 744–747.
17. MONACO, J.J. *et al.* 1990. Transport protein genes in the murine MHC: possible implications for antigen processing. Science **250**: 1723–1726.

18. LIVINGSTONE, A.M. *et al.* 1989. A transacting major histocompatibility complex-linked gene whose alleles determine gain and loss changes in the antigenic structure of a classical class I molecule. J. Exp. Med. **170:** 777–795.
19. NEEFJES, J.J. & H.L. PLOEGH. 1992. Inhibition of endosomal proteolytic activity by leupeptin blocks surface expression of MHC class II molecules and their conversion to SDS resistant αβ heterodimers in endosomes. EMBO J. **11:** 411–416.
20. SHEPHERD, J.C. *et al.* 1993. TAP1-dependent peptide translocation *in vitro* is ATP dependent and peptide selective. Cell **74:** 577–584.
21. MONACO, J.J. & H.O. MCDEVITT. 1982. Identification of a fourth class of proteins linked to the murine major histocompatibility complex. Proc. Natl. Acad. Sci. USA **79:** 3001–3005.
22. PARHAM, P. 1990. Antigen processing. Transporters of delight. Nature **348:** 674–675.
23. GOLDBERG, A.L. & K.L. ROCK. 1992. Proteolysis, proteasomes and antigen presentation. Nature **357:** 375–379.
24. GLYNNE, R. *et al.* 1991. A proteasome-related gene between the two ABC transporter loci in the class II region of the human MHC. Nature **353:** 357–360.
25. KELLY, A. *et al.* 1991. Second proteasome-related gene in the human MHC class II region. Nature **353:** 667–668.
26. ORTIZ-NAVARETTE, V. *et al.* 1991. Subunit of the '20S' proteasome (multicatalytic proteinase) encoded by the major histocompatibility complex. Nature **353:** 662–664.
27. LI, F. *et al.* 1994. Abnormal class I assembly and peptide presentation in the diabetic NOD mouse. Proc. Natl. Acad. Sci. USA **91:** 11128–11132.
28. PEARCE, R.B. *et al.* 1993. Polymorphism in the mouse Tap-1 gene. Association with abnormal CD8+ T cell development in the nonobese nondiabetic mouse. J. Immunol. **151:** 5338–5347.
29. WICKER, L.S. *et al.* 1992. Expression of intra-MHC transporter (Ham) genes and class I antigens in diabetes-susceptible NOD mice. Science **256:** 1826–1831.
30. SERREZE, D.V. *et al.* 1996. MHC class I-mediated antigen presentation and induction of CD8+ cytotoxic T-cell responses in autoimmune diabetes-prone NOD mice. Diabetes **45:** 902–908.
31. HUANG, R. *et al.* 1995. Elimination of self-peptide major histocompatibility complex class I reactivity in NOD and beta$_2$-microglobulin-negative mice. Diabetes **44:** 1114–1120.
32. TAKEI, I. *et al.* 1992. Suppression of development of diabetes in NOD mice by lactate dehydrogenase virus infection. J. Autoimmunity **5:** 665–674.
33. SATOH, J. *et al.* 1988. Treatment with streptococcal preparation (OK0432) suppresses anti-islet autoimmunity and prevents diabetes in BB rats. Diabetes **37:** 1188–1194.
34. AKI, M. *et al.* 1994. Interferon-γ induces different subunit organizations and functional diversity of proteasomes. J. Biochem. **115:** 257–269.
35. VAN KAER, L. *et al.* 1994. Altered peptidase and viral-specific T cell response in LMP-2 mutant mice. Immunity **1:** 533–541.
36. WILBERZ, S. *et al.* 1991. Persistent MHV (mouse hepatitis virus) infection reduces the incidence of diabetes mellitus in non-obese diabetic mice. Diabetologia **34:** 2–5.
37. HERMITTE, L. *et al.* 1990. Paradoxical lessening of autoimmune processes in nonobese diabetic mice after infection with the diabetogenic variant of encephalomyocarditis virus. Eur. J. Immunol. **20:** 1297–1303.
38. KAWAMURA, T. *et al.* 1993. Prevention of autoimmune type I diabetes by CD4+ suppressor T cells in superantigen-treated nonobese diabetic mice. J. Immunol. **151:** 4362–4370.
39. KINO, K. *et al.* 1990. An immunomodulating protein Ling Zhi-8 (LZ-8) prevents insulitis in nonobese diabetic mice. Diabetologia **33:** 713–718.
40. ELIAS, D. *et al.* 1990. Induction and therapy of autoimmune diabetes in the nonobese diabetic (NOD/lt) mouse by a 65-kDa heat shock protein. Proc. Natl. Acad. Sci. USA **87:** 1576–1580.
41. SADELAIN, M.W.J. *et al.* 1990. Prevention of type I diabetes in NOD mice by adjuvant immunotherapy. Diabetes **39:** 583–589.
42. MCINERNEY, M.F. *et al.* 1991. Prevention of insulitis and diabetes onset by treatment with complete Freund's adjuvant in NOD mice. Diabetes **40:** 715–725.
43. HUANG, R. *et al.* 1995. Elimination of self-peptide major histocompatibility complex class I reactivity in NOD and β2-microglobulin-negative mice. Diabetes **44:** 1114–1120.

44. MUIR, A. & N.K. MACLAREN. 1991. Autoimmune diseases of the adrenal glands, parathyroid glands, gonads, and hypothalamicpituitary axis. Endocrinol. Metab. Clin. North Am. **20:** 619–644.
45. AHOHEN, P. *et al.* 1988. The expression of autoimmune polyglandular disease Type I appears associated with several HLA-A antigens but now with HLA-DR. J. Clin. Endocrinol. Metab. **66:** 1152–1157.
46. MCKUSICK, V.A. 1992. Mendelian Inheritance in Man. Johns Hopkins University Press. Baltimore.
47. MACLAREN, N.K. & W.J. RILEY. 1986. Inherited susceptibility to autoimmune Addison's disease is linked to human leukocyte antigens-DR3 and/or DR4, except when associated with type I autoimmune polyglandular syndrome. J. Clin. Endocrin. Metab. **62:** 455–459.
48. RABINOWE, S.L. & G.S. EISENBARTH. 1986. Polyglandular autoimmunity. Adv. Intern. Med. **31:** 293–307.
49. AALTONEN, J. *et al.* 1994. An autosomal locus causing autoimmune disease: autoimmune polyglandular disease type I assigned to chromosome 21. Nat. Genet. **8:** 83–87.
50. AHONEN, P. 1985. Autoimmune polyendocrinopathy-candidosis-ectodermal-dystrophy (APECED): Autosomal recessive inheritance. Clin. Genet. **27:** 535–542.
51. AALTONEN, J. *et al.* 1993. Autoimmune polyglandular disease type I. Exclusion map using amplifiable multiallelic markers in a microtiter well format. Eur. J. Hum. Genet. **1:** 164–171.
52. AHOHEN, P. *et al.* 1990. Clinical variation of autoimmune polyendocrinopathy-candidiasis-ectodermal dystrophy (APECED) in a series of 68 patients. N. Engl. J. Med. **322:** 1829–1836.
53. WAGNER, R. et al. 1994. Lack of immunohistological changes in the islets of non-diabetic, autoimmune, polyendocrine patients with beta-selective GAD-specific islet cell antibodies. Diabetes **43:** 851–856.
54. BOTTAZZO, G.F. *et al.* 1974. Islet-cell antibodies in diabetes mellitus with autoimmune polyendocrine deficiencies. Lancet **2:** 1279–1283.
54a. CECIL: Textbook of Medicine, 19th Ed. 1988. J.B. Wyngaarden & L.H. Smith, Eds. W.B. Saunders Company. Philadelphia, PA.
55. GACZYNSKA, M. *et al.* 1994. Peptidase activities of proteasomes are differentially regulated by the major histocompatibility complex-encoded genes for LMP-2 and LMP-7. Proc. Natl. Acad. Sci. USA **91:** 9213–9217.
56. FEHLING, H.J. *et al.* 1994. MHC class I expression in mice lacking the proteasome subunit LMP-7. Science **265:** 1234–1237.

Clinical Implications of the Dry Mouth
Oral Mucosal Diseases

J.L. JENSEN[a] AND P. BARKVOLL

Department of Oral Surgery and Oral Medicine, Faculty of Dentistry, University of Oslo, P.O. Box 1109 Blindern, 0317 Oslo, Norway

ABSTRACT: Salivary hypofunction caused by salivary gland disease, medication, or radiation may predispose for secondary oral mucosal diseases. In these patients the protective coating of saliva is reduced or absent, leaving the oral mucosa more vulnerable. Candidiasis, burning mouth syndrome, and white lesions of the oral mucosa are increased in frequency. The aim of management is to prevent oral pathological changes. The management procedure may include proper oral hygiene, saliva-stimulating agents, or saliva substitutes, depending on the severity of the salivary dysfunction. Treatment includes antifungal therapy if candidiasis is diagnosed. In severely distressed patients, local or systemic corticosteroids may be indicated. Precautions, like refraining from smoking and avoiding toothpastes containing sodium lauryl sulfate, should also be taken. In the future, agents combining antibacterial and antiinflammatory actions, like triclosan, may show promising effects in patients with oral mucosal diseases secondary to salivary hypofunction.

INTRODUCTION

Salivary hypofunction, defined as a true reduction in the amount of saliva produced by the salivary glands, is most frequently caused by drugs with anticholinergic side effects, by diseases like Sjögren's syndrome, or it is a sequel of radiation to the head or neck area. Xerostomia, the subjective feeling of dry mouth, is a common complaint in the population, especially among elderly women.[1,2] The degree of xerostomia and salivary hypofunction do not always correlate.[3] In this presentation, the clinical consequences of salivary hypofunction are discussed.

Saliva has many functions in the oral cavity.[4] Among them are the formation of a mucin layer on the oral mucosa and pellicle formation of the teeth. This allows for facilitated movements during speech, eating, and swallowing. The mucin layer is the most important nonimmune defence mechanisms of the oral cavity.[5] In a patient suffering from severe salivary hypofunction, oral functions are associated with pain or discomfort, and the quality of life may be reduced. The most prevalent oral mucosal diseases in patients with dry mouth are outlined below.

ORAL MUCOSAL DISEASES

Oral candidiasis is a common finding in dry mouth patients (FIG. 1). Reduced salivary secretion is one of the predisposing factors for oral candidiasis, as are diabetes, smoking, dentures, reduced immune responsiveness, and treatment with antibiotics. Frequently, one or more of the predisposing factors are seen in one patient. Various

---

[a] Tel: +47 22 85 22 05; fax: +47 22 85 23 41; e-mail: jljensen@odont.uio.no

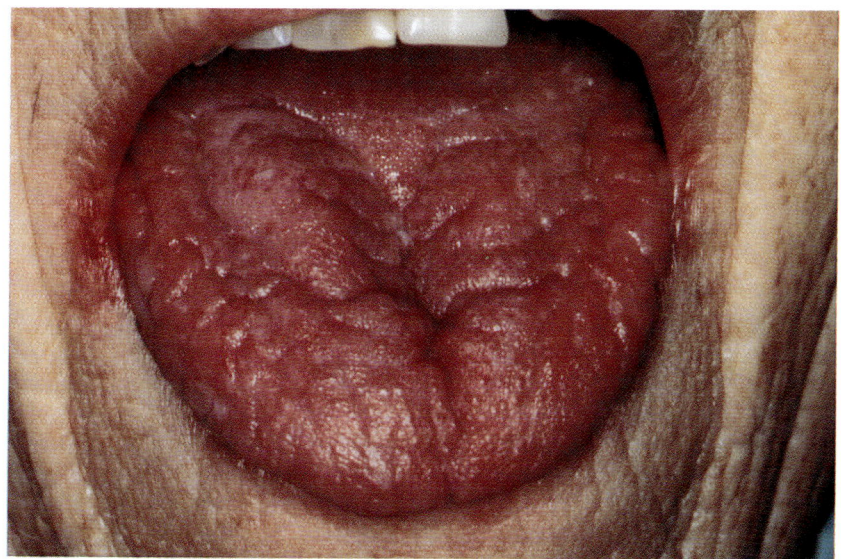

FIGURE 1. Oral candidiasis in a patient with dry mouth.

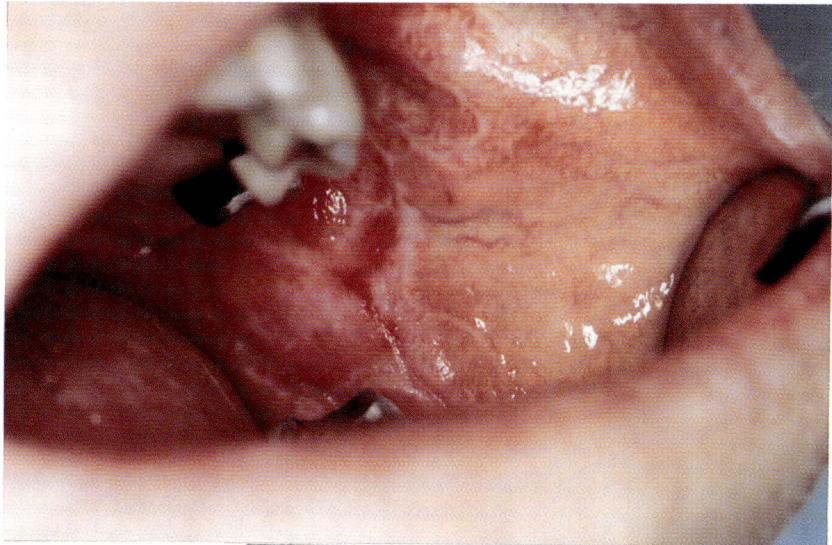

FIGURE 2. Oral lichen planus in a patient with salivary hypofunction. Both erosive and atrophic forms are present.

forms of oral candidiasis exist, and the fungal infection may be associated with burning and itching of the oral mucosa. The infection should be diagnosed to ensure proper treatment. For diagnosis, commercial kits (Oricult N, Orion Diagnostica) or Sabouraud's medium can be used. Other diagnostic possibilities include biopsy with PAS staining or cytological smears.

In a patient with dry mouth, it is important to bear in mind that severely reduced salivary secretion does not allow the solubilization of antifungal tablets, so that drugs in liquid form should be used. Second, treatment should last for four weeks, not one to two as in normal patients. Third, the predisposing factors often remain, and the patients may experience a new infection with time. Therefore, patient compliance is of great importance and patient information is time consuming.

Lichen planus is a common disease of the skin that also may be seen in the oral cavity. Oral lichen planus (OLP) is a benign, inflammatory condition of the oral mucous membranes affecting between 0.1% and 2% of the population. OLP appears to be more frequent in dry mouth patients. Many variants of lichen planus exist: reticular, plaque, and papular forms are associated with an unbroken epithelium, whereas the erosive/ulcerative, atrophic, and bullous forms are associated with destruction of the epithelial surface. In a patient with dry mouth, the forms of lichen planus disrupting the mucosa are painful, as the mucosa is devoid of the protective mucin layer. In FIGURE 2, the oral mucosa of a patient with a mixed OLP condition is demonstrated.

Fungal infections are frequently superimposed on these OLP lesions, increasing the discomfort of the patient. Actually, many patients benefit greatly from antifungal therapy alone. The use of local or systemic corticosteroid treatment is indicated if the patient is severely distressed. Saliva stimulation regimens may also be helpful in increasing the patient's comfort. Detailed treatment procedures of OLP are outlined in "Meeting Report, Third European Congress of Oral Medicine."[6]

BURNING MOUTH SYNDROME (BMS)

In this condition, the oral mucosa appears normal, but the patient complains of a burning sensation from certain areas of the mouth, the tongue being the most common site. Salivary hypofunction is one of the precipitating factors for BMS, cancerphobia, social distress, diabetes, and oral *Candida* infection being others. A management protocol for BMS is given by Lamey,[7] including hemantinic assays, evaluation of vitamin B and blood glucose, saliva tests, antifungal treatment, psychological assessment, as well as assessment of denture status and parafunctional habits. This regimen was claimed to render 70% of the patients asymptomatic.

STUDIES OF SOME COMPONENTS OF ORAL HYGIENE PRODUCTS AFFECTING THE ORAL MUCOSA

At the faculty of dentistry of the University of Oslo, there is a long tradition for studying effects of various toothpaste and mouthrinse ingredients on the oral mucosa tissue. In these studies recurrent aphthous ulcers (RAU) is used as an oral mucosal disease model. RAU is characterized by the development of painful, recurring single or multiple necrotizing ulcers of the nonkeratinized oral and pharyngeal mucosa, and the tongue. Sodium lauryl sulfate (SLS) is the foaming agent in most commercial toothpastes. SLS is a strong denaturing agent with high affinity for proteins, thereby increasing epithelial permeability. In a double-blind cross-over study, a significantly

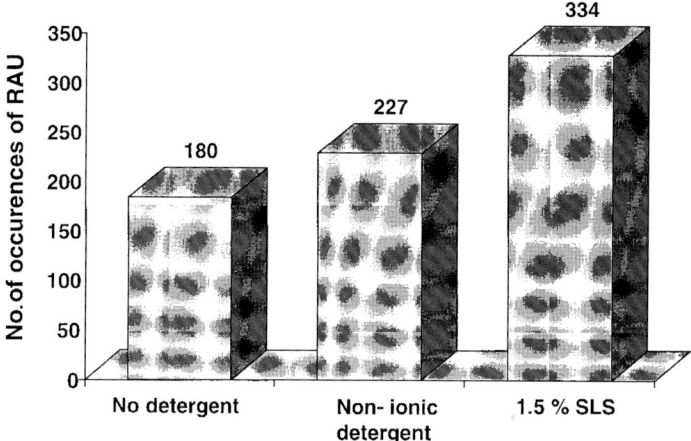

FIGURE 3. Effect of avoiding SLS on the number of occurrences of recurrent aphthous ulcers in 25 patients.[8]

higher frequency of aphthous ulcers was demonstrated when patients brushed with an SLS-containing versus a detergent-free toothpaste (FIG. 3).[8] Also patients with OLP who avoided SLS-containing toothpaste benefited greatly.[9] It therefore seems reasonable to claim that a detergent-free toothpaste is well suited for patients with oral mucosal diseases.

In the future, agents with a combined antibacterial and antiinflammatory potential may be of interest for patients suffering from various oral mucosal diseases. Triclosan, (2,4,4'-trichloro-2'-hydroxydiphenyl ether), a lipid soluble antimicrobial agent, present in toothpastes and mouthrinses, has recently been shown to exhibit antiinflammatory properties.[10,11] Furthermore, it has been shown that triclosan prevents chemical cytotoxicity by SLS to human gingival fibroblasts, and that it also may have a specific inhibiting effect on prostaglandin and leukotriene production.[12] Triclosan is also known to exhibit a certain analgesic effect[13] and to penetrate skin and oral mucosa.[14] Triclosan has been shown to effectively reduce the occurrences of ulcers in patients suffering from RAU.[15] Furthermore, it has been demonstrated that triclosan may reduce the oral mucosal desquamation provoked by SLS.[16]

TREATMENT

In drug-induced salivary hypofunction, any alternative medication, dose reduction or drug withdrawal should be discussed with the patient's physician. If the cause of salivary dysfunction cannot be eliminated, treatment is multifactorial. A clinical management scheme has been prepared regarding subjective and objective findings in patients suffering from oral discomfort (FIG. 4). Treatment includes antifungal therapy if candidiasis is diagnosed. In severely distressed patients, local or systemic corticosteroids may be indicated. Precautions, like refraining from smoking and avoiding toothpastes containing SLS should also be taken. The management procedure may include proper oral hygiene, saliva-stimulating agents, or saliva substitutes, depending on the severity of the salivary dysfunction.

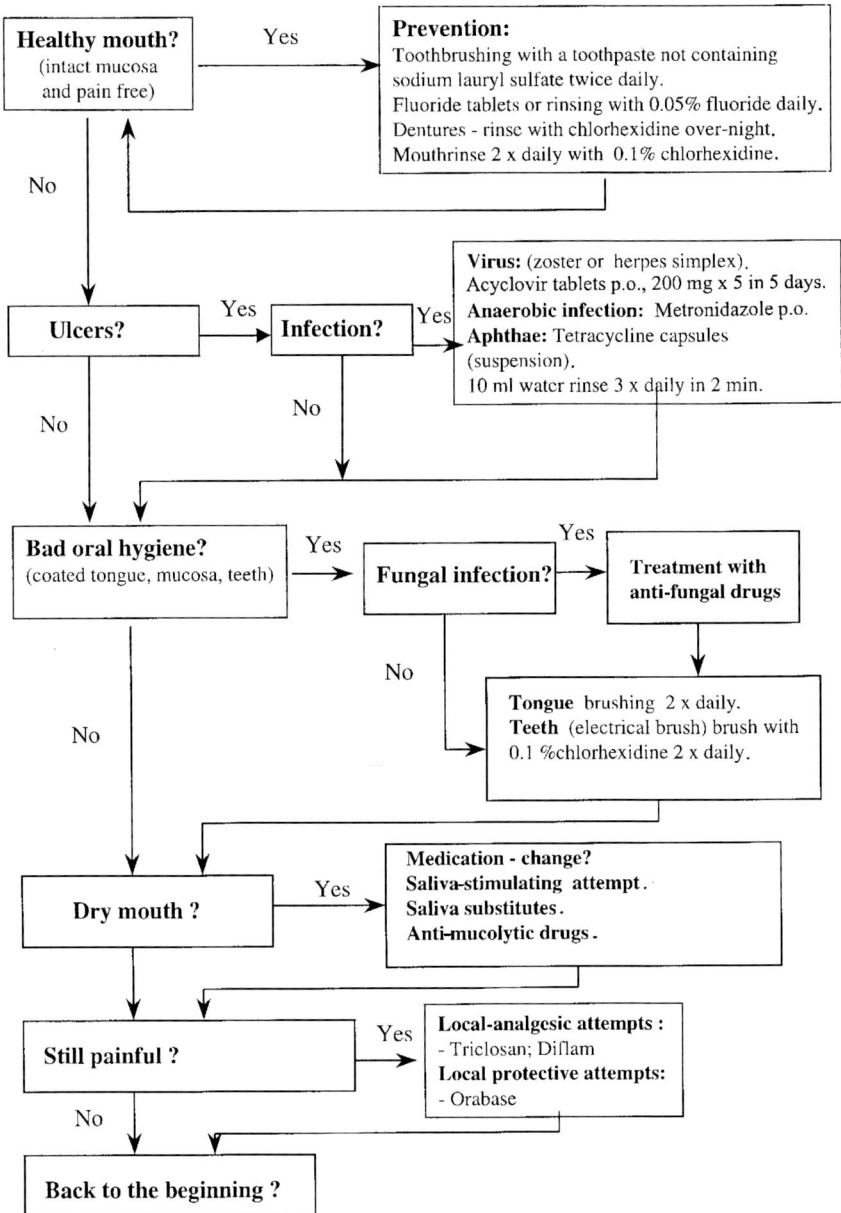

FIGURE 4. Clinical management scheme for patients with oral discomfort.

The degree of salivary dysfunction should be assessed by performing salivary tests. Salivary secretory rates in both resting and stimulating conditions should be measured.[17] Obtaining the values of the quantity of unstimulated and stimulated whole saliva may be used to ensure that the patient has a capacity to stimulate the salivary secretion and for future comparisons. Unfortunately, tests of the quality of saliva are not available in the clinic. Studies in patients with rheumatoid arthritis and severe sicca complaints from eyes and mouth have demonstrated reduced secretion of selected salivary proteins like proline-rich proteins, statherin, and histatins from the submandibular gland.[18] A reduced salivary protein secretion may further compromise salivary functions.

Saliva stimulation is achieved by chewing gum and lozenges, preferably sweetened by xylitol because of its antibacterial effects. Other available treatment modalities include such parasympathomimetic agents as pilocarpine,[19] marketed as Salagen in the United States. If the patient has no saliva stimulatory potential, saliva substitutes may be used, but water rinses and the use of various oils seem to be as helpful. This paper has focused on oral mucosal diseases in patients with salivary hypofunction. However, another oral health hazard in dry mouth patients is the increased risk of caries. Use of topical fluorides is therefore mandatory.

REFERENCES

1. ÖSTERBERG, T., S. LANDAHL & B. HEDEGARD. 1984. Salivary flow, saliva, pH and buffering capacity in 70-year-old men and women. J. Oral Rehabil. **11:** 157–170.
2. NEDERFORS, T. 1996. Xerostomia: Prevalence and pharmacotherapy with special reference to β-adrenoceptor antagonists. Thesis, University of Gothenburg, Sweden.
3. FOX, P.C., K.A. BUSCH & B.J. BAUM. 1987. Subjective reports of xerostomia and objective measures of salivary gland performance. JADA **115:** 581–4.
4. MANDEL, I.D. 1989. The role of saliva in maintaining oral homeostasis. JADA **119:** 298–304.
5. TABAK, L.A., M.J. LEVINE, I.W. MANDEL & S.A. ELLISON. 1982. Role of salivary mucins in the protection of the oral cavity. J. Oral Pathol. **11:** 1–17.
6. Meeting report. Third European Congress of Oral Medicine. 1997. Oral Dis. **3:** 43–48.
7. LAMEY, P-J. 1996. Burning mouth syndrome. Dermatol. Clin. **14:** 339–354.
8. HERLOFSON, B.B. & P. BARKVOLL. 1996. The effect of two toothpaste detergents on the frequency of recurrent aphthous ulcers. Acta Odontol. Scand. **54:** 150–153.
9. BARKVOLL, P. 1992. Considerations concerning the sodium lauryl sulfate content of dentifrices as an ingredient of dentifrices. *In* Oxford Press, London. G. Embery & G. Rølla, Eds. Clinical and Biological Aspects of Dentifrices.
10. BARKVOLL, P. & G. RÖLLA. 1994. Triclosan protects the skin against dermatitis caused by sodium lauryl sulphate exposure. J. Clin. Periodontol. **21:** 717–719.
11. KJÆRHEIM, V., P. BARKVOLL, S.M. WAALER & G. RÖLLA. 1995. Triclosan inhibits histamine-induced inflammation in human skin J. Clin. Periodontol. **22:** 423–426.
12. GAFFAR, A., D. SCHERL, J. AFFLITTO & E.J. COLEMAN. 1995. The effect of triclosan on mediators of gingival inflammation. J. Clin. Periodontol. **22:** 480–484.
13. KJAERHEIM, V., A. ROED, P. BRODIN & G. ROLLA. 1995. Effects of triclosan on the rat phrenic nerve-diaphragm preparation. J. Clin. Periodontol. **22:** 488–493.
14. BLACK, J.G., D. HOWES & T. RUTHERFORD. 1975. Percutaneous absorption and metabolism of Irgasan® DP300. Toxicology **3:** 33–47.
15. SKAARE, A.B., G. EIDE, B.B. HERLOFSON & P. BARKVOLL. 1996. The effect of toothpaste containing *triclosan* on oral mucosal desquamation—A model study. J. Clin. Periodontol. **23:** 1100–1103.
16. SKAARE, A.B., B.B. HERLOFSON & P. BARKVOLL. 1996. Mouthrinses containing triclosan reduce the incidence of recurrent aphthous ulcers. J. Clin. Periodontol. **23:** 778–781.
17. ATKINSON, J.C., C. DAWES, T. ERICSON, P.C. FOX, B.K. GANDARA, D. MALAMUD, I.D. MANDEL, M. NAVAZESH & L.A. TABAK. 1993. Guidelines for saliva nomenclature and collection. *In* Saliva as a Diagnostic Fluid. D. Malamud & L. Tabak, Eds.: **694:** xi–xii. Annals of the New York Academy of Sciences. New York.

18. JENSEN, J.L., T. UHLIG, T.K. KVIEN & T. AXELL. 1997. Characteristics of rheumatoid arthritis patients with self-reported sicca symptoms: Evaluation of medical, salivary and oral parameters. Oral Dis. **3**: 254–261.
19. FOX, P.C., J.C. ATKINSON, A.A. MACYNSKI, A. WOLF, D.S. KUNG, I.H. VALDEZ, W. JACKSON, R.A. DELAPHENA, J. SHIROKY & B.J. BAUM. 1991. Pilocarpine treatment of salivary gland hypofunction and dry mouth (xerostomia). Arch. Intern. Med. **151**: 1149–1152.

Combination Gene Therapy for Salivary Gland Cancer

BERT W. O'MALLEY JR.[a] AND DAQING LI

Department of Otolaryngology-HNS, Johns Hopkins University, P.O. Box 41402, Johns Hopkins University, Baltimore, Maryland 21203-6402, USA

> ABSTRACT: An established combination gene therapy strategy involving adenovirus vector delivery of the herpes thymidine kinase (tk) and murine interleukin-2 genes was adapted to treat salivary gland cancer in a murine model. Salivary tumors were generated by transcutaneous injection of 5×10^5 murine squamous carcinoma cells into the submandibular gland of syngeneic C3H/HeJ mice. After one week, established submandibular gland tumors were injected with a recombinant adenovirus containing therapeutic and control genes. Animals were subsequently administered ganciclovir twice daily (25 mg/kg) for six days. All animals receiving tk and ganciclovir demonstrated tumor regression, however a significantly greater response was seen in mice that were treated with both tk + mIL-2. Residual tumors from all treatment and control groups were harvested for microscopic evaluation and immunohistochemistry staining. Specific immunostaining revealed a predominance of $CD8^+$ lymphocytes in the tumor beds of the animals treated with IL-2, suggesting a preferential immune response resulting from the local IL-2 expression. Although still in its infancy, the concept of using adenoviral gene therapy strategies to provide less invasive means of treating salivary tumors is promising.

INTRODUCTION

Approximately 20% of parotid gland neoplasms and 50% of submandibular gland neoplasms are malignant.[1] In minor salivary gland neoplasms malignancies are present in up to 75% of the cases. Although benign lesions can usually be controlled with surgical excision in most cases, the malignant lesions remain a therapeutic challenge. Aside from surgical morbidity, malignant lesions have a high rate of local recurrence.[2] Novel therapeutic approaches on the horizon include using tumor vaccines and gene therapies to treat primary neoplasms or enhance standard treatment. The modern concept of a tumor vaccine presently involves the transplantation of irradiated and genetically modified tumor cells that have been engineered to secrete such immune modulators as interleukin-2 (IL-2) and granulocyte-macrophage colony-stimulating factor (GM-CSF).[3–5] With a desire to circumvent the *"ex vivo"* step in tumor vaccines and to avoid tumor cell transplantation, the application of direct gene therapy strategies for treating established tumors holds promise. One of the most effective gene therapy strategies to date involves the transfer of the "suicide gene" herpes thymidine kinase (tk) followed by systemic ganciclovir (GCV) administration.[6,7] This tk system preferentially kills actively dividing cells found in a tumor by interrupting DNA synthesis. As direct gene transfer strategies evolve, a natural merger is occurring with the principles and methods of the classic tumor vaccine strategy to create new combination therapy schemes. Based on our previous work in an oral cancer murine model,[8,9] we have developed a

---

[a] Tel: (410) 955-8409; fax: (410) 955-0465; e-mail: bomalle@gwgate1.jhmi.jhu.edu

murine salivary cancer model and demonstrated a response to novel combination gene therapy. Recombinant adenovirus vectors carrying the tk and the mIL-2 gene are used to treat established submandibular gland (SMG) tumors. The delivery of tk results in direct tumor cell killing (in the presence of GCV), whereas the mIL-2 acts synergistically to induce an antitumor immune response. We will evaluate tumor regression, histopathologic findings, and the presence and content of immune infiltrates in this new model for salivary gland cancer.

MATERIAL AND METHODS

Construction of Recombinant Adenoviral Vectors

The original adenoviral vectors were generously provided by Dr. Savio L.C. Woo and were subsequently amplified and purified in our laboratory. Construction replication-defective Ad5 adenoviral vectors containing the tk and mIL-2 genes under transcriptional controls of the Rous sarcoma virus (RSV) long-terminal repeat have been reported previously.[9,10] The viral titer (plaque-forming units (pfu)/mL) was determined by standard plaque assay.

Establishing Salivary Tumors and Adenovirus Treatment

All animal experiments were performed on C3H/HeJ mice (Jackson Laboratories) using sterile technique under a laminar flow hood. The squamous carcinoma cell line SCC VII[11,12] was delivered directly into the (SMG) of 8-week-old C3H/HeJ mice to create the salivary cancers. Mice were anesthetized using the inhalational agent, Metophane, and a 0.1 cc suspension of 5×10^5 SCC VII cells in Hank's buffered saline solution was injected directly into the SMG. The animals were then maintained in standard housing conditions.

Six days after tumor cell implantation, mice were anesthetized with 0.5 cc of Avertin at a concentration of 20 mg/mL. A skin incision was made in the lower neck, and surgical dissection revealed the established SMG tumors. Tumors were measured in three dimensions with calipers. Using a 100 µL syringe (Hamilton, Reno, NV) and 26 gauge needle, 1.0×10^9 total pfu of either ADV/RSV-tk, ADV/RSV-b-gal control, ADV/RSV-tk + ADV/RSV-mIL-2 (2.0×10^8), or ADV/RSV-mIL-2 in 50 µL solution were injected directly into the tumors. Neck incisions were closed with 4-0 silk suture (Ethicon). Eighteen hours after adenoviral injection, the mice were administered GCV ip at a regimen of 25 mg/kg twice daily. On the seventh day, mice were sacrificed, residual tumor masses were measured, and specimens including normal surrounding tissues were processed for routine histology. Significance of outcomes was determined by Mann-Whitney analysis.

Histology

At the time of necropsy, harvested tumor, surrounding tissues, and distant organs were placed in 10% buffered formalin for fixation. The specimens were then embedded in paraffin, sectioned, and stained with hematoxylin and eosin (H&E).

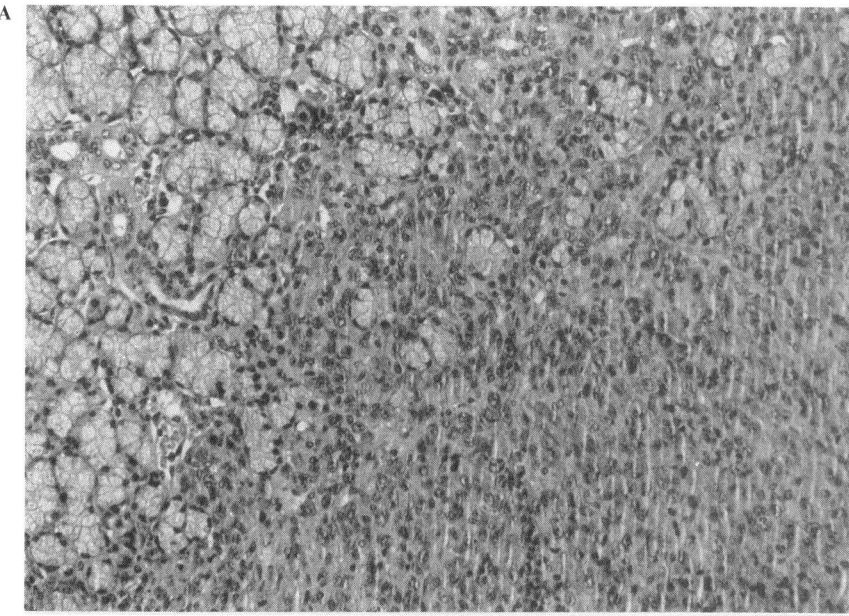

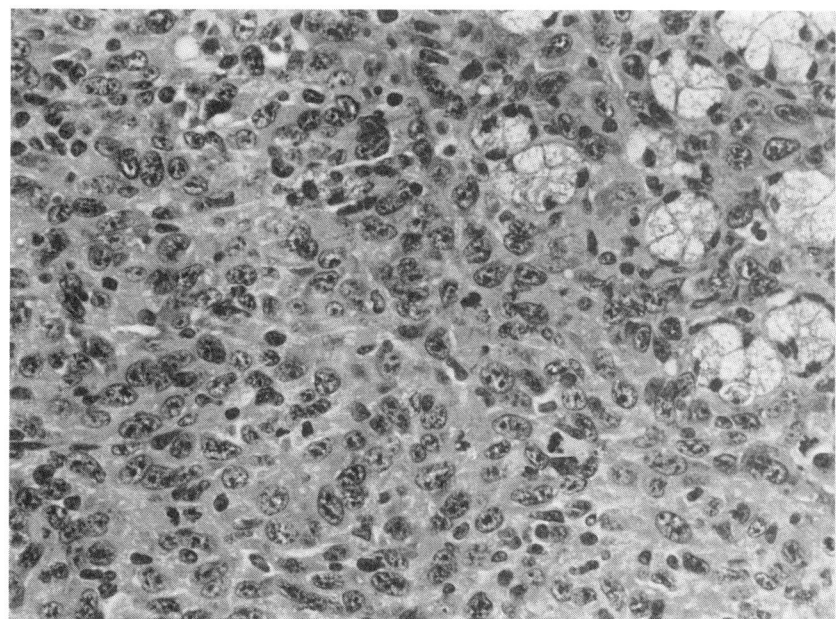

FIGURE 1. Microscopic examination of tumor specimens growing *in vivo* in the submandibular gland of C3H/HeJ mice. **A:** Poorly differentiated squamous cell carcinoma with invasion throughout the gland (× 200, reduced here by 36%). **B:** High-power view of invasion within mucous glands. Note the large number of mitotic figures (× 400, reduced here by 36%).

Immunohistochemistry

Residual tumor masses were harvested and one half of the mass was frozen in liquid nitrogen. Frozen tissues were sectioned at 4 µm and placed on saline-coated slides. Endogenous peroxidase activity in the tissue was blocked by H_2O_2 treatment. Nonspecific binding was blocked with phosphate-buffered saline (PBS) containing 0.3% bovine serum albumin. Fluorescein-conjugated primary monoclonal antibodies used in the assay were as follows: rat anti-mouse CD4 (L3T4) (Gibco BRL, Grand Island, NY), rat anti-mouse CD8a (Ly-2) (Gibco, BRL), mouse anti-mouse NK (5E6) (Pharmingen, San Diego, CA). After reaction with primary antibodies, the sections were rinsed and incubated with peroxidase-conjugated rabbit antifluorescein isothiocyanate (FITC) (Dako, Carpinteria, CA) for 2 hours at room temperature. After rinsing, the slides were incubated in chromogen solution (DAB 3 mg, PBS 10 mL, 8% NiCl 50 µL, 30% H_2O_2 1 µL) for 10 minutes. The reaction was stopped in running distilled water for 1 minute, and the slides were counterstained with Nuclear Fast Red for 5 minutes.

RESULTS

Tumor Growth in Submandibular Glands

After implantation of 5×10^5 tumor cells into 32 animals, the mice showed rapid tumor growth in the SMG over five days. At the time of adenovirus injection, four animals were sacrificed, and the SMG glands (containing tumor) were harvested and evaluated microscopically. A poorly differentiated squamous cell carcinoma was pre-

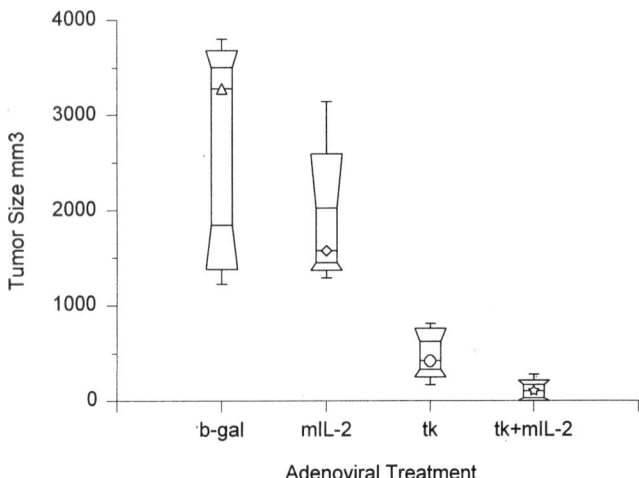

FIGURE 2. Box and Whisker plot of residual tumor sizes after various adenoviral treatments in 28 C3H/HeJ mice (4 groups of seven) with established SMG tumors. The full range of data points is depicted by the vertical lines, and each subsequent horizontal line depicts percentiles in descending order of 90, 75, 50, 25, and 10th percentile, where applicable. The geometric shape within the box represents the median. Both the tk + mIL-2 and tk alone groups demonstrate a significant antitumor response, as compared to both the b-gal and the mIL-2 alone groups (p = .002).

sent within the gland, and invasion was noted throughout the serous and mucous alveoli (FIG. 1).

Submandibular Gland Tumor Response to Combination Gene Therapy

In all four experimental groups (b-gal control, mIL-2 alone, tk alone, and tk + mIL-2), pretreatment tumor volumes ranged from 60–120 mm^3. There were no significant variations in pretreatment tumor sizes between each tumor group as determined by Mann-Whitney analysis (data not shown). After adenoviral treatment, no animals displayed a change in eating habits or evidence of cachexia at one week. Animals treated with either tk or the combination tk + mIL-2 demonstrated significant tumor regression as compared to the large tumors found in mIL-2 alone or b-gal control injection mice (p = .002) (FIG. 2). Although there were some animals that showed a limited antitumor response to the mIL-2 alone, the group as a whole did not respond significantly compared to the b-gal alone control animals (p = .160). The synergistic response to tk + mIL-2 treatment is evident by its superior response even when compared to the tk alone group (p = .004).

Microscopic and Immunohistochemical Analysis

Routine H&E staining revealed poorly differentiated squamous cell carcinoma in residual tumors. Of note, the larger tumors present in both the mIL-2 alone group and b-gal control groups showed tumor invasion into the mandible (FIG. 3). There was no such invasion seen in residual tumors of the tk alone or the mIL-2 + tk combination–treated groups. There were areas of tumor necrosis that were more pronounced in the tk + mIL-2 and tk alone treatment groups. Immunohistochemical staining was performed on four of seven tumor specimens (chosen at random), and positive staining cells were counted per 10 high-powered fields (hpf). Total lymphocyte staining in each specimen was evaluated and designated as follows: –, no lymphocytes / 10 hpf; +/–, 10 or less; +, 10 to 30; ++, 30 to 100; +++, greater than 100 positive-staining lymphocytes. Average total staining for each experimental group is depicted in TABLE 1. All the tumor specimens showed a minimum staining for both CD4 and CD8 lymphocytes, but there was a strong increase in CD8 response in groups treated with the mIL-2 vector. The residual tumors that received combination mIL-2 + tk or mIL-2 alone showed up to four times more positive CD8 cells. It appears that the presence of increased CD8 lymphocyte tumor infiltration is specific to treatment with adenoviral gene transfer of vectors containing IL-2. Although there was a strong increase in CD8 lymphocytes in the mIL-2 alone group, there was no significant therapeutic benefit from this treatment. This finding suggests that despite recruitment of CD8 cells, there is no significant tumor recognition without the presence of the tk suicide gene. There was a strong macrophage infiltrate in all tumor specimens, which suggests a general response to the adenovirus vector itself. This macrophage infiltrate, however, does not result in any antitumor activity. Previous experiments *in vitro* and *in vivo* in a murine oral cancer model have demonstrated no significant antitumor effects of adenovirus b-gal control–treated tumors versus nontreatment or saline-injected controls (data not shown).

DISCUSSION

The adenoviral tk gene therapy strategy has been used in many tumor models including our oral cancer immunocompetent animal model.[9] Although initially promis-

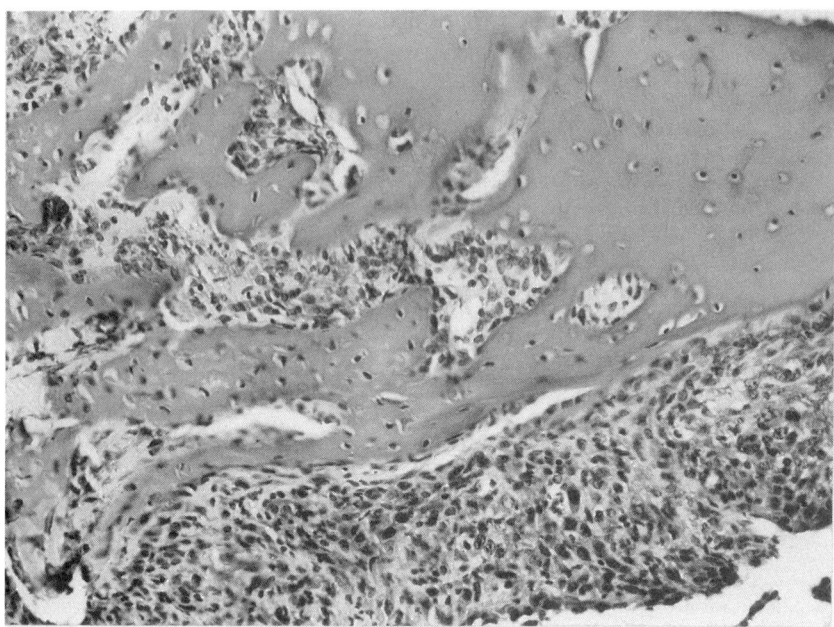

FIGURE 3. Direct invasion of the advanced tumors in the b-gal and mIL-2 alone control animal groups. Note the direct invasion of the squamous cell carcinoma into the mandibular bone (× 200, reduced here by 36%).

ing, the use of tk (and GCV) gene therapy has not met with great clinical success in human clinical trials to date.[13] Because of this limited efficacy, the combination tk and cytokine (IL-2) strategy was developed to provide a powerful but limited direct cytotoxic effect coupled with a local and systemic immune stimulator. Previous combination gene therapy application to both metastatic colon cancers and primary oral cancers in animal models has shown a benefit in both tumor regression and animal survival.[9,14] The purpose of this work was to develop a model for studying salivary cancer and evaluate the potential application of combination gene therapy.

TABLE 1. Summary of Immunohistochemical Staining on Residual Tumors One Week after Adenoviral Treatment[a]

Treatment	CD4	CD8	Mac
tk + mIL-2	+/−	++	+++
tk	+/−	+	+++
mIL-2	+	++	+++
β-gal	+/−	+	+++

[a] Four tumors from each animal group were randomly selected and stained for CD8 and CD4 lymphocytes and macrophage infiltrate. The average total positive staining is depicted. +/−, 10 or less lymphocytes/10 hpf (× 400 for each hpf); +, 10–30/10 hpf; ++, 30–100/10 hpf; +++, greater than 100/10 hpf.

Although more extensive studies are required to completely evaluate the biology of this tumor model, there are important similarities to human salivary gland neoplasms. The submandibular tumors showed notable glandular invasion, and after 12 days untreated or control tumors showed invasion beyond the gland. The mandible was the primary site of extraglandular extension. This invasive tumor behavior resembles the natural biology of SMG tumors and provides a relatively realistic orthotopic model for squamous cell cancer of the SMG. Longer intervals of tumor growth and the presence of local lymph node and distant metastases will be the focus of future work.

Although not unexpected, the SMG tumors did respond to the tk and combination tk + mIL-2 gene therapy in a similar fashion as in other previously reported tumor models.[9,14] We hypothesize that this apparent synergism requires both tumor necrosis and a local expression of cytokine. The transfer of the suicide tk gene along with systemic GCV administration directly kills infected tumor cells and also results in killing to bystander cells that were not infected with the virus. This "bystander effect" is well known to the tk strategy and is a major advantage that obviates the need to infect every tumor cell in order to achieve significant antitumor responses.[15,16] The tumor killing and release of tumor antigens provides an important medium in which the concurrent local mIL-2 expression can stimulate and enhance a tumor-specific immune response. The need for both of these genes in concert is supported by the lack of significant antitumor response in the tumors treated with mIL-2 alone, despite a prominent CD8 infiltration.

Although these studies are not complete, they do introduce the concept of studying the effects of novel gene therapies on salivary gland cancer. Although carcinomas of the parotid gland are more common, malignant submandibular tumors have the worst prognosis with an overall five-year survival of approximately 40 percent.[17] Of the SMG malignancies, squamous cell cancer has the poorest prognosis, with reports ranging from 5 to 40% survival over five years. Because of its invasive and aggressive nature, it also has a high rate of local failure despite surgical and radiation intervention. The overall poor control and cure rates for this salivary neoplasm make it an ideal candidate for the development of new therapies to be used both primarily and in conjunction with standard surgery and radiation.

ACKNOWLEDGMENTS

We would like to thank Dr. Candace S. Johnson, Dr. Savio L.C. Woo, and Dr. Shu-Hsia Chen for their valuable support that has enabled us to develop new animal models and investigate novel gene therapy strategies for treating malignancies.

REFERENCES

1. KAPLAN, M.J. & M.E. JOHNS. 1993. Salivary Glands: Malignant neoplasms. *In* Otolaryngology-Head and Neck Surgery, second edition. Mosby-Year Book, Inc. St. Louis, Missouri.
2. FRIEDMAN, M. *et al.* 1986. Malignant tumors of the major salivary glands. Otolaryngol. Clin. North. Am. **19:** 625–630.
3. FEARON, E.R., D.M. PARDOLL, R. ITAYA, P. GOLUMBEK, H. LEVITSKY & J. SIMONS. 1990. Interleukin-2 production by tumor cells bypasses T helper function in the generation of an antitumor response. Cell **60:** 397–403.
4. DRANOFF, G., E. JAFFEE, A. LAZENBY, P. GOLUMBEK, H. LEVITSKY, K. BROSE, V. JACKSON, H. HIROFUMI, D.M. PARDOLL & R.C. MULLIGAN. 1993. Vaccination with irradiated tumor cells engineered to secrete murine granulocyte-macrophage colony-stimulating factor stim-

ulates potent, specific, and long lasting anti-tumor immunity. Proc. Natl. Acad. Sci. USA **90:** 3539–3543.
5. GANSBACJER, B., K. ZIER, B. DANIELS, K. CRONIN, R. BANNERJI & E. GILBOA. 1990. Interleukin-2 gene transfer into tumor cells abrogates tumorigenicity and induces protective immunity. J. Exp. Med. **172:** 1217–1224.
6. MOOLTEN, F.L. 1986. Tumor chemosensitivity conferred by inserted herpes thymidine kinase genes: paradigm for a prospective cancer control strategy. Cancer. Res. **46:** 5276–5281.
7. MOOLTEN, F.L. & J.M. WELLS. 1990. Curability of tumors bearing herpes thymidine kinase genes transferred by retroviral vectors. J. Natl. Cancer Inst. **82:** 297–300.
8. O'MALLEY, B.W. JR., S.-H. CHEN, M.R. SCHWARTZ & S.L.C. WOO. 1995. Adenovirus-mediated gene therapy for human head and neck squamous cell cancer in a nude mouse model. Cancer Res. **55:** 1080–1085.
9. O'MALLEY, B.W. JR, K.A. COPE, S.-H. CHEN, D. LI, M.R. SCHWARTZ & S.L.C. WOO. 1996. Combination gene therapy for oral cancer in a murine model. Cancer Res. **56:** 1737–1741.
10. CHEN, S.-H., D. SHINE, J.C. GOODMAN, R.G. GROSSMAN & S.L.C. WOO. 1994. Gene therapy for brain tumors: Regression of experimental gliomas by adenovirus-mediated gene transfer. Proc. Natl. Acad. Sci. USA **91:** 3054–3057.
11. GRANDIS, J.R., M.-J. CHANG, W.-D. YU & C.S. JOHNSON. 1995. Antitumor activity of interleukin-1a and Cisplatin in a murine model system. Arch. Otolaryngol. Head & Neck Surg. **121:** 197–200.
12. O'MALLEY, B.W. JR., K.A. COPE, C.S. JOHNSON & M.R. SCHWARTZ. 1997. A new immunocompetent murine model for oral cancer. Arch. Otolaryngol. Head Neck Surg. **123:** 20–24.
13. ROTH, J.A. & R.J. CRISTIANO. 1997. Gene therapy for cancer: What have we done and where are we going? J. Natl. Cancer. Inst. **89**(1): 21–39.
14. CHEN, S-H., X.H. LI CHEN, Y. WANG, K.-I. KOSAI, M.J. FINEGOLD, S.S. RICH & S.L.C. WOO. 1995. Combination gene therapy for liver metastasis of colon carcinoma in vivo. Proc. Natl. Acad. Sci. USA **92:** 2577–2581.
15. WAN, L.B., L.M. PARYSEK, R. WARNICK & P.J. STAMBROOK. 1993. *In vitro* evidence that metabolic cooperation is responsible for the bystander effect observed with HSV tk retroviral gene therapy. Hum. Gene Ther. **4:** 725–731.
16. FREEMAN, S.M., C.N. ABBOUD, K.A. WHARTENBY, D.S. KOEPLIN, F.L. MOOLTEN & G.N. ABRAHAM. 1993. The "bystander effect": Tumor regression when a fraction of the tumor mass is genetically modified. Cancer Res. **53:** 5274–5283.
17. YU, G.Y. & D.Q. MA. 1987. Carcinoma of the salivary gland: A clinicopathologic study of 405 cases. Semin. Surg. Oncol. **3:** 240–244.

Somatic Gene Transfer to Salivary Glands

BRIAN C. O'CONNELL,[b] C. DAVID LILLIBRIDGE, INDU AMBUDKAR, AND DAVID KRUSE[a]

Gene Therapy and Therapeutics Branch, National Institute of Dental Research, Building 10/1N113, 10 Center Drive, National Institutes of Health, Bethesda, Maryland 20892-1190

[a]*Oral Pathology Research Laboratory, Veterans Administration Medical Center, Washington, DC 20422*

> ABSTRACT: Recent developments in gene transfer technology have expanded the range of *in vivo* experimentation and provided new insights that might be applicable to the treatment of human diseases. Somatic gene transfer may complement conventional transgenic animal experiments by allowing for more restricted gene expression. Salivary glands of rats are readily transduced *in vivo* by adenovirus vectors. This model has been used to demonstrate the effects of transferring a water channel (aquaporin) gene to glands that have been damaged by radiation. Submandibular glands that receive the aquaporin vector increase the stimulated salivary flow close to normal levels. The possible role of E2F1 in promoting cell regeneration *in vivo* was also explored. A vector expressing E2F1 was capable of increasing DNA synthesis in rat salivary glands, though complete mitosis was not observed. Future generations of vectors must overcome current limitations of efficiency, immunogenicity, and transient expression.

USE OF GENE TRANSFER FOR *IN VIVO* EXPERIMENTS

Over the past five years there has been a dramatic expansion of the field of *in vivo* gene transfer.[1] This has gone hand in hand with the development of clinical gene therapy, which is a specific application of gene transfer.[2,3] Gene transfer refers to any technique by which new genetic information is transferred to an individual. Gene therapy implies that the transfer is to a human subject and that there is a therapeutic intent. Although many aspects of these experiments remain rudimentary, the rapid improvements in viral and nonviral systems of gene transfer suggest that the technology is far from reaching its potential.[4,5]

In principle, gene transfer opens new possibilities for the study of gene regulation and protein function.[6] Using a variety of methods, native or exogenous proteins may be expressed in a particular tissue. This may include gain-of-function or replacement experiments. Increasingly, strategies are being developed to perform "knockout" experiments also.[7] By these means it is hoped that physiological and pathological mechanisms may be better understood and that the functions of newly discovered genes may be elucidated.[8] *In vivo* gene transfer can now be considered an alternative or complement to conventional transgenic or knockout animal experiments.[9,10] As such, gene transfer has different characteristics that can prove to be useful in some cases or a distinct disadvantage in other cases. For example, transgenic animals will contain copies of the transgene in every cell, whereas gene transfer typically affects only a particular organ or tissue. Therefore, somatic gene transfer makes it easier to distinguish among the effects of protein expression in different sites. On the other hand, gene transfer to

---

[b] Tel: (301) 496 8328; fax: (301) 402 1228; e-mail: oconnell@yoda.nidr.nih.gov

somatic cells is sometimes inefficient, so only some cells in an organ may be transduced. Unless the exogenous protein has a dominant effect, it can be difficult to measure its activity. Because transgenic animals contain the foreign gene within their chromosomes, the gene persists throughout the life of the animal. However, it can sometimes be difficult to strictly regulate the temporal and spatial expression of an integrated transgene—this can be a problem if the product is toxic. By contrast, gene transfer is frequently short-lived, so expression of the transgene is lost after a period.[11] This may be appropriate if one wants to study the transient expression of a protein, for example, to ask the question, What happens after the protein is removed? When studying exogenous proteins expressed by somatic gene transfer, an immune response may develop to the protein and limit its persistence or intereferek with its effects.[12–14] Repeated administration of vectors presents a particular challenge.[15–17] Germline transmission, however, ensures that there is tolerance to the transgene product.

Perhaps the main reason that gene transfer has gained in popularity is that experiments can often be performed more rapidly and cheaply than with a conventional approach. These reagents are also convenient to store and to distribute among investigators. Once a vector or other transfer reagent (*e.g.,* liposome) is developed, it can frequently be used in several *in vivo* and *in vitro* systems. In some cases, it is a distinct advantage to be able to work with primates or other animals.[18–20] The availability of gene transfer technology makes it possible to perform animal studies that are a closer simulation of a clinical situation than could be achieved with traditional means.[21] Nonetheless, gene transfer experiments should be viewed with the same caution as those in transgenic or knockout animals. Frequently, biological redundancy means that no change in phenotype is seen following gene transfer. Alternately, the transferred gene may cause effects through indirect actions that are poorly understood.

PRINCIPLES OF GENE TRANSFER TO SALIVARY GLANDS

The salivary glands have been the subject of gene transfer experiments, both to understand their physiology and also to explore novel approaches to the treatment of salivary disorders. Currently, there is no gene transfer system that is close to optimal for the salivary glands. Ideally, a vector would be safe, efficient, and effective *in vivo.*[22] Hence the vector should be simple and inexpensive to produce, should not elicit a host immune response, should transduce a high percentage of the cells it targets, and should persist for as long as it is required. In some cases it would be desirable to regulate the expression of the transgene in response to functional requirements (*e.g.,* hormones).[23] It would also be useful to target expression to specific subsets of cells in the major glands (*e.g.,* acinar or ductal cells). TABLE 1 shows the characteristics of the major transfer systems as they relate to the salivary glands. Because of their efficiency and ease of delivery, adenoviruses have been the main vector system used in the salivary glands.[24–27]

RESTORATION OF FUNCTION TO SALIVARY GLANDS

It has been known for some time that when salivary glands are exposed to ionizing radiation, for example, during treatment for head and neck cancer, there follows a dose-dependent decrease in salivary flow.[28] This is thought to be primarily due to the loss of acinar cells.[29] It is not clear why there is a relative preservation of salivary ductal cells following radiation. Baum and colleagues proposed that increasing the water permeability of residual ductal cells might allow water movement through the cells into the lumen and increase the flow of fluid into the oral cavity (FIG. 1).[30,31] Although

TABLE 1. Nominal Characteristics of Various Methods for Gene Transfer to Salivary Glands

	Efficacy in Salivary Gland	Cell Specificity	Stability of Expression
Adenovirus[a]	++	–	T[b]
Retrovirus[c]	+/–	–	S[d]
Adeno-associated virus[e]	+/–	–	?
SV40 virus	?		
Vaccinia virus	?		
Lentivirus	?		
DNA[e]	+/–	–	T
Ligand-DNA complexes[e]	+/–	?	T
Liposomes[e]	+/–	–	T

[a] See Mastrangeli et al.[24]
[b] T; transient expression.
[c] See Barka and Van der Noen.[25]
[d] S; stable expression.
[e] Unpublished observations.

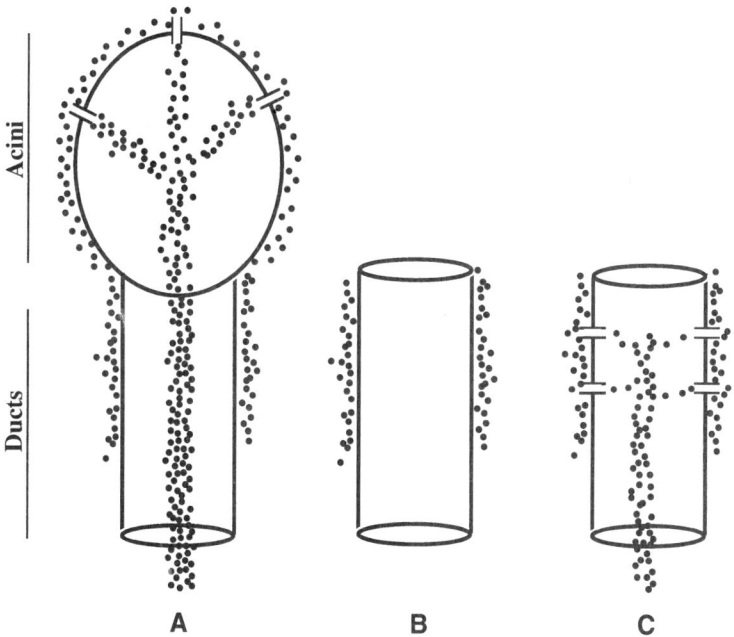

FIGURE 1. Simplified concept of increasing fluid flow in damaged salivary glands. Diagram shows water passing through acinar cells into duct lumen in normal salivary gland (A). When acinar cells are lost, there is no salivary flow (B). Addition of a facilitated water transport pathway in ductal cells may allow for fluid to reach the duct lumen (C).

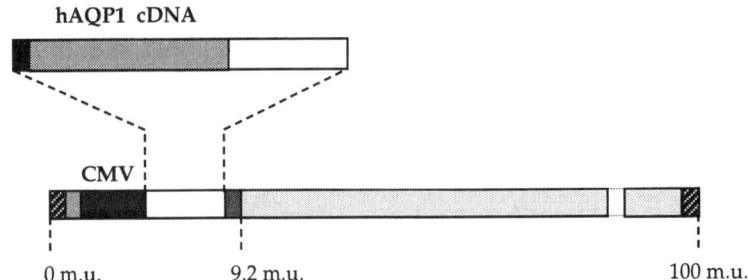

FIGURE 2. Structure of adenovirus vector. First generation vector has a deletion in the E1 region (1.3 to 9.2 map units (m.u.)), which makes the virus replication deficient. An expression cassette contains the gene of interest (hAQP1 cDNA) and a heterologous promoter (CMV).

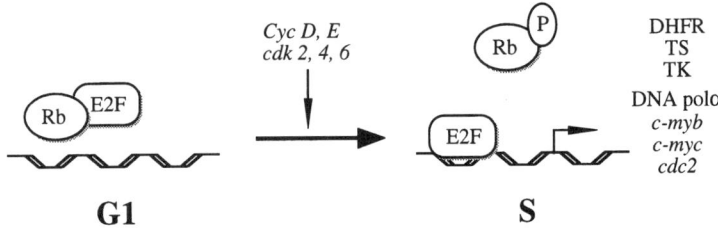

FIGURE 3. E2F is a key regulator of the G1 to S-phase transition. In G1 phase E2F is bound to the retinoblastoma protein, Rb. During S-phase progression Rb is phosphorylated (RbP), and E2F is released and binds to its DNA recognition sequence. E2F transactivates a number of genes that are required for DNA synthesis. Exogenous E2F in excess is presumed to saturate the available Rb, thereby promoting entry into S phase.

TABLE 2. Effect of Adenovirus-mediated E2F1 Overexpression on Growth-arrested HSG Cells[a]

	Percent of Cells in S Phase		
	0 hpi[b]	24 hpi	48 hpi
Untreated	12.7	11.9	8.0
Cytokines + no virus	3.5	2.9	3.1
Cytokines + Adα1AT	6.0	3.8	3.1
Cytokines + AdE2F1	5.0	6.7	14.4

[a] Cells treated with cytokines were grown in the presence of 1000 U/mL IFN-γ and 20 U/mL of TNF-α for 72 hours before infection. Cells were infected with 10 plaque-forming units/cell of control virus (Adα1AT) or E2F1-producing virus (AdE2F1). At subsequent time points, cells were harvested and analyzed by flow cytometry. The percentage (mean of triplicate experiment) of cells in the S-phase gate is shown.

[b] hpi, hours postinfection.

the composition of this fluid may differ from that of saliva, it is believed that the fluid would alleviate some of the consequences of salivary hypofunction. In order to test this hypothesis, a gene transfer experiment was proposed. The gene encoding a membrane water channel protein, aquaporin 1, was delivered to the submandibular glands of rats that had received γ-radiation.[27] The gene was transferred to the glands using an adenovirus vector. Adenovirus vectors are modified viruses that have at least part of their genome removed to make them replication deficient (FIG. 2).[32] In place of the virus genes, the exogenous gene of interest is inserted in an expression cassette. When the rats were given 21 Gy of radiation, their salivary flow was decreased by 64% after four months. Administration of a control vector to the animals did not change their salivary flow rate. However, when the aquaporin 1 vector was instilled into the submandibular glands, the flow rates returned to 91% of normal (unirradiated) values. This experiment demonstrates the usefulness of an *in vivo* gene transfer approach. Indeed, it would be very difficult to test the above hypothesis using conventional approaches. It is important to note that adenovirus-mediated gene expression in the salivary glands is quite transient, typically lasting from one to two weeks.[24,33] These vectors are also known to cause significant host immune responses.[34] Hence, the current technology is more suited to these "proof of principle" experiments than practical clinical applications. However, such experiments increase our understanding of salivary function and suggest possible strategies for the future.

SALIVARY GLAND REGENERATION

It has already been noted that the loss of salivary tissue causes significant clinical morbidity. The replacement of damaged salivary tissue would be a rational strategy for treatment. However, the glands consist mainly of terminally differentiated epithelial cells with a limited capacity for regeneration. As the events governing cell-cycle regulation are better understood, we can expand the opportunities to control cell proliferation. This may include the inhibition of cell division for the treatment of neoplasms, or the controlled expansion of cell numbers for regeneration. Hence, one approach to the restoration of salivary function would be to enable salivary parenchymal cells to complete a few rounds of mitosis in order to restore cell numbers in the gland. An initial attempt at salivary cell replacement involved the expression of the transcription factor, E2F1, in rat salivary glands. Extensive *in vitro* studies with E2F1 have demonstrated that it is capable of pushing quiescent cells into S phase (FIG. 3).[35,36] In addition, salivary epithelial cells (HSG cells) that were growth arrested by cytokine treatment were able to overcome this growth arrest when they overexpressed E2F1 (TABLE 2).[37] Using an adenovirus vector that contained the E2F1 cDNA (AdE2F1), it was shown that E2F1 could be overexpressed in rat submandibular glands. Moreover, following infection of the glands with AdE2F1, there was a significant increase in DNA synthesis both in acinar and ductal cells (FIG. 4). One concern with stimulating DNA synthesis *in vivo* is that dysregulation of the process could lead to tumor formation. However, in the case of E2F1 expression, it appears that DNA synthesis peaked and then decreased in parallel with the known kinetics of adenovirus-based gene expression (TABLE 3). The DNA content of the submandibular gland cells was determined by flow cytometry of control and AdE2F1-infected animals (FIG. 5). The data are consistent with the expected effects of E2F1 overexpression: there was an increase in the percentage of cells in S phase, and no evidence of polyploidy. This is also consistent with the observation that E2F1 may act as a tumor suppressor in salivary glands.[38] Nonetheless, there is no convincing data that E2F1 alone predictably facilitates complete mitosis. In fact, *in vitro,* the inappropriate expression of E2F1 often leads to DNA synthesis followed by

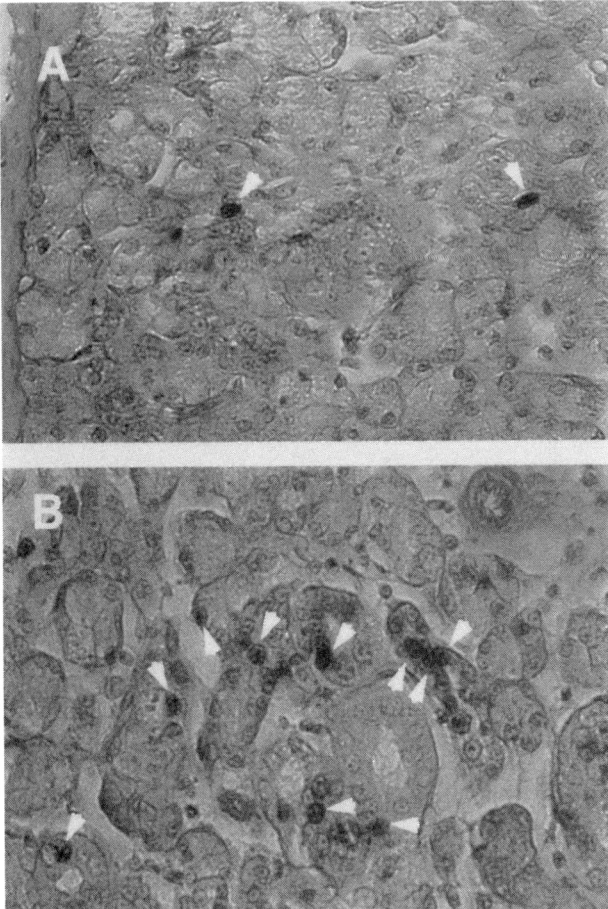

FIGURE 4. E2F1 overexpression in rat submandibular glands increases DNA synthesis. Animals received buffer **(A)** or 5×10^9 pfu of AdE2F1 **(B)** by retrograde infusion into their submandibular glands. Before sacrifice, BrdU (100 mg/kg) was given by intraperitoneal injection. Sections were stained for BrdU-labeled cells, some of which are indicated by the white arrows.

apoptosis.[37,39] The fate of the cells in AdE2F1-infected salivary glands remains to be elucidated. It is very possible that other members of the E2F protein family may be more suited to facilitating mitosis than E2F1. Alternately, other cell cycle regulatory proteins may be needed for completion of the cycle.

CELL-SPECIFIC EXPRESSION IN SALIVARY GLANDS

The salivary glands have several anatomical advantages for gene transfer *in situ*. The salivary ducts provide convenient access for the retrograde delivery of vectors to the

TABLE 3. Level of DNA Synthesis in Rat Submandibular Glands Infected with AdE2F1[a]

	Percent of Cells BrdU Positive		
Hours postinfection	Uninfected	Adα1AT infected	AdE2F1 infected
24	0.05 ± 0.02	0.23 ± 0.02	5.6 ± 1.5
48	ND[b]	0.34 ± 0.36	2.1 ± 0.53

[a] Animals received buffer, or were infected with Adα1AT or AdE2F1 by retrograde ductal infusion. Ninety minutes before sacrifice, each rat was injected with 100 mg/kg of BrdU. The submandibular glands were sectioned, stained with an antibody to BrdU, and counterstained with methyl green. BrdU-positive and unstained nuclei were counted in 6 separate fields (~ 1200 cells/field) from different gland sections (n=4 glands for each group). The mean ± SEM of BrdU-positive cells is shown for each group.
[b] ND, not determined.

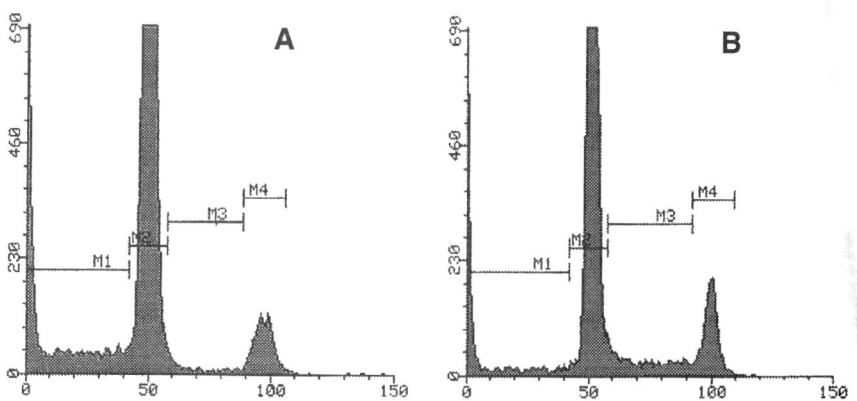

FIGURE 5. Flow cytometry of rat submandibular gland cells. Glands were infected with Adα1AT **(A)** or AdE2F1 **(B)** and removed after 24 hours. The tissue was cleaned and minced repeatedly with a scissors, followed by sequential digestion with trypsin, collagenase, and hyaluronidase. At intervals the cells were passed through progressively smaller pipette tips. Finally, the cells were passed through a nylon mesh and prepared for flow cytometry. At this time point, AdE2F1 increased the percentage of cells in S phase (M3) from 0.8% to 3.0%.

glands. In a similar clinical procedure, sialography, contrast medium is introduced to the gland without anesthesia, and there is minimal discomfort to the patient. The extensively branched duct system allows a vector to contact all the epithelial cells within the gland. It seems likely that any genetic material introduced into the salivary gland by retrograde ductal infusion will remain confined to the glands.[33] Although targeting the salivary glands themselves is not difficult, current gene delivery systems are not capable of gene transfer to specific cell types within the glands. In some instances, such as the regeneration strategy, it would clearly be desirable to effect transgene expression in particular cell populations. This may become feasible as we learn more about receptors that may be present on the apical surfaces of salivary acinar and ductal cells. In other systems, considerable progress has been made in using cell-selective receptors to target gene delivery.[40–42] An alternative approach has been to put the transgene under the control of cell-specific promoters. In this way, the DNA may be transferred to any cell type within the salivary gland but will only be expressed in certain cell populations. For example, the salivary amylase promoter was able to direct adenovirus-mediated gene expression specifically in the acinar cells of rat submandibular glands. One challenge for the future will be to increase the activity of cell-specific promoters closer to that of viral promoters while maintaining their fidelity *in vivo*.

PERSPECTIVES FOR THE FUTURE

Gene transfer experiments are already capable of providing useful insights into cell biology, protein function, and pathological mechanisms. However, it is important to interpret gene transfer experiments with the same caution used in conventional transgenic animal models. At present, the usefullness of gene transfer is limited by the technology of transfer itself. In particular, improved delivery systems will be needed for safe and practical clinical applications.

REFERENCES

1. Ross, G., R. Erickson, D. Knorr *et al.* 1996. Gene therapy in the United States: a five-year status report. Hum. Gene Ther. **7:** 1781–1790.
2. Marcel, T. & J.D. Grausz. 1996. The TMC Worldwide Gene Therapy Enrollment Report (June 1996). Hum. Gene Ther. **7:** 2025–2046.
3. Leiden, J.M. 1995. Gene therapy—promise, pitfalls, and prognosis [editorial; comment]. N. Engl. J. Med. **333:** 871–873.
4. Touchette, N. 1996. Gene therapy: Not ready for prime time. Nature Med. **2:** 7–8.
5. Flotte, T.R. & T.W. Ferkol. 1997. Genetic therapy. Past, present, and future. Pediatr. Clin. North Am. **44:** 153–178.
6. Ledley, F.D. 1996. "Our study is man" (and woman) [editorial]. Hum. Gene Ther. **7:** 1193–1195.
7. Rohlmann, A., M. Gotthardt, T.E. Willnow, R.E. Hammer & J. Herz. 1996. Sustained somatic gene inactivation by viral transfer of Cre recombinase. Nat. Biotechnol. **14:** 1562–1565.
8. Collins, F.S. 1997. Sequencing the human genome. Hosp. Pract. **32:** 35–43, 46–39, 53–34.
9. Tsukui, T., Y. Kanegae, I. Saito & Y. Toyoda. 1996. Transgenesis by adenovirus-mediated gene transfer into mouse zona-free eggs. Nat. Biotechnol. **14:** 982–985.
10. Wilson, J.M. 1996. Animal models of human disease for gene therapy. J. Clin. Invest. **97:** 1138–1141.
11. Kaplan, J.M., D. Armentano, T.E. Sparer *et al.* 1997. Characterization of factors involved in modulating persistence of transgene expression from recombinant adenovirus in the mouse lung. Hum. Gene Ther. **8:** 45–56.
12. Yang, Y., Q. Li, H.C. Ertl & J.M. Wilson. 1995. Cellular and humoral immune responses to viral antigens create barriers to lung-directed gene therapy with recombinant adenoviruses. J Virol. **69:** 2004–2015.
13. Worgall, S., G. Wolff, E. Falck-Pedersen & R.G. Crystal. 1997. Innate immune mechanisms dominate elimination of adenoviral vectors following *in vivo* administration. Hum. Gene Ther. **8:** 37–44.
14. Gilgenkrantz, H., D. Duboc, V. Juillard *et al.* 1995. Transient expression of genes transferred in vivo into heart using first-generation adenoviral vectors: role of the immune response. Hum. Gene Ther. **6:** 1265–1274.
15. Smith, T.A.G., B.D. White, J.M. Gardner, M. Kaleko & A. McClelland. 1996. Transient immunosuppression permits successful repetitive intravenous administration of an adenovirus vector. Gene Ther. **3:** 496–502.
16. Tripathy, S.K., H.B. Black, E. Goldwasser & J.M. Leiden. 1996. Immune responses to

transgene-encoded proteins limit the stability of gene expression after injection of replication-defective adenovirus vectors. Nature Med. **2:** 545–550.
17. YANG, Y., K. GREENOUGH & J.M. WILSON. 1996. Transient immune blockade prevents formation of neutralizing antibody to recombinant adenovirus and allows repeated gene transfer to mouse liver. Gene Ther. **3:** 412–420.
18. SIMON, R.H., J.F. ENGELHARDT, Y. YANG et al. 1993. Adenovirus-mediated transfer of the CFTR gene to lung of nonhuman primates: toxicity study. Hum. Gene Ther. **4:** 771–780.
19. OHNO, T., D. GORDON, H. SAN et al. 1994. Gene therapy for vascular smooth muscle cell proliferation after arterial injury [see comments]. Science **265:** 781–784.
20. KOZARSKY, K.F., D.R. MCKINLEY, L.L. AUSTIN et al. 1994. In vivo correction of low density lipoprotein receptor deficiency in the Watanabe heritable hyperlipidemic rabbit with recombinant adenoviruses. J. Biol. Chem. **269:** 13695–13702.
21. MORSY, M.A., J.Z. ZHAO, T.T. NGO et al. 1996. Patient selection may affect gene therapy success. Dominant negative effects observed for ornithine transcarbamylase in mouse and human hepatocytes. J. Clin. Invest. **97:** 826–832.
22. KESSLER, D.A., J.P. SIEGEL, P.D. NOGUCHI et al. 1993. Regulation of somatic-cell therapy and gene therapy by the food and drug administration. N. Engl. J. Med. **329:** 1169–1173.
23. RIVERA, V.M., T. CLACKSON, S. NATESAN et al. 1996. A humanized system for pharmacologic control of gene expression. Nature Med. **2:** 1028–1032.
24. MASTRANGELI, A., B. O'CONNELL, W. ALADIB et al. 1994. Direct in vivo adenovirus-mediated gene transfer to salivary glands. Am. J. Physiol. **266:** G1146–G1155.
25. BARKA, T. & H.M. VAN DER NOEN. 1996. Retrovirus-mediated gene transfer into salivary glands in vivo. Hum. Gene Ther. **7:** 613–618.
26. O'CONNELL, B.C., T. XU, T.J. WALSH et al. 1996. Transfer of a gene encoding the anticandidal protein histatin 3 to salivary glands. Hum. Gene Ther. **7:** 225–2261.
27. DELPORTE, C., B.C. O'CONNELL, X. HE et al. 1997. Increased fluid secretion after adenoviral-mediated transfer of the aquaporin-1 cDNA to irradiated rat salivary glands. Proc. Natl. Acad. Sci. USA. **94:** 3268–3273.
28. FRANZEN, L., U. FUNEGARD, T. ERICSON & R. HENRIKSSON. 1992. Parotid gland function during and following radiotherapy of malignancies in the head and neck. A consecutive study of salivary flow and patient discomfort. Eur. J. Cancer. **28:** 457–462.
29. PRICE, R.E., K.K. ANG, L.C. STEPHENS & L.J. PETERS. 1995. Effects of continuous hyperfractionated accelerated and conventionally fractionated radiotherapy on the parotid and submandibular salivary glands of rhesus monkeys. Radiother. Oncol. **34:** 39–46.
30. BAUM, B.J. & B.C. O'CONNELL. 1995. The impact of gene therapy on dentistry. J. Am. Dent. Assoc. **126:** 179–189.
31. DELPORTE, C., B.C. O'CONNELL, X. HE et al. 1996. Adenovirus-mediated expression of aquaporin-5 in epithelial cells. J. Biol. Chem. **271:** 22070–22075.
32. BECKER, T.C., R.J. NOEL, W.S. COATS et al. 1994. Use of recombinant adenovirus for metabolic engineering of mammalian cells. Methods Cell Biol. **43 Pt A:** 161–189.
33. KAGAMI, H., B.C. O'CONNELL & B.J. BAUM. 1996. Evidence for the systemic delivery of a transgene product from salivary glands. Hum. Gene Ther. **7:** 2177–2184.
34. ADESANYA, M.R., R.S. REDMAN, B.J. BAUM & B.C. O'CONNELL. 1996. Immediate inflammatory responses to adenovirus-mediated gene transfer in rat salivary glands. Hum. Gene Ther. **7:** 1085–1093.
35. JOHNSON, D.G., J.K. SCHWARZ, W.D. CRESS & J.R. NEVINS. 1993. Expression of transcription factor E2F1 induces quiescent cells to enter S phase. Nature **365:** 349–352.
36. SCHWARZ, J.K., C.H. BASSING, I. KOVESDI et al. 1995. Expression of the E2F1 transcription factor overcomes type beta transforming growth factor-mediated growth suppression. Proc. Natl. Acad. Sci. U S A **92:** 483–487.
37. LILLIBRIDGE, C.D. & B.C. O'CONNELL. 1997. In human salivary gland cells, overexpression of E2F1 overcomes an interferon-γ and tumor necrosis factor-α induced growth arrest but does not result in complete mitosis. In press.
38. YAMASAKI, L., T. JACKS, R. BRONSON, et al. 1996. Tumor induction and tissue atrophy in mice lacking E2F-1. Cell **85:** 537–548.
39. KOWALIK, T.F., J. DEGREGORI, J.K. SCHWARZ & J.R. NEVINS. 1995. E2F1 overexpression in

quiescent fibroblasts leads to induction of cellular DNA synthesis and apoptosis. J. Virol. **69:** 2491–2500.
40. COTTEN, M. 1995. Adenovirus-augmented, receptor-mediated gene delivery and some solutions to the common toxicity problems. Curr. Top. Microbiol. Immunol. **199:** 283–295.
41. DOUGLAS, J.T., B.E. ROGERS, M.E. ROSENFELD, et al. 1996. Targeted gene delivery by tropism-modified adenoviral vectors. Nat Biotechnol. **14:** 1574–1578.
42. WICKHAM, T.J., P.W. ROELVINK, D.E. BROUGH & I. KOVESDI. 1996. Adenovirus targeted to heparan-containing receptors increases its gene delivery efficiency to multiple cell layers. Nat. Biotechnol. **14:** 1570–1573.

Studying Development of Disease Through Temporally Controlled Gene Expression in the Salivary Gland[a]

PRISCILLA A. FURTH,[b,c,e] MINGLIN LI,[b] AND LOTHAR HENNIGHAUSEN[d]

[b] *Division of Infectious Diseases, Department of Medicine, University of Maryland Medical School; the Baltimore Veterans Affairs Medical Center; and the Institute of Human Virology, Baltimore, Maryland 21201, USA*

[c] *Department of Physiology, University of Maryland Medical School, Baltimore, Maryland 21201, USA*

[d] *Laboratory of Biochemistry and Metabolism, National Institute of Diabetes and Digestive Diseases, National Institutes of Health, Bethesda, Maryland 20892, USA*

ABSTRACT: Multistep tumorigenesis proceeds through activation of oncogenes and inactivation of tumor suppressor genes. Initiating oncoproteins induce secondary changes that maintain transformation in the absence of original stimuli. Time-dependent reversal of SV40 T antigen (TAg)–induced hyperplasia was studied using temporally controlled gene expression. Targeting TAg expression to the submandibular salivary gland of transgenic mice produces focal hyperplasias at age two weeks, which extend through large areas of the gland by four months. At twelve months, fibrosis and tumor foci accompany hyperplasia. Hyperplasia reverses when TAg expression is discontinued at four months but not at seven months. Secondary changes that maintain transformation appear to be time dependent. The system can be used to identify genetic events resulting in phenotypic reversal at four months and to expose factors preventing its occurrence at seven months. Expression of other proteins can be targeted to the salivary gland, and temporally controlled gene deletions can also be made using this system.

INTRODUCTION

Conditional gene expression systems can be used to study time-dependent factors in development, physiology, and oncogenesis.[1] A tetracycline-responsive gene expression system adapted to transgenic mice[2] has been employed to examine time-sensitive reversal of simian virus 40 (SV40) T antigen (TAg)–induced hyperplasia in the submandibular salivary gland.[3] The same system can be used to explore additional questions in salivary gland biology and disease.

THE TETRACYCLINE-RESPONSIVE TRANSACTIVATOR SYSTEM IN TRANSGENIC MICE

Use of the tetracycline-responsive transactivator system in transgenic mice enables an investigator to temporally control gene expression in the intact animal.[2,4–9] In this

---

[a] This work was supported in part by a Pangborn Award from the University of Maryland Medical School (to P.A.Furth) and by the Veterans Administration Research Service.

[e] Address for correspondence: Priscilla A. Furth, Institute of Human Virology, Medical Biotechnology Center, 725 West Lombard Street, Room 545, Baltimore, Maryland 21201-1192, USA. Tel: (410) 706-4606; fax: (410) 706-1992; e-mail: furth@umbi.umd.edu

system, transgene expression is controlled by the administration or withdrawal of tetracycline.[10,11] The tetracycline-transactivator system has three components: one, a genetic construct that controls expression of the targeted protein using the tet-op promoter; two, a gene that encodes a tetracycline-responsive transactivator (tTA); and three, a tetracycline derivative. Expression of the sequences encoding the targeted protein are controlled by a promoter containing seven DNA operator sequences from the *E. coli* transposon 10 (Tn 10). The bacterial operator sequences are linked to a minimal promoter derived from the human cytomegalovirus immediate early gene 1 promoter creating the tet-op promoter. This promoter exhibits very low levels of basal transcription when integrated into a mammalian genome.[2,10] Expression from the tet-op promoter is activated by binding of a tTA to the operator sequences. tTA is a hybrid transactivator composed of the tetracycline repressor protein from TN10 fused to the viral protein 16 (VP16) activation domain from the herpes simplex virus. Fusion of the repressor sequences to VP16 creates a eukaryotic transactivator protein from what was a bacterial repressor protein. Binding of tTA to the operator sequences is controlled by the administration or withdrawal of tetracycline. Tetracycline binds to tTA and, in doing so, modifies its conformation[12] and ability to bind to DNA operator sequences. In the transgenic system described here, tTA binds to operator sequences in the absence of tetracycline. When tetracycline is complexed with tTA, it is unable to recognize operator sequences, and gene expression is turned off. A reverse tetracycline system also has been developed.[11] In that system a mutated tetracycline repressor domain was used to make a reverse transactivator (rtTA). rtTA binds operator sequences only when tetracycline is complexed to it. In this reverse system gene expression is turned on by tetracycline. The two tetracycline transactivator systems are diagrammed in FIGURE 1.

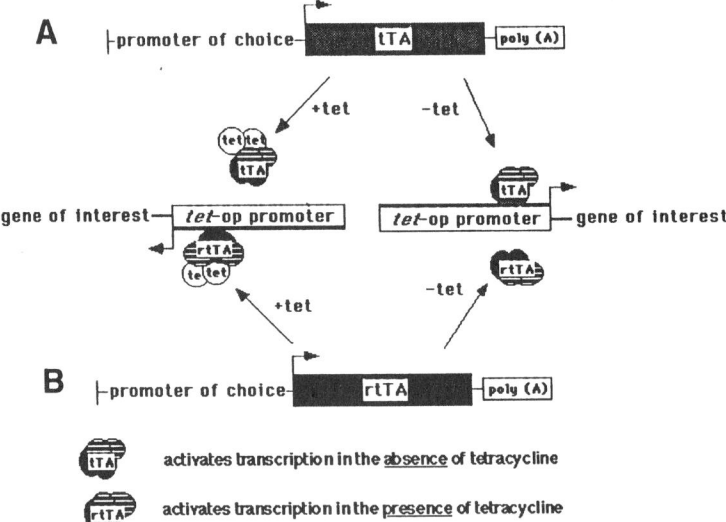

FIGURE 1. Diagram of the tetracycline-responsive transactivator systems. A: When tTA is present, there is no gene transcription in the presence of tetracycline. B: When the reverse transactivator (rtTA) is present, gene transcription is activated by tetracycline.

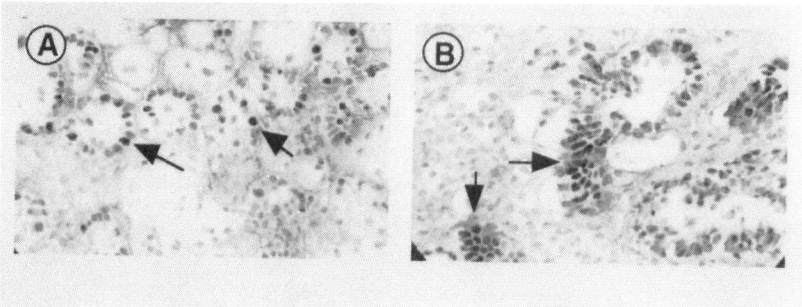

FIGURE 2. Immunohistochemical analysis of TAg expression in the submandibular salivary gland (**A**) and parotid gland (**B**) from a double transgenic mouse carrying MMTV-tTA and tet-op-TAg transgenes. Salivary gland specimens were frozen in OTC medium, and 7.5 micron sections were prepared. TAg protein was detected using the monoclonal antibody Pab 101 (Santa Cruz Biotechnology, Inc., Santa Cruz, CA). Arrows point to nuclei exhibiting TAg staining. Original magnification: ×60.

TEMPORALLY CONTROLLED GENE EXPRESSION IN THE SUBMANDIBULAR SALIVARY GLAND

The tetracycline-responsive transactivator system has been used to temporally control gene expression in striated duct cells of the submandibular salivary gland.[3,9] The mouse mammary tumor virus long-terminal repeat (MMTV-LTR) targets near homogeneous expression of SV40 T antigen (TAg) to these cells (FIG. 2A). Scattered areas of focal TAg expression are seen in the parotid gland (FIG. 2B). When luciferase and beta-galactosidase reporter genes are used, heterogeneous expression is detected in the mammary gland, testicular Leydig's cells, seminal vesicle, and basal cells of the skin.[9]

SV40 TAG EXPRESSION IN TISSUES OF TRANSGENIC MICE LEADS TO HYPERPLASIA AND TUMOR FORMATION

TAg has been expressed in a broad range of tissues in transgenic mice.[3,13–29] In most examples studied, TAg expression leads to transformation and tumor development. In the mammary gland, initial expression of TAg in mammary epithelial cells induces p53-independent apoptosis.[29] This suggests that there are cellular defense mechanisms that operate at very early stages in TAg-induced transformation to reduce the number of TAg-expressing cells. In the mammary gland, resistance to p53-independent apoptosis develops over time. Development of resistance to p53-independent apoptosis contributes to tumor development in both the mammary gland[30] and pancreas.[27,28]

Targeting TAg expression to the striated duct cells of the submandibular salivary gland leads to the early appearance of hyperplasia and the late development of fibrosis and tumors. Hyperplastic ductal structures are evident by two weeks of age (FIG. 3A). Hyperplastic histologic changes persist and progress. By four months of age, large areas of the gland are involved (FIG. 3B). Areas of hyperplasia are surrounded by fibrosis at 12 months (FIG. 3C), and tumors appear (FIGURES 3E and F).

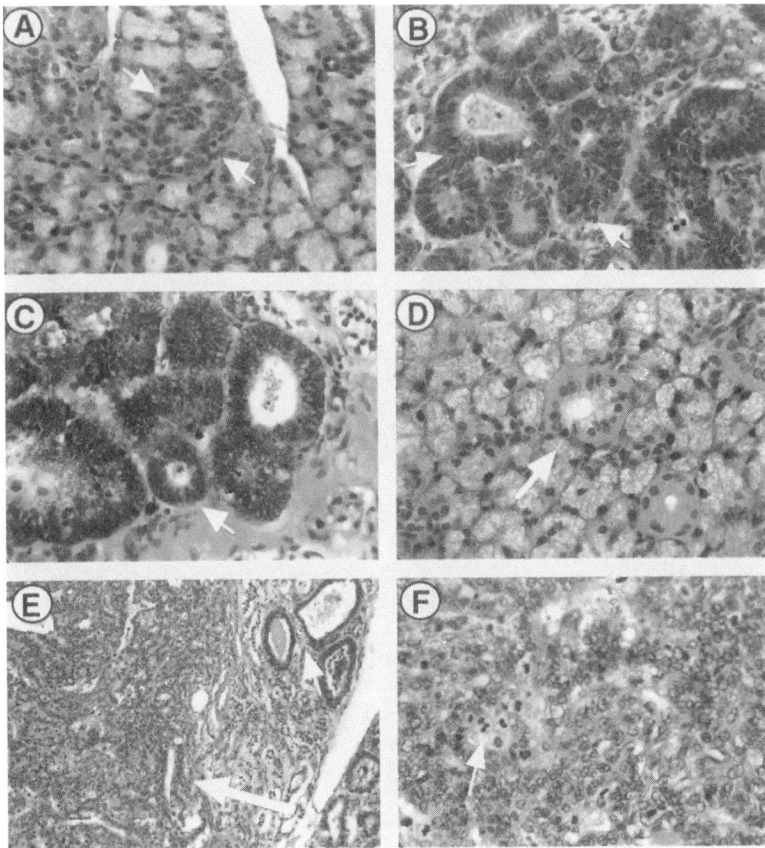

FIGURE 3. Histological analysis of submandibular salivary gland tissue from 2-week-old (**A**), 4-month-old (**B**), and 12-month-old (**C**) double transgenic mice carrying MMTV-tTA and tet-op-TAg transgenes in the absence of tetracycline exposure, and submandibular salivary gland tissue from 4-month-old double transgenic mice carrying MMTV-tTA and tet-op-TAg transgenes after a two-week exposure to tetracycline (**D**). Salivary gland tumor tissue from a 12-month-old double transgenic mouse at low power in **E** and high power in **F**. Arrows in **A, B,** and **C** point to areas of ductal hyperplasia. The arrow in **D** points to normal-appearing striated duct cells. The large arrow in **E** points to the tumor. The small arrow indicates an area of ductal hyperplasia. Mitotic figures (shown by the arrow in **F**) can be see in the tumor at high magnification. Tissues were fixed in 10% neutral formalin and embedded in paraffin. Five micron sections were prepared and stained with hematoxylin and eosin. Original magnification, A, B, C, D, F: ×60; original magnification, E: ×20.

TIME-SENSITIVE REVERSAL OF TAG-INDUCED HYPERPLASIA IN THE SALIVARY GLAND

Temporally controlled expression of TAg in the submandibular salivary gland is used to study the reversibility of hyperplastic change as a function of time.[3] At four months of age, hyperplastic changes reverse when TAg expression is turned off. Reversal is seen as early as two weeks after tetracycline treatment is initiated (FIG. 3D). When TAg expression is turned off at seven months of age, a time when there is also extensive fibrosis, hyperplasia is not reversed. Transformed cells that do not revert remain polyploid. This suggests that TAg-induced changes in these cells are able to maintain the transformed phenotype in the absence of Tag protein. The temporally controlled model offers unique opportunities to study genetic and physiological mechanisms induced by changing viral oncoprotein expression. For example, genetic events that govern reversal of the transformed phenotype can be examined. Specifically, the mechanism and role of apoptosis in removal of transformed cells and function of precursor and stem cells in reconstitution of the gland can be addressed. The nonrevertant phenotype at seven months of age can be used to identify the specific genetic changes triggered by viral oncoprotein expression which result in maintenance of the transformed phenotype. It is likely that some, if not all, critical genetic changes found in striated ductal cells will generalize to other cell types.

THE USE OF TEMPORALLY CONTROLLED GENE EXPRESSION TO STUDY SALIVARY GLAND BIOLOGY AND DISEASE

The tetracycline-responsive transactivator system described here can be used to study both normal development and physiology as well as specific disease states in the salivary gland. Temporally controlled expression of other gene products can be targeted to striated ductal cells by placing their coding sequences under control of the tet-op promoter and the MMTV-LTR. Gene deletions can be targeted to striated ductal cells by combining the Cre-lox gene recombination system with the MMTV-LTR–driven tetracycline transactivator system.[1,3,9,31] The use of alternative promoters to target tTA expression to different cell populations in the salivary glands, or other tissues, enables investigators to extend the use of temporally controlled gene expression to other cell types.[2,4,6–8,32]

ACKNOWLEDGMENT

The authors thank Jiadi Hu for performing TAg immunohistochemistry.

REFERENCES

1. FURTH, P.A. 1997. Conditional control of gene expression in the mammary gland. Mammary Gland Biol. Neoplasia. **2:** 373–383.
2. FURTH, P.A., L. ST.ONGE, H. BOGER, P. GRUSS, M. GOSSEN, A. KISTNER, H. BUJARD & L. HENNINGHAUSEN. 1994. Temporal control of gene expression in transgenic mice by a tetracycline responsive promoter. Proc. Natl. Acad. Sci. USA **91:** 9302–9306.
3. EWALD, D., M. LI, S. EFRAT, G. AUER, R.J. WALL, P.A. FURTH & L. HENNINGHAUSEN. 1996. Time-sensitive reversal of hyperplasia in transgenic mice expressing SV40 T antigen. Science **273:** 1384–1386.
4. MAYFORD, M., M.E. BACH, Y.-Y. HUANG, L. WANG, R.D. HAWKINS & E.R. KANDEL. 1996. Controlling memory formation using regulated expression of a CaMKII transgene. Science **274:** 1678–1683.
5. SCHULTZE, N., Y. BURKI, Y. LANG, U. CERTA & H. BLUETHMANN. 1996. Efficient control of gene expression by single step integration of the tetracycline system in transgenic mice. Nature Biotechnol. **14:** 499–503.
6. KISTNER, A., M. GOSSEN, F. ZIMMERMAN, J. JERECIC, C. ULLMER, H. LUBBERT & H. BU-

JARD. 1996. Doxycycline-mediated quantitative and tissue-specific control of gene expression in transgenic mice. Proc. Natl. Acad. Sci. USA **93:** 10933–10938.
7. FISHMAN, G.I., M.L. KAPLAN & P.M. BUTTRICK. 1994. Tetracycline-regulated cardiac gene expression *in vivo*. J. Clin. Invest. **93:** 1864–1868.
8. YU, Z., C.S. REDFERN & G.I. FISHMAN. 1996. Conditional transgene expression in the heart. Circ. Res. **79:** 691–697.
9. HENNINGHAUSEN, L., R. WALL, U. TILLMANN, M. LI & P.A. FURTH. 1995. Conditional gene expression in secretory tissues and skin of transgenic mice using the MMTV-LTR and the tetracycline responsive system. J. Cell. Biochem. **59:** 463–472.
10. GOSSEN, M. & H. BUJARD. 1992. Tight control of gene expression in mammalian cells by tetracycline-responsive promoters. Proc. Natl. Acad. Sci. USA **89:** 5547–5551.
11. GOSSEN, M., S. FREUNDLIB, G. BENDER, G. MULLER, W. HILLEN & H. BUJARD. 1995. Transcriptional activation by tetracyclines in mammalian cells. Science **268:** 1766–1769.
12. HINRICHS, W., C. KISKER, M. DUVEL, A. MULLER, K. TOVAR, W. HILLEN & W. SAENGER. 1994. Structure of the Tet repressor-tetracycline complex and regulation of antibiotic resistance. Science **264:** 418–420.
13. TZENG, Y.-J., E. GUHL, M. GRAESSMANN & A. GRAESSMANN. 1993. Breast cancer formation in transgenic animals induced by the whey acidic protein SV40 T antigen (WAP-SV-T) hybrid gene. Oncogene **8:** 1965–1971.
14. KUHLMANN, E., P.G. TERHUNE & D.S. LONGNECKER. 1993. Evaluation of c-K-*ras* in pancreatic carcinoma from Ela-1, SV40E transgenic mice. Carcinogenesis **14:** 2649–2651.
15. INOUE, T., Y. HIRABAYASHI, H. MITSUI, Y. FURUTA, Y. SUDA, S. AIZAWA & Y. IKAWA. 1994. Experimental model for MDS-like myelodysplasia in transgenic mice harboring the SV40 large-T antigen under an immunoglobulin enhancer. Leukemia **8**(Suppl. 1): S202–S205.
16. MAXWELL, P.H., M.K. OSMOND, C.W. PUGH, A. HERYET, L.G. NICHOLLS, C.C. TAN, B.G. DOE, D.J.P. FERGUSON, M.H. JOHNSON & P.J. RATCLIFFE. 1994. Erythropoietin-producing cells in transgenic mice expressing SV40 T antigen directed by erythropoietin control sequences. Ann. N.Y. Acad. Sci. **718:** 356–358.
17. TEITZ, T., T.S.B. YEN, J.C. CHANG & Y.W. KAN. 1994. SV40 T antigen directed by a powerful erythroid enhancer-promoter produced sarcomas and pancreatic tumors but not erythroid-specific tumors in transgenic mice. DNA Cell Biol. **13:** 705–710.
18. SANDMÖLLER, A., R. HALTER, E. GÓMEZ-LA-HOZ, H.-J. GRÖNE, G. SUSKE, D. PAUL & M. BEATO. 1994. The uteroglobin promoter targets expression of the SV40 T antigen to a variety of secretory epithelial cells in transgenic mice. Oncogene **9:** 2805–2815.
19. WILKIE, T.M., R.A. SCHMIDT, M. BAETSCHER & A. MESSING. 1994. Smooth muscle and bone neoplasms in transgenic mice expressing SV40 T antigen. Oncogene **9:** 2889–2895.
20. SERVENIUS, B., J. VERNACHIO, J. PRICE, L.C. ANDERSSON & P.A. PETERSON. 1994. Metastasizing neuroblastomas in mice transgenic for simian virus 40 large T (SV40T) under the olfactory marker protein gene promoter. Cancer Res. **54:** 5198–5205.
21. HINO, O., T. KITAGAWA, K. NOMURA, K. OHTAKE, L. CUI, Y. FURUTA & S. AIZAWA. 1991. Hepatocarcinogenesis in transgenic mice carrying albumin-promoter SV40 T antigen gene. J. Cancer Res. **82:** 1226–1233.
22. SCHIRMACHER, P., W.A. HELD, D. YONG, L. BIENPICA & C.E. ROGLER. 1991. Selective amplification of periportal transitional cells precedes formation of hepatocellular carcinoma in SV40 large T antigen transgenic mice. Am. J. Pathol. **139:** 231–241.
23. HELD, W.A., J. PAZIK, J.G. O'BRIEN, K. KERNS, M. GOBEY, R. MEIS, L. KENNY & Y. RUSTUM. 1994. Genetic analysis of liver tumorigenesis in SV40 T antigen transgenic mice implies a role for imprinted genes. Cancer Res. **54:** 6489–6495.
24. DRUCKER, D.J. 1994. Molecular pathophysiology of glucagon-SV40 T antigen transgenic mice. Am. J. Physiol. Endocrinol. Metab. **267:** E629–E635.
25. CHEAH, K.S.E., A. LEVY, P.A. TRAINOR, A.W. WAI, T. KUFFNER, C.L. SO, K.K.H. LEUNG, R.H. LOVELL-BADGE & P.P.L. TAM. 1995. Human COL2A1-directed SV40T antigen expression in transgenic and chimeric mice results in abnormal skeletal development. J. Cell Biol. **128:** 223–237.
26. SYMONDS, H., L. KRALL, L. REMINGTON, M. SAENZ-ROBLES, S. LOWE, T. JACKS & T. VAN DYKE. 1994. p53-dependent apoptosis suppresses tumor growth and progression *in vivo*. Cell **78:** 703–711.

27. CHRISTOFORI, G., P. NAIK & D. HANAHAN. 1994. A second signal supplied by insulin-like growth factor II in oncogene-induced tumorigenesis. Science **369:** 414–417.
28. NAIK, P., J. KARRIM & D. HANAHAN. 1996. The rise and fall of apoptosis during multistage tumorigenesis: down-modulation contributes to tumor progression from angiogenic progenitors. Genes & Dev. **10:** 2105–2116.
29. LI, M., J. HU, K. HEERMEIER, L. HENNIGHAUSEN & P.A. FURTH. 1996. Expression of a viral oncoprotein during development of the mammary gland alters cell fate and function: induction of p53 independent apoptosis is followed by impairment of milk protein production in surviving cells. Cell Growth & Differ **7:** 3–11.
30. BAR-PELED, U., M. LI, M., R. JAEGER, L. HENNIGHAUSEN, H. WEIHER & P.A. FURTH. Unpublished observations.
31. ST.ONGE, L., P.A. FURTH & P. GRUSS. 1996. Temporal control of Cre recombinase in transgenic mice by a tetracycline responsive promoter. Nucleic Acids Res. **24:** 3875–3877.
32. EFRAT, S., D. FUSCO-DEMANE, H. LEMBERG, O. AL EMRAN & X. WANG. 1995. Targeting conditional expression of TAg to pancreatic acinar cells using the tetracycline responsive system in transgenic mice. Proc. Natl. Acad. Sci. USA **92:** 3576–3580.

In Vitro and In Vivo Models for the Reconstruction of Intercellular Signaling[a]

KAMAL H. BOUHADIR AND DAVID J. MOONEY[b]

Departments of Chemical Engineering and Biological and Materials Sciences, University of Michigan, Ann Arbor, Michigan 48109, USA

ABSTRACT: A critical need in both tissue-engineering applications and basic cell culture studies is the development of synthetic extracellular matrices (ECMs) and experimental systems that reconstitute three-dimensional cell–cell interactions and control tissue formation *in vitro* and *in vivo*. We have fabricated synthetic ECMs in the form of fiber-based fabrics, highly porous sponges, and hydrogels from biodegradable polymers (*e.g.*, polyglycolic acid) and tested their ability to regulate tissue formation. Both cell seeding onto these synthetic ECMs and subsequent culture conditions can be varied to control initial cell–cell interactions and subsequent cell growth and tissue development. Three-dimensional tissues composed of cells of interest, matrix produced by these cells, and the synthetic ECM (until it degrades) can be created with these systems. For example, smooth muscle cells can be grown on polyglycolic acid fiber-based synthetic ECMs to produce tissues with cell densities in excess of 10^8 cells/mL. These tissues contain extensive elastin and collagen, and the smooth muscle cells within the tissue express the contractile phenotype (*e.g.*, α-actin staining). Similar approaches can be used to grow a number of other tissues (*e.g.*, dental pulp) that resemble the native tissue. These engineered tissues may provide novel experimental systems to study the role of three-dimensional intercellular signaling in tissue development and may also find clinical application as replacements to lost or damaged tissues.

INTRODUCTION

Clinicians faced with replacing tissue lost to disease, trauma, or congenital defects currently have two options. The first, use of synthetic materials as a prosthesis, has a long history. The prosthesis typically does not replace the entire range of tissue functions and can serve as a site for infections and other chronic problems. The other option, use of autologous or allogenic tissue/organ transplantation is often very effective at replacing lost tissue structure and function. However, there exists a significant shortage of donor tissues available for tissue reconstruction and organ transplantation. For example, in 1988, only around 10% of the number of patients suffering from liver failure received a liver transplant.[1] This is mainly due to the limited number of organs available for transplantation every year. These limitations have led to the development of the tissue-engineering field, in which new tissues are created from cultured cells and biomaterial matrices.[2] This field has been defined as a "combination of the principles and methods of the life sciences with those of engineering to elucidate fundamental understanding of structure-function relationships in normal and diseased tissues, to develop materials and methods to repair damaged or diseased tissues, and to create en-

---

[a] Research in the authors' laboratories is supported by Reprogenesis, the National Science Foundation, the National Institutes of Health, and the Whitaker Foundation.

[b] Corresponding author: David J. Mooney, Department of Chemical Engineering, University of Michigan, Ann Arbor, MI 48109-2136, USA. Tel: (313) 763-4816; fax: (313) 764-7453; e-mail: mooneyd@engin.umich.edu

tire tissue replacement."[3] It may be possible to treat a large number of patients by developing tissue-engineering strategies that use cell transplantation. One such strategy uses a combination of synthetic polymer matrices and cells to recreate three-dimensional cell–cell interactions and, hence, tissue formation. These matrices serve as both a transplant delivery system for the cells and templates guiding tissue proliferation and organization. In addition, these systems may provide new models to study tissue development and disease progression in well-controlled, *in vitro* experiments. There is a critical need for cell-culture models that, in contrast to standard tissue culture models, create three-dimensional cell interactions.

Natural extracellular matrices (ECMs) are used as a model for the development of synthetic matrices for tissue engineering. The natural ECM is composed of a complex network of macromolecules that hold cells together in an organized fashion to form tissues. These organized networks allow cells within to migrate and interact with one another. Moreover, nutrients, metabolites, and hormones from neighboring blood vessels diffuse into the ECM to provide nourishment and communication to the cells. The two main classes of extracellular macromolecules that form ECMs are proteoglycans (PG) and fibrous proteins. Proteoglycans contain long unbranched polysaccharide side chains (glycosaminoglycans) covalently tethered to a protein backbone. Proteoglycans form networks of hydrated gels in which cells are embedded, thus providing a three-dimensional space for tissue formation. Structural fibrous proteins like collagen provide the tensile strength of ECMs, whereas proteoglycans provide compressive strength. Hence, critical functions of ECMs include providing potential space for tissue development and mechanical support during this process. Recently, it has been become clear that the ECM also plays an essential role in such cellular functions as growth, differentiation, and motility. The cell–ECM interactions are mediated by the affinity of cell-membrane receptors for specific peptide sequences present in ECM molecules. The best-studied sequence is the tripeptide Arg-Gly-Asp (RGD), which is responsible for cell adhesion of many ECM proteins.[4] Cell adhesion to ECMs by way of ligand-receptor affinity is the first step in a series of biological reactions, and communications between cells and the ECM, and between cells. Cell–ECM interactions ultimately guide the generation of new tissues.

SYNTHETIC BIODEGRADABLE MATRICES

A variety of synthetic ECMs have shown promise in tissue-engineering applications. Natural biodegradable matrices (collagen, fibrin) have been widely used as cell immobilization matrices; however, they suffers from batch to batch inconsistency, which is a major concern in production scale-up. As a result, synthetic polymers have been alternatively used as cell-delivery devices due to their well-controlled structures and properties. It is particularly attractive if these matrices are biodegradable. This eliminates the need to remove the matrix following tissue development. The rate at which the matrix degrades should be compatible with the rate of new tissue development and regeneration. In addition, the degradation products should be biocompatible. In this paper, we will discuss several examples where biodegradable synthetic matrices have been successfully used for tissue engineering.

Polyglycolic acid (PGA), poly-L-lactic acid (PLLA), and copolymers of lactic and glycolic acid (PLGA) are the most widely used biodegradable polymers to fabricate synthetic ECMs. These synthetic polymers have been used in a variety of biomedical applications (*e.g.*, suture materials) for over twenty years.[5] PGA, PLLA, and PLGA contain ester linkages (FIG. 1) and are susceptible to hydrolysis in aqueous environments. Hydrolytic cleavage of the ester linkage yields naturally occurring metabolic by-products that are biocompatible and cause minimal inflammatory responses. PGA is a highly crystalline polymer with a high melting point and low solubility in organic solvents and is relatively hydrophilic. PGA implants lose their structural integrity within two weeks and are absorbed after about four weeks of implantation.[6,7] PLLA, on the other hand, is more hydrophobic and more soluble in organic solvents. As a result, PLLA is less labile to aqueous hydrolysis and degrades at a much slower rate compared to PGA.[8] Copolymers of varying ratios of L-lactic acid and glycolic acid yield polymers with a wide range of degradation rates and mechanical properties, making them more attractive candidates for cell-delivery devices in tissue engineering.[12]

Several techniques have been developed to process these polymers into devices suitable for tissue-engineering applications.[9] PGA is typically processed by melting and extruding into fibers (diameter, 10–15 μm) that are used to construct woven and nonwoven fiber-based meshes.[20,21] Nonwoven meshes of PGA fibers are highly porous, permitting diffusion of nutrients throughout the scaffold, and are capable of delivering high densities of cells. However, such constructs lack the structural stability to withstand compressive forces *in vivo*. To improve upon their mechanical properties, PGA fibers in these matrices have been physically bonded with PLLA and PLGA.[21] A wide range of mechanical strengths and rates of degradation can be achieved by varying the amount of physical bonding.

To further improve upon the mechanical strength of synthetic ECMs, highly porous sponges have been fabricated from PLLA and poly-D,L-lactic-co-glycolic acid (PLGA). These polymers are commonly processed into sponges with various pore sizes by a variety of methods involving a phase transition. Typical methods include solvent casting

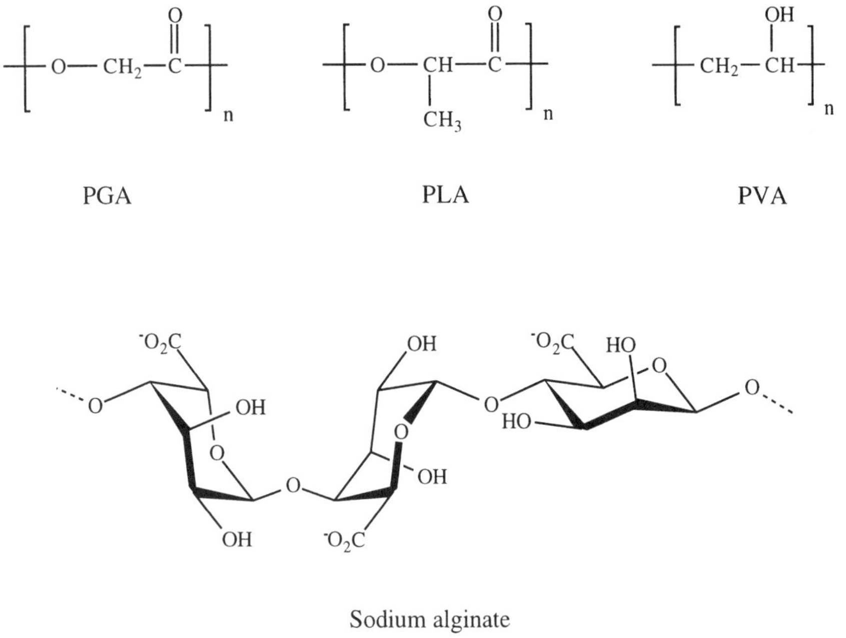

FIGURE 1. Chemical structures of polyglycolic acid (PGA), poly-L-lactic acid (PLLA), polyvinyl alcohol (PVA), and sodium alginate.

and particulate leaching or a gas-foaming method.[10–13] In the former method, the polymer is dissolved in an organic solvent and cast into cylindrical molds packed with sodium chloride particles of a desired size range. The organic solvent is evaporated, and the entrapped salt particles are leached out in aqueous solutions. The dimensions of the sponge can be controlled by the size and shape of the mold. Moreover, the pore size distribution can be controlled by the size of the salt particles used in packing the mold, and the porosity of the sponges can be varied by altering the ratio of polymer/salt particles.[10–12] To avoid the use of organic solvents, another approach to fabricate highly porous sponges was developed using high-pressure gases to induce nucleation and growth of gas cells within the polymer matrix. Highly porous matrices (up to 93%) can be fabricated with this approach.[13]

Other materials that are promising for cell immobilization matrices in tissue engineering include alginates. Algal alginate, a naturally occurring polysaccharide isolated from seaweed, has been extensively used in the chemical and food industry as a thickening, emulsifying, and stabilizing agent. Biomedical applications of alginates include wound dressings, dental impression materials, and, more recently, cell immobilization matrices.[14,22,23] Alginates are linear polysaccharides that contains variable amounts of the uronic acids D-mannuronic acid (M) and L-guluronic acid (G) (FIG. 1). The two monosaccharides present are in random sequences of poly-mannuronate (M-M-M-M), poly-guluronate (G-G-G-G), and an alternating sequence of both uronic acids (-M-G-M-G).[15] An attractive feature of alginates is their ability to form hydrogels in the presence of divalent cations (*e.g.*, Ca^{2+}, Sr^{2+}, and Ba^{2+}). It is well established that this affinity and selectivity for divalent cations is related to the poly-guluronate content of the polymer. Sodium alginates with a wide range of G and M content are commercially available. Hydrogels of alginates seeded with cells have the potential to be transplanted endoscopically into a patient, thus providing a minimally invasive method for cell transplantation.[17,18]

IN VITRO TISSUE DEVELOPMENT

The development of cell seeding and cell-culture conditions for the cell-polymer constructs is essential to efficiently engineer tissues. To optimize the number of adherent cells onto fiber-based polymer constructs, different methods for cell seeding have been investigated.[16] Dynamic seeding methods (*e.g.*, seeding in stirred bioreactors) produces a higher number of adherent cells as compared to static seeding methods.[16] Cell seeding can also be enhanced by surface modifications of matrices.[17] The importance of culture conditions has been demonstrated by studies comparing the development of smooth muscle tissue in static and stirred culture conditions. Optimal tissue development is typically achieved in bioreactors with nutrient flow, as indicated by higher cell densities and matrix compositions. Tissues developed in bioreactors contained more elastin and collagen, and the amount of elastin was comparable to that of native tissue.[6] Similar results have been found when engineering dental pulp tissue (unpublished data). Tissues (*e.g.*, dental pulp) developed under appropriate conditions (FIG. 2) can resemble the native tissues.[18] Nonwoven PGA fiber-based scaffolds have also been seeded with bovine chondrocytes and used to engineer new cartilage *in vitro*.[19]

IN VIVO EVALUATION OF CELL-POLYMER CONSTRUCTS

The potential of tissue engineering to create tissues *in vivo* has also been demonstrated with a number of tissue types. Cartilage in various sizes and shapes (*e.g.*, nasal

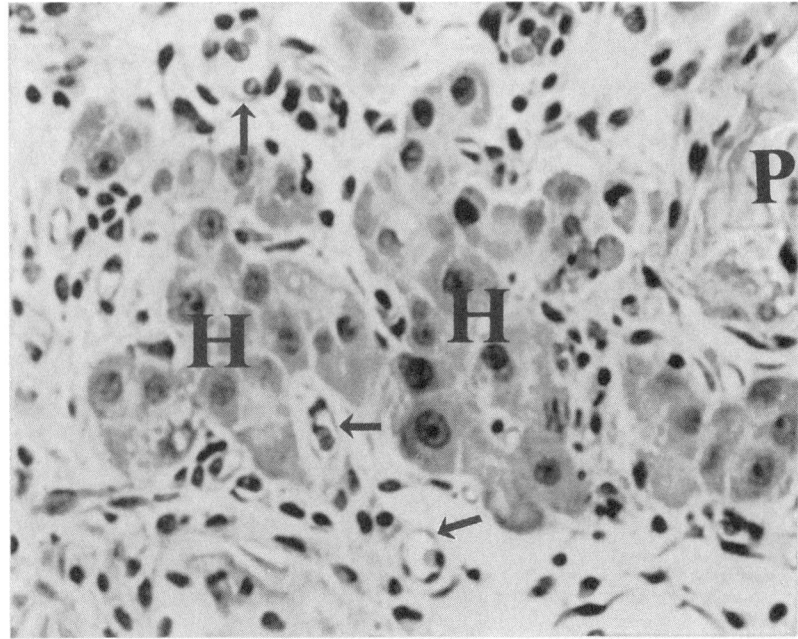

FIGURE 2. Photomicrograph of new liver-like tissue engineered *in vivo*.[17] Hepatocytes (H), residual polymer matrix (P), and new capillaries (arrows) are visible in the photomicrograph (D. J. Mooney, unpublished data).

septal cartilage) has been engineered in various animal models using polyglycolic acid matrices.[20,21] Cartilage regeneration has also been demonstrated with such other biodegradable polymer materials as the sodium alginates.[22] The newly formed cartilage in these studies resembled native cartilage biochemically and structurally.[23] The feasibility of using injectable chondrocyte-alginate gel suspensions has also been demonstrated in the treatment of vesicoureteral reflux in pigs.[24,25] Sponge-based matrices have been used to transplant hepatocytes and engineer new liver-like tissues.[17] A variety of other tissues, including intestine, have also been partially engineered with this type of matrix.[26,27] Implantation of these highly porous matrices typically leads to the ingrowth of blood vessels that support the metabolic needs of the new tissue (FIG. 3).

APPLICATION TO SALIVARY TISSUE

The principles of tissue engineering have not yet been applied to salivary tissue. However, the matrices and systems developed with other tissues will likely be directly applicable to salivary tissue. Matrices developed to transplant hepatocytes, another secretory cell type, will likely be useful for *in vitro* and *in vivo* models of salivary tissue engineering. Matrices to create tubular structures, which would be a critical component of engineered salivary tissue, have also been demonstrated.[26,27] Creation of three-

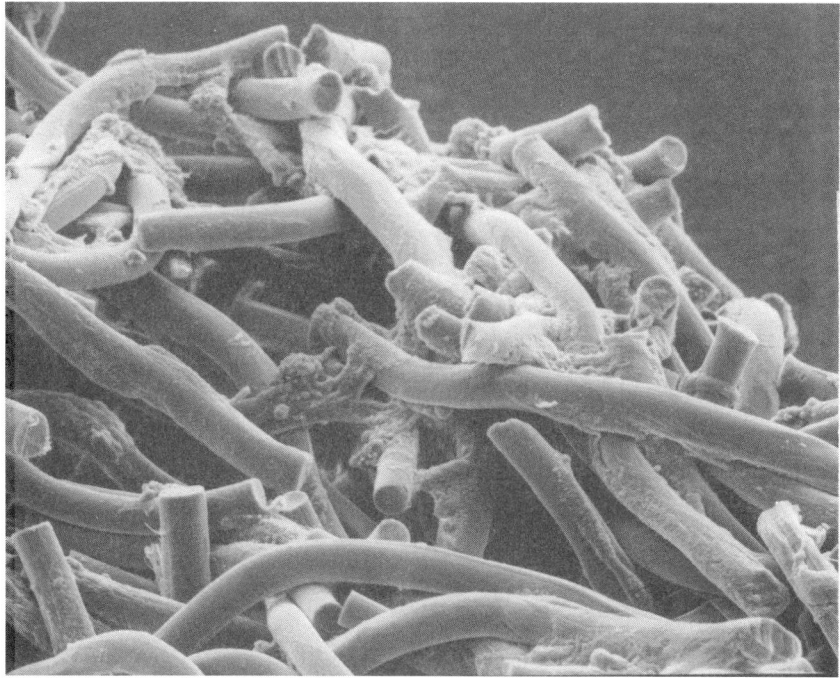

FIGURE 3. Human pulp-derived fibroblasts adherent to fibers of a polyglycolic acid matrix. The cells will proliferate, secrete extracellular matrix, and fill the pores while the matrix degrades. A new, pulp-like tissue will result.[18]

dimensional salivary tissue culture systems may also lead to an improved understanding of the role of cell–cell interactions in salivary development, function, and dysfunction in various disease states.

REFERENCES

1. AMERICAN LIVER FOUNDATION. 1988. Vital statistics of the United States 2, part A. New Jersey: ALF.
2. LANGER, R. & J.P. VACANTI. 1993. Tissue engineering. Science **260:** 920–926.
3. NEREM, R.M. & A. SAMBANIS. 1995. Tissue engineering: From biology to biological substitutes. Tissue Eng. **1:** 3–13.
4. RUOSLABTI, E. & M.D. PIERSCHBACKER. 1987. Science **238:** 491–497.
5. HUANG, S.J. 1989. Biodegradable Polymers. *In* Polymers-Biomaterials and Medical Applications. J. I. Kroschwitz, Ed.: 5–28. Wiley & Sons. New York.
6. FRAZZA, E. J. & E.E. SCMITT. 1971. A new absorbable suture. J. Biomed. Mater. Res. Symp. **1:** 43–48.
7. KATZ, A.R. & R. TURNER. 1970. Evaluation of tensile strength and absorption properties of polyglycolic acid sutures. Surg. Gynecol. & Obstet. **131:** 701–716.
8. REED, A.M. & D.K. GIDDING. 1981. Biodegradable polymers for use in surgerypoly(glycolic)/poly(lactic acid) homo and copolymers. Polymer **22:** 494–498.
9. MOONEY, D.J. & R.S. LANGER. 1995. Engineering Biomaterials for tissue engineering: The

10–100 micron size scale. *In* The Biomedical Engineering Handbook. J. D. Bronzino, Ed.: 1609–1618. Boca Raton: CRC Press.
10. MOONEY, D.J., G. ORGAN, J. VACANTI & R. LANGER. 1994. Design and fabrication of cell delivery devices to engineer tubular tissues. Cell Transplant. **3:** 203–210.
11. MOONEY, D.J., S. PARK, P.M. KAUFMAN, K. SANO, K. MCNAMARA, P. VACANTI & R. LANGER. 1995. Transplantation of hepatocytes using porous, biodegradable sponges. Transplant. Proc. **26:** 4025–4026.
12. MOONEY, D.J., C. BREUER, K. MCNAMARA, P. VACANTI & R. LANGER. 1995. Fabricating tubular devices from polymers of lactic and glycolic acid for tissue engineering. Tissue Eng. **1:** 107–118.
13. MOONEY, D.J., D.F. BALDWIN, N.P. SUH, J.P. VACANTI & R. LANGER. 1996. Novel approach to fabricate porous sponges of poly(D,L-lactic-co-glycolic acid) without the use of organic solvents. Biomaterials **17:** 1417–1422.
14. SCHMIDT, R.J., L.Y. CHUNG, A.M. ANDREWS, O. SPYRATOU & T.D. TURNER. 1992. Biocompatibility of wound management products: A study of the effects of various polysaccharides on murine L929 fibroblasts proliferation and macrophage respiratory burst. J. Pharm. Pharmacol. **45:** 508–513.
15. SUTHERLAND, I.W. 1991. Alginates. *In* Biomaterials: Novel materials from biological sources. D. Byron, Ed. Stockton Press. New York.
16. KIM, B-S., A.J. PUTMAN, T.J. KULIK & D.J. MOONEY. Submitted.
17. MOONEY, D.J., S. PARK, P.M. KAUFMAN, K. SANO, K. MCNAMARA, P.J. VACANTI & R. LANGER. 1995. Biodegradable sponges for hepatocyte transplantation. J. Biomed. Mater. Res. **29:** 959–965.
18. MOONEY, D.J., C. POWELL, J. PIANA & B. RUTHERFORD. 1996. Engineering dental pulp-like tissue in vitro. Biotechnol. Prog. **12:** 865–868.
19. MA, P.X., B. SCHLOO, D.J. MOONEY & R. LANGER. 1995. Development of biomechanical properties and morphogenesis of *in vitro* tissue engineered cartilage. J. Biomed. Mater. Res. **29:** 1587–1595.
20. PUELACHER, W.C., D.J. MOONEY, R. LANGER, J.P. VACANTI & C.A. VACANTI. 1994. Design of nasoseptal cartilage replacements synthesized from biodegradable polymers and chondrocytes **15:** 774–778.
21. MOONEY, D.J., C.L. MAZZONI, C. BREUER, K. MCNAMARA, D. HERN, J.P. VACANTI & R. LANGER. 1996. Stabilized polyglycolic acid fiber-based tubes for tissue engineering. Biomaterials **17:** 115–124.
22. PAIGE, K.T., L.G. CIMA, M.J. YAREMCHUK, B.L. SCLOO, J.V. VACANTI & C.A. VACANTI. 1995. De novo cartilage generation using calcium alginate-chondrocyte constructs. Plast. Reconstr. Surg. **97:** 168–178.
23. PAIGE, K.T., L.G. CIMA, M.J. YAREMCHUK & J.V. VACANTI. 1995. Injectable cartilage. Plast. Reconstr. Surg. **96:** 1390–1398.
24. ATALA, A., L.G. CIMA, W. KIM, K.T. PAIGE, J.V. VACANTI, A.B. RETIK & C.A. VACANTI. 1993. Injectable alginate seeded with chondrocytes as a potential treatment for vesicoureteral reflux. J. Urol. **150:** 745–747.
25. ATALA, A., W. KIM, K.T. PAIGE, C.A. VACANTI & A.B. RETIK. 1994. Endoscopic treatment of vesicoureteral reflux with a chondrocyte-alginate suspension. J. Urol. **152:** 641–643.
26. ORGAN, G.M., D.J. MOONEY & L.K. HANSEN. 1992. Enterocyte transplantation using cell polymer devices to produce a neointestine. Transplant. Proc. **24:** 3009–3011.
27. ORGAN, G.M., D.J. MOONEY & L.K. HANSEN. 1993. Enterocyte transplantation using cell polymer devices to create epithelial-lined tubes. Transplant. Proc. **25:** 998–1001.

Molecular Dissection of the Genetic Targets of ALG7 in the Serpentine Receptor-mediated Signal Transduction Pathway in Yeast

KELLEY LENNON, ALBERTO BIRD, AND MARIA A. KUKURUZINSKA[a]

Division of Oral Biology, Boston University Goldman School of Dental Medicine, Center for Advanced Biomedical Research, 700 Albany Street, Boston, Massachusetts 02118, USA

INTRODUCTION

Salivary gland development comprises several highly regulated genetic programs that include cell proliferation, differentiation, morphogenesis, migration, and apoptosis. Although many of the key factors involved in the development of salivary glands have yet to be determined, we have identified one evolutionarily conserved gene, ALG7, that plays a role in the development of diverse biological systems, ranging from yeast to mammals. ALG7, the first gene in, and the regulator of, the dolichol pathway of protein N-glycosylation, is a tightly regulated, early growth response gene[1] whose expression has been shown to be modulated with proliferation, at two major control points of the yeast cell cycle: G0/G1 and G1/S.[2] Furthermore, unwarranted changes in ALG7 expression in yeast result in defects in proliferation and differentiation.[2,3] Recent studies with higher eukaryotes have shown that levels of the ALG7 protein product, GPT, are regulated with proliferation in Chinese hamster ovary cells[4] and with the differentiation of the murine mammary gland[5] and the hamster submandibular gland.[4]

Much of the current understanding of development comes from the dissection of events in the life cycle of yeast. Therefore, we have used the yeast-mating response pathway, a model for both a multicomponent signal transduction cascade and a multistep developmental program, to decipher the developmentally relevant cellular functions affected by ALG7 in order to identify potential genetic targets for this gene (FIG. 1). Specifically, we have examined mRNA levels of critical components of the yeast α-factor response pathway that act at the cell surface, within the phosphorylation cascade, and at the branch points that lead to G1 arrest, the induction of differentiation and cell polarization in *alg7 3'UTR* mutant cells.[3] Inasmuch as mammalian homologues of many proteins involved in the yeast-mating response have been identified, insight gained from this study is relevant to the understanding of similar signaling mechanisms in salivary cells.

METHODS

Saccharomyces cerevisiae strains used in this study were wild type SMKY14 *(MATa lys2-801 his-619 alg7::URA/pMK14)* and an *alg7 3'UTR* mutant strain, SMKY44 *(MATa alg7::URA/pMKΔ44)*. Cells were grown to $OD_{660}=1$, and the mating

---

[a] To whom correspondence should be addressed. Tel: (617) 638-4859; fax: (617) 638-4924; e-mail: mkukuruz@bu.edu

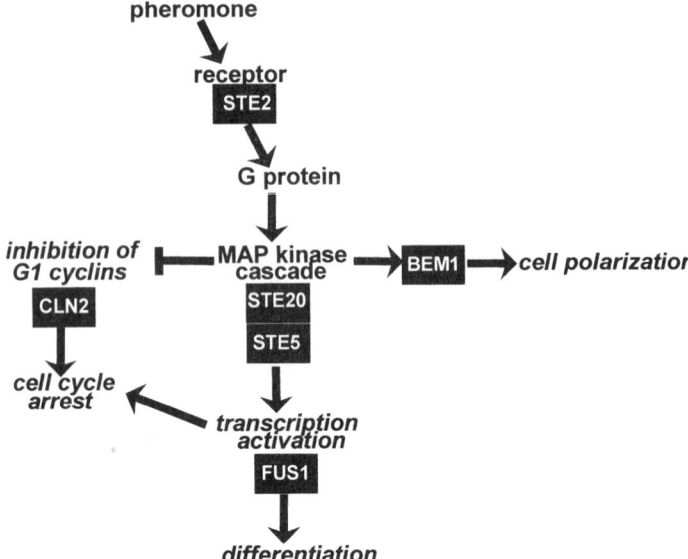

FIGURE 1. The pheromone response pathway of *Saccharomyces cerevisiae*. Haploid yeast cells, of either a or α mating type, secrete pheromones to induce the conjugation of cells with the opposite mating type. These pheromones bind to serpentine receptors at the cell surface, transmit a signal through a heterotrimeric G protein, and trigger a MAP kinase cascade that ultimately results in cell-cycle arrest in G1, the induction of differentiation, and reorganization of the actin cytoskeleton. Genes assayed for expression are shown in black boxes.

pheromone α-factor was added to 10 μM. At t0 and 1, 2.5, 4.5, and 8 h after treatment, cells were removed for RNA isolations and blotting assays, as described previously.[1] Blots were hybridized sequentially with probes specific for STE2, STE5, STE20, CLN2, FUS1, and BEM1 at high stringency. Autoradiography was performed at −80°C with DuPont X-ray film and intensifying screens.

RESULTS/CONCLUSIONS

Expression of the STE2 Receptor in alg7 3'UTR Mutants

The results from our study are summarized in TABLE 1. As predicted, STE2 mRNA expression in wild-type cells increased following treatment with α-factor. Interestingly, STE2 transcript levels were induced to even higher levels than the wild type, albeit the time course for the induction was slower; the significance of this result is unclear but may reflect a compensatory response to the lower GPT activity in these cells.

Effect of Deregulated ALG7 Expression on Proliferation

Cell-cycle progression in yeast is controlled by cyclin-dependent kinase complexes: Cdc28 associates with both G1 and G2 cyclins to facilitate G1/S and G2/M transition,

TABLE 1. Transcript Levels of Pheromone-response Pathway Components in Wild-type vs. *alg7 3'UTR* Mutant Cells

Component	Function of Protein Product	Wild Type	*alg7 3'UTR* Mutant
STE2	receptor	upregulated within 1 h of treatment; declined with recovery	slower upregulation than wild type; induced to higher levels
STE20	phosphorylation cascade	levels unaffected by treatment	same as wild type
STE5	phosphorylation cascade	levels unaffected by treatment	same as wild type
CLN2	G1 cyclin	downregulated to undetectable levels within 1 h of treatment	slightly downregulated, but effect is transient; induced to > t0 at 4.5 h
FUS1	differentiation-specific gene necessary for cell fusion	greatly induced within 1 h of treatment; declined with recovery	slower induction than wild type
BEM1	interacts with actin cytoskeleton in polarization	upregulated within 1 h of treatment; declined with recovery	levels only slightly affected by treatment

respectively. As expected, treatment of wild-type cells with α-factor resulted in a rapid inhibition of CLN2 transcript abundance, to barely detectable levels, consistent with cell-cycle arrest. In the *alg7 3'UTR* mutant cells, however, CLN2 mRNAs were not significantly attenuated following pheromone treatment; in fact, CLN2 transcripts were induced 4.5 h after treatment. These results suggest that the mutant cells do not effectively arrest in response to the mating pheromone. Moreover, they are consistent with the flow cytometric analyses of DNA profiles of *alg7 3'UTR* mutants that show a significant percentage of cells still cycling following treatment with α-factor (data not shown).

Effect of Unwarranted Changes in ALG7 Expression on Differentiation

Conjugation in yeast requires the expression of genes that promote cell and nuclear fusion. One such differentiation-specific gene is FUS1. Although in both wild-type and *alg7 3'UTR* mutant cells, FUS1 transcript levels rose sharply following pheromone treatment, the time course for induction was slower in the mutants, resembling the effects observed with STE2 expression.

Cytoskeletal Reorganization in alg7 3'UTR Mutants

Cells responding to α-factor adopt a polarized shape termed "shmoos," with projections directed toward the source of the pheromone. This reorganization of the actin cytoskeleton requires the function of Bem1p. In wild-type cells, BEM1 mRNA expression was induced within 1 h of treatment and declined to the original levels within 4.5 hours. Cells with deregulated expression of ALG7, however, showed no significant induction of BEM1 transcript levels, which remained fairly constant throughout the time course, being only slightly downregulated at 8 h after α-factor treatment. These results suggest that deregulation of ALG7 expression causes an aberrant polarization response in yeast.

SUMMARY

These initial studies show that deregulated expression of ALG7 affects diverse cellular functions crucial to development, including proliferation, differentiation, and morphogenesis. Furthermore, the data suggest multiple genetic targets for ALG7 and provide the basis for future dissection of these developmentally relevant pathways.

REFERENCES

1. KUKURUZINSKA, M.A. & K. LENNON. 1994. Growth-related coordinate regulation of the early N-glycosylation genes in yeast. Glycobiology **4:** 437–443.
2. PRETEL, R., K. LENNON, A. BIRD & M.A. KUKURUZINSKA. 1995. Expression of the first N-glycosylation gene in the dolichol pathway, ALG7, is regulated at two control points in the G1 phase of the *Saccharomyces cerevisiae* cell cycle. Exp. Cell Res. **219:** 477–486.
3. KUKURUZINSKA, M.A. & K. LENNON. 1995. Diminished activity of the first N-glycosylation enzyme, dolichol-P-dependent N-acetylglucosamine-1-P transferase (GPT) gives rise to mutant phenotypes in yeast. Biochim. Biophys. Acta **1247:** 51–59.
4. FERNANDES, R., M. FOX, D. COTANCHE, K. LENNON & M.A. KUKURUZINSKA. 1998. Changes in the expression of the first dolichol pathway gene, ALG7, mark salivary cell differentiation. Submitted.
5. MA, J., H. SAITO, T. OKA & I.K. VIJAY. 1996. Negative regulatory element involved in the hormonal regulation of GlcNAc-1-P transferase gene in mouse mammary gland. J. Biol. Chem. **271:** 11197–11203.

Cholecystokinin as Neurotransmitter and Neuromodulator in Parasympathetic Secretion in the Rat Submandibular Gland

NORIYASU TAKAI,[a,c] TORU SHIDA,[b] KENJI UCHIHASHI,[a] YUTAKA UEDA,[b] AND YO YOSHIDA[a]

Departments of [a]Physiology and [b]Anesthesiology, Osaka Dental University, 8-1, Kuzuha-hanazono-cho, Hirakata, Osaka 573-0021, Japan

INTRODUCTION

The main regulatory factors controlling salivary secretion are such autonomic neurotransmitters as norepinephrine and acetylcholine released by the innervating parasympathetic and sympathetic nerves. In recent years, various peptides, for example, substance P, calcitonin gene-related peptide, neuropeptide Y, and vasoactive intestinal peptide (VIP), have been considered to play important roles in the regulatory mechanism as neurotransmitters or neuromodulators.[1]

Cholecystokinin (CCK) is a peptide thought to act as both a hormone and a neurotransmitter, centrally in the brain and peripherally in the enteric nervous system and in various gastrointestinal organs.[2] In the salivary gland, Ruellan et al.[3] reported that CCK octapeptide (CCK-8) caused lipase secretion from the rat Ebner gland. On the other hand, Habara[4] has shown that there is no comparable change in rat parotid gland amylase to the treatment of CCK-8. Recently, Purushotham et al.[5] also showed that CCK-8 alone does not influence the activities of amylase, protein kinase C, and 3-kinase phosphatidylinositol 3-kinase in the parotid gland. Although there are some data reported on the effect of CCK-8 on the glandular enzyme activity in the salivary gland, the effect of this peptide on salivary fluid secretion has not been reported. In the present study using rat submandibular gland, we examined the functional evidence of CCK as neurotransmitter or modulator in parasympathetic salivary secretion.

MATERIAL AND METHODS

Male Wistar rats (200–250 g) were anesthetized with sodium pentobarbital (50 mg/kg, ip). A saliva sample from the submandibular gland was collected through a polyethylene cannula (Intramedic PE-10, Becton Dickinson) inserted into the oral opening of the the duct. The saliva was collected into a micropipette connected to the cannula to measure the volume. At the end of the experiment, the gland was dissected out and weighed. The amount of the secreted saliva was expressed in microliters of saliva per minute per 100 mg wet weight of the gland (µL/min/100 mg gland).

For the parasympathetic secretory stimulation, the chorda tympani on the excretory duct was stimulated electrically with 3.0–3.5 V pulses of 5.0 ms duration for 2 minutes. For the sympathetic secretory stimulation, the superior cervical ganglion was stimulated with 4.5–5.0 V pulses of 5.0 ms duration for 2 minutes.

---

[c] Tel: 81-720-64-3054; fax: 81-720-64-3154; e-mail: takai@cc.osaka-dent.ac.jp

As agonist and antagonist, sulfated CCK-8 (Peptide Institute Inc., Japan) and CR-1409 (Peninsula Lab., USA) were used, respectively. The CCK antagonist (10^{-4} M) or various doses of CCK-8 were dissolved in Ringer's solution and administered by the partial perfusion technique described by Takai et al.[6] to avoid systemic influences. Close-arterial infusion into the glandular branch of the facial artery was performed using a syringe pump at a rate of 20 µL/min, and venous efferent was discarded through the cannula inserted into the anterior facial vein. Ringer's solution, infused at 20 µL/min, had no effect on salivatory function induced by chorda stimulation. Atropine sulfate (Sigma, USA), a cholinergic muscarinic antagonist, was dissolved in Ringer's solution and administered intravenously (1 mg/kg) 10 min prior to stimulation.

RESULTS AND DISCUSSION

In the present study using the rat submandibular gland, we demonstrated that CCK-8 alone employs a modest action to stimulate salivary secretion after a rather long latency (>3 min). The salivary effect of CCK-8 on the secretory cell was direct because we employed the vascular isolated method for peptide administration. There was no spontaneous secretion from the submandibular gland, and the infusion of CCK-8 (10^{-12}–10^{-8} M) evoked salivary flow, the maximal response being about 3.8 µL/min/100 mg gw of saliva at 10^{-10} M of CCK-8. Atropine inhibited the salivary secretion evoked by CCK-8 at 10^{-12}–10^{-10} M, but not at 10^{-9} and 10^{-8} M (FIG. 1). Thus, CCK-8 may affect the submandibular acinar cell through at least two distinct pathways: CCK-8 stimulates secretory response directly through the CCK receptor at the acinar cell (as a neuro-

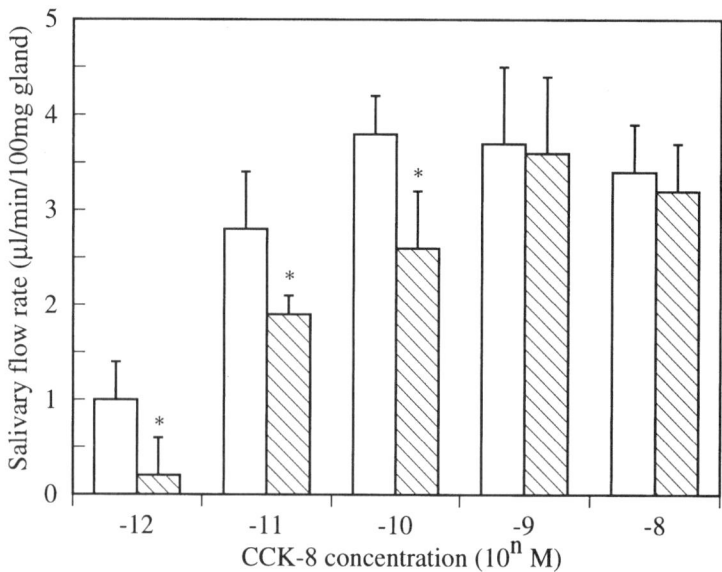

FIGURE 1. Effect of atropine on the salivary flow evoked by exogenous CCK-8 at various doses. *, Significantly different (p < 0.05, paired *t*-test) from CCK-8 stimulation alone (mean ± SE, n=12). ☐, control; ◪, with atropine.

transmitter), and the effect of CCK-8 is modulated by interactions with the cholinergic receptor (as a neuromodulator). In the latter pathway, it is reported that the inhibitory effect of atropine on the CCK-8 induced an enzyme secretory response in the exocrine pancreas,[7] and CCK-8 evoked the release of acetylcholine in rat pancreas.[8]

When the chorda was stimulated at low frequencies (less than 10 Hz), the inhibitory effects of the CCK antagonist were never seen. However, the CCK antagonist partially inhibited the salivary secretion elicited by chorda stimulation at high frequency (over 20 Hz). Additionally, the salivary secretion evoked by stimulation of the superior cervical ganglion (sympathetic secretory nerve) was not significantly affected by the CCK antagonist. Thus, these findings clearly show that endogenous CCK plays a role in regulation of parasympathetic nerve-induced salivary secretion in the submandibular gland, and high-frequency stimulation is needed to release endogenous CCK from nerve terminals of the chorda. It has been reported that several neuropeptides and acetylcholine coexist in postganglionic parasympathetic nerve fibers, and their corelease from the same nerve terminals was also in the submandibular glands.[9] Although it is not known whether the neurons within the rat submandibular gland contain CCK, Lindh and Hökfelt[10] reported that some cholinergic secretomotor neurons contain CCK in the enteric nervous system.

Stimulation of the chorda (parasympathetic secretory nerve) at various frequencies (0.5–60 Hz) increased the salivary flow in a frequency-dependent manner, and maximal responses were obtained at 20–40 Hz. As shown in FIGURE 2, the inhibitory effects of the CCK antagonist on salivary flow were not seen when the chorda was stimulated at a low frequency (less than 10 Hz). However, the inhibitory effects of the antagonist were observed with stimulation at 20–60 Hz, showing that high-frequency stimulation is

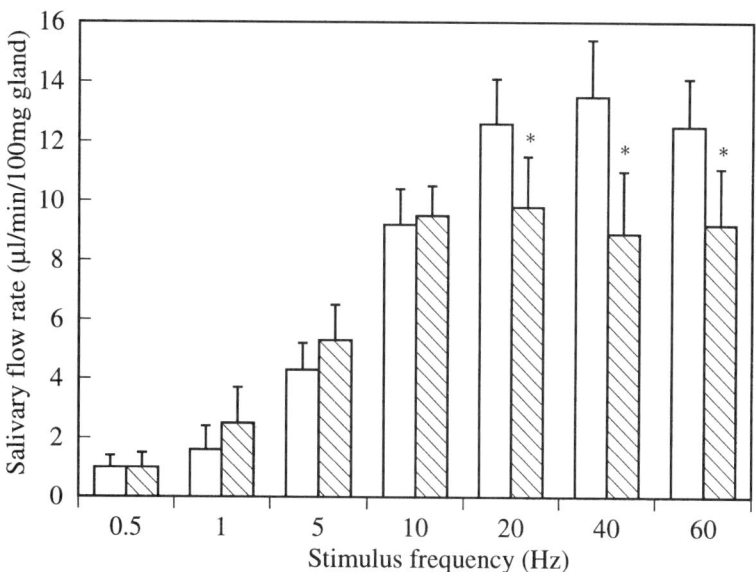

FIGURE 2. Effect of the CCK antagonist on the salivary flow rate evoked by chorda stimulation at various frequencies in the submandibular gland. *, Significantly different ($p < 0.05$, paired t-test) from chorda stimulation alone (mean ± SE, n=12). ☐, control; ▨, with CCK antagonist.

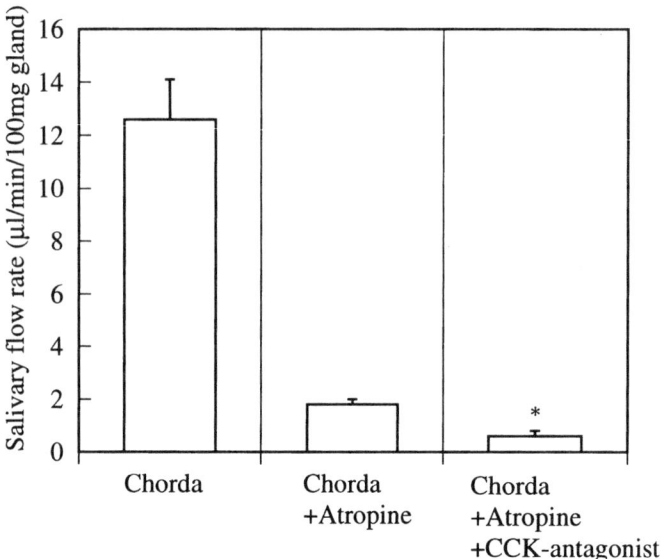

FIGURE 3. Effect of the CCK antagonist on atropine-resistant parasympathetic secretion (chorda + atropine). *, Significantly different ($p < 0.05$, paired t-test) from atropine-resistant secretion (mean ± SE, n=12).

needed to release an adequate amount to elicit flow of saliva of endogenous CCK from nerve terminals of the chorda. The salivary secretion evoked by stimulation of the superior cervical ganglion (sympathetic secretory nerve) was not significantly affected by the CCK antagonist (control; 2.0± 0.2, CCK antagonist; 2.1± 0.2 mL/min/100 mg gland). Thus, endogenous CCK plays a complementary role with acetylcholine in the regulation of parasympathetic nerve-induced salivary secretion in the submandibular gland.

Atropine-resistant parasympathetic secretion has been reported in the sheep parotid,[11] ferret submandibular,[12] and rat submandibular[13] glands. Our study confirmed this phenomenon and further showed that the CCK antagonist significantly reduced the atropine-resistant secretion by approximately 18% (FIG. 3). The atropine-resistant salivary secretion is nonadrenergic, noncholinergic, and was explained to be due to the release of several neuropeptides from postganglionic parasympathetic nerve terminals.[1] CCK is strongly suggested to be one of these neuropeptides in the rat submandibular gland.

REFERENCES

1. TITCHEN, D.A. & A.M. REID. 1990. Non-adrenergic, non-cholinergic control of salivary gland function. *In* Epithelial Secretion of Water and Electrolytes. J.A. Young & P.Y. Wong, Eds.: 219–228. Springer-Verlag. Berlin.
2. WANK, S.A. 1995. Cholecystokinin receptors. Am. J. Physiol. 269: G628–G646.
3. RUELLAN, C. *et al.* 1988. The Ebner glands: A pancreatic-like gland secreting an acid lipase. Secretory regulation *in vitro.* Int. J. Pancreotol. 3: 293–300.

4. HABARA, Y. 1989. Suppression of secretagogue-induced amylase secretion in pancreatic acini of cold-exposed rats. J. Physiol. **414:** 73–87.
5. PURUSHOTHAM, K. R. *et al.* 1993. Cholecystokinin modulates isoproterenol induced changes in rat parotid gland. Comp. Biochem. Physiol. **106C:** 249–254.
6. TAKAI, N. *et al.* 1983. Secretion and re-absorption of glucose in rat submandibular and sublingual saliva. J. Dent. Res. **62:** 1022–1025.
7. ADLER, G. *et al.* 1991. Interaction of the cholinergic system and cholecystokinin in the regulation of endogenous and exogenous stimulation of pancreatic secretion in humans. Gastroenterology **100:** 537–543.
8. SOUDAH, H.C. *et al.* 1992. Cholecystokinin at physiological levels evokes pancreatic enzyme secretion via a cholinergic pathway. Am. J. Physiol. **263:** G102–G107.
9. LUNDBERG, J.M. 1989. Peptidergic control of the autonomic regulation system in the orofacial region. Proc. Finn. Dent. Soc. **85:** 239–250.
10. LINDH, B & T. HÖKFELT. 1990. Structural functional aspects of acetylcholine peptide coexistence in the autonomic nervous system. Prog. Brain Res. **84:** 175–191.
11. REID, A.M. & D.A. TITCHEN. 1988. Atropine-resistant secretory responses of the ovine parotid gland to reflex and direct parasympathetic stimulation. Q. J. Exp. Physiol. **73:** 413–424.
12. TOBIN, G. *et al.* 1991. Atropine-resistant submandibular responses to stimulation of the parasympathetic innervation in the anaesthetized ferret. J. Physiol. **437:** 327–339.
13. EKSTRÖM, J. *et al.* 1987. Non-adrenergic, non-cholinergic parasympathetic secretion in the rat submaxillary and sublingual glands. Pharmacol. Toxicol. **60:** 284–287.

Transfection of COS Cells with Human Cystatin cDNA and Its Effect on HSV-1 Replication[a]

TARA R. WEAVER-HILTKE AND LIBUSE A. BOBEK[b]

Department of Oral Biology, School of Dental Medicine, State University of New York at Buffalo, Buffalo, New York 14214, USA

INTRODUCTION

The cystatin (Csn) superfamily of proteins are natural cysteine proteinase (CysP) inhibitors; however, their rate of inhibition of known CysP varies greatly among the different members. These variations may allow for a more vast defense mechanism against diseases of bacterial and/or viral origin. Several Csns have been shown to possess viral inhibitory properties. These include chicken egg white (CEW) Csn and oryzacystatin (rice Csn) and the ability to inhibit poliovirus replication.[1,2] Oryzacystatin has also been shown to inhibit herpes simplex virus Type 1 (HSV-1) *in vitro* and *in vivo*.[3] Human cystatin C (CsnC) has the ability to inhibit HSV-1 and coronavirus replication.[4,5] Human whole saliva and salivary fractions containing CsnSN have been shown to inhibit HSV-1 replication.[6,7] Thus we are interested in determining the mechanism of inhibition of HSV-1 by CsnC and CsnSN. We have shown that rCsnSN, and confirmed that rCsnC, reduce the viral yield of HSV-1 when these proteins are added exogenously to CV-1 cells at the start of HSV-1 infection.[8] It is thought that the Csns may enter the cells after the cell membranes become permeable as a result of the viral infection[4] and are thus able to inhibit viral and/or host cell CysP necessary for the viral replication. Poliovirus replication is inhibited by CEW Csn through a CysP necessary for polyprotein processing and essential for viral replication and propagation.[1] Also, a serine proteinase encoded by HSV-1 has been identified and found to be necessary for the packaging of the mature virions.[9] Therefore, it is plausible that CsnC and/or CsnSN inhibit HSV-1 replication through a CysP.

We hypothesize that if Csn is produced in large amounts by the cells prior to or during the viral infection, then it may more effectively inhibit HSV-1 replication. Our hypothesis is supported by a recent study that showed that the introduction of the corn Csn gene into rice plants resulted in high levels of expression of the corn Csn mRNA and protein. The corn Csn produced in rice served as an effective inhibitor of insect pest gut CysP.[10] To evaluate our hypothesis, we are using transfection technology for establishing CV-1 cell lines that will continuously produce CsnSN and CsnC mRNA and protein, with a goal of using these cell lines for HSV-1 inhibition studies. These studies will allow us to better understand the mechanism of interaction and thereby inhibition of HSV-1 by Csns.

RESULTS AND DISCUSSION

In order to establish cell lines expressing high levels of Csn for HSV-1 inhibition studies, we have initially cloned cDNA fragments encoding the secreted peptide of

---

[a] This work was supported by USPHS Grants DE09820 and DE07034.

[b] Corresponding author: Libuse A. Bobek, Ph.D., Department of Oral Biology, 202 Foster Hall, School of Dental Medicine, State University of New York at Buffalo, 3435 Main Street, Buffalo, NY 14214, USA. Tel: (716) 829-2465; fax: (716) 829-3942; e-mail: libuse_bobek@sdm.buffalo.edu

CsnC and CsnSN (120 and 121 amino acids, respectively) into the eukaryotic expression vector pcDNA 3.0, under the control of the CMV promoter. The recombinant plasmids were transfected into COS-1 cells. Stable clones were selected with G418 and isolated onto 24-well plates. Simultaneous to individual clone selection, we analyzed a heterogeneous population of cells for mRNA and protein production. The Northern blot analysis showed a very large increase in mRNA of both CsnC and CsnSN (refer to FIG. 1A), whereas the Western blot analysis was inconclusive (data not shown). Upon evaluation of individual clones (>20 for each of CsnC and SN), we found no increase in the Csn mRNA or protein production in any of the clones. These results indicate that even though the individual clones were antibiotic resistant, they were false positive.

In order to better evaluate the ability to transfect eukaryotic cells with CsnC or CsnSN, we used transient transfections. We examined both lipofectamine and calcium phosphate transfection methods, as well as CV-1 and NIH-293 cells. We found that both CV-1 and NIH-293 transfected best with lipofectamine and that the NIH-293 cells have little or no endogenous CsnC (refer to FIG. 1B). As compared to CV-1 cells, NIH-293 cells were less infectable by HSV-1; therefore, in subsequent transfections and HSV-1 infections we used CV-1 cells. We have successfully transiently transfected CV-1 cells with untargeted CsnC cDNA, as documented by an increase in CsnC protein production by Western blot analysis of total cell protein (as shown in FIG. 2A). However, transiently transfected CV-1 cells with untargeted CsnSN cDNA have shown no increase in CsnSN protein production (data not shown); the reason for this remains un-

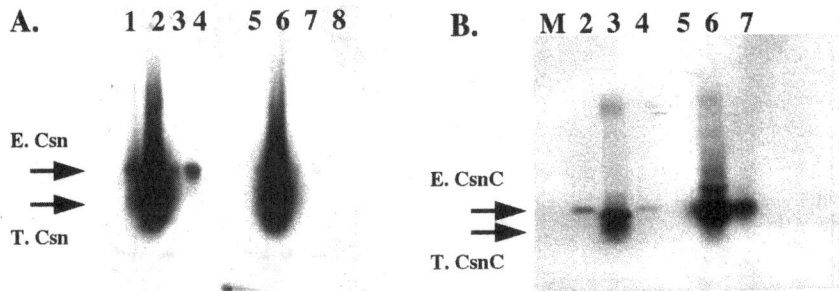

FIGURE 1. Northern blot analyses of CsnC and CsnSN mRNAs in transfected cells. A: Analysis of Csn mRNAs in a heterogeneous population of stably transfected COS-1 cells. Lanes 1 and 5: cells transfected with pcDNA 3.0 vector only; lanes 2 and 6: transfected cells with CsnC and CsnSN, respectively; lane 3: human ovary RNA (CsnC positive control); lane 7: human submandibular gland RNA (CsnSN positive control); lanes 4 and 8: untransfected COS-1 cells. Lanes 1–4 were probed with a CsnC probe, and lanes 5–8 with a CsnSN probe. E. Csn represents endogenous Csn, 360 b; T. Csn represents transfected Csn, ~750 b. B: Analysis of CsnC mRNA in transiently transfected CV-1 cells (lanes 2–4) and NIH-293 cells (lanes 5–7). Lane 1: RNA marker; lanes 2 and 5: untransfected cells; lanes 3 and 6: cells transfected with CsnC using the lipofectamine method; lanes 4 and 7: cells transfected with CsnC using calcium phosphate method. Cells were harvested 48 h after transfections. Methods: The cells were transfected using either the lipofectamine-mediated transfer (20 mg) or the calcium phosphate method with CsnSN or CsnC cDNA (10 mg). Stable transfectants were selected with 800 mg/mL G418 (Geneticin). One plate containing transfected cells was used for extraction of total RNA. The RNA concentration was determined spectrophotometrically and confirmed by gel electrophoresis. The RNA (10 μg) was separated on a 1.0% agarose gel containing 2.0% formaldehyde, and a capillary transferred overnight onto a BA85 nitrocellulose membrane (Schleicher and Schuell, Keene, NH). The blots were probed with a ^{32}P-labeled CsnC or CsnSN cDNA probe (360 bp fragment encoding the translated region).

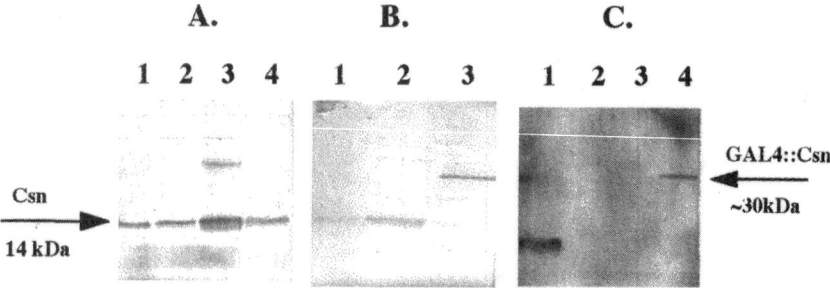

FIGURE 2. Western blot analyses of proteins from transiently transfected CV-1 cells. **A:** Analysis of cells transfected with untargeted CsnC. Lane 1: rCsnC (positive control); lane 2: untransfected cells; lane 3: cells transfected with CsnC using the lipofectamine method; lane 4: cells transfected with CsnC using the calcium phosphate method. **B:** Analysis of cells transfected with CsnC + GAL4 nuclear signal. Transfections were done using the lipofectamine method. Lane 1: rCsnC (positive control); lane 2: untransfected cells; lane 3: cells transfected with CsnC + GAL4 nuclear signal. **C:** Analysis of cells transfected with CsnSN +/– GAL4 nuclear signal. Transfections were done using the lipofectamine method. Lane 1: CsnSN (positive control); lane 2: untransfected cells; lane 3: cells transfected with untargeted CsnSN; lane 4: cells transfected with CsnSN + GAL4 nuclear signal. Methods: CV-1 cells were transfected with the lipofectamine or the calcium phosphate method, followed by incubation for 48 h. The total protein was then extracted in a 1× SDS-PAGE sample buffer containing 5.0% β-mercaptoethanol. Protein concentration was determined by a BIORAD protein assay. Proteins (50 μg) were separated on a 0.1% SDS-13% PAGE and transferred onto an Immobilon-P membrane (Millipore Corp. Bedford, MA) using semidry apparatus (Hoefer Scientific Instruments, San Francisco, CA). The membranes in panels A and B were probed with a rabbit anti-CsnC (Dako Corp, Carpinteria, CA, 1:1000) and with rabbit anti-CsnSN (#221, 1:500, gift from Dr. Michael Levine, SUNY Buffalo) in panel C. Goat anti-rabbit IgG conjugated to alkaline phosphatase (Promega Corp., Madison, WI, 1:7500) was used as a secondary antibody.

clear. Further, we have successfully transiently transfected CV-1 cells with CsnC and CsnSN cDNA containing a nuclear retention signal (147 aa residues of GAL4-encoding sequence[11] added to the 5′ end of the Csns), as reflected by a production of GAL4/CsnSN and GAL4/CsnC proteins, shown in FIGURE 2B and C, respectively. We targeted the nucleus because most HSV-1 functions (*i.e.,* transcription, replication, and packaging) occur within the host cell nucleus.

Currently, we are in the process of reselecting stable clones expressing high levels of rCsnC and rCsnSN ± nuclear signal. However, for these experiments we have subcloned CsnC and CsnSN cDNA fragments into the pcDNA 3.1 eukaryotic expression vector because the stable clones are selected with zeocin (250 μg/mL), which should yield less false positives and shorten the selection time.

We have also explored the possibility of HSV-1 inhibition using the transiently transfected CV-1 cells with CsnSN. The cells were infected with HSV-1 (m.o.i. of 0.1) at 24, 36, and 48 h posttransfection (p.t.). The results indicate that at 48 h p.t. we have achieved a similar degree of HSV-1 inhibition as compared with the exogenously added rCsnSN (~ 1 log of HSV-1 virus yield reduction, data not shown). This is probably because in transient transfections, only a small fraction of the cells become transfected, and the level of transfection is not consistent between each transfection. Therefore, it is necessary to obtain stable cell lines that express high amounts of CsnC or CsnSN in order to evaluate the mechanism of HSV-1 inhibition by Csns.

In conclusion, our first attempt to establish stable cell lines producing CsnSN or CsnC were unsuccessful. This may be due to a large incidence of false positives, or perhaps because it is not possible to produce stable cell lines expressing high levels of Csns (CysP inhibitors). In fact, it has been shown that it is very difficult to obtain transfected cells with expression levels of calpain (CysP) and/or its natural inhibitor, calpastatin, significantly different from that of control cells. Large deviations from the normal level seem to be lethal.[12] It is also documented that rice plants transfected with the rice Csn gene did not express high levels of rice Csn mRNA or protein (insufficient for the effective protection against insect pests).[13] On the other hand, the study by Irie *et al.*[10] has shown that transfection of the rice plants with the corn Csn gene yielded transgenic rice plants with levels of corn Csn protein more than 20 times higher than that of the intrinsic oryzacystatin. More importantly the corn Csn protein effectively inhibited insect pest gut CysP. Therefore, we remain optimistic that we will be successful in establishing cell lines that will produce high levels of CsnSN and CsnC that can be used to determine the mechanism of HSV-1 inhibition by cystatins.

ACKNOWLEDGMENTS

We thank Dr. Te Chung Lee for the GAL4 nuclear signal plasmid; Dr. Michael J. Levine for the CsnSN #221 antibody, and use of his facilities; and Dr. E. James Bergey for help with the HSV-1 plaque-reduction assay.

REFERENCES

1. KORANT, B.D., J. BRZIN & V. TURK. 1985. Cystatin, a protein inhibitor of cysteine proteases alters viral protein cleavages in infected human cells. Biochem. Biophys. Res. Commun. **127:** 1072–1076.
2. KONDO, H., S. IJIRI, K. ABE, H. MAEDA & S. ARAI. 1992. Inhibitory effect of oryzacystatin and a truncation mutant on the replication of poliovirus in infected vero cells. FEBS Lett. **299:** 48–50.
3. AOKI, H., T. AKAIKE, K. ABE, M. KURODA, S. ARAI, R. OKAMUA, A. NEGI & H. MAEDA. 1995. Antiviral effect of oryzacystatin, a proteinase inhibitor in rice, against herpes simplex virus type 1 *in vitro* and *in vivo*. Antimicrob. Agents Chemother. **39:** 846–849.
4. BJORCK, L., A. GRUBB & L. KJELLEN. 1990. Cystatin C, a human proteinase inhibitor, blocks replication of herpes simplex virus. J. Virol. **64:** 941–943.
5. COLLINS, A. & A. GRUBB. 1991. Inhibitory effects of recombinant human cystatin C on human coronaviruses. Antimicrob. Agents Chemother. **35:** 2444–2446.
6. BERGEY, E.J., M. GU, A. COLLINS, S. BRADWAY & M. LEVINE. 1993. Modulation of herpes simplex virus type 1 replication by human salivary secretions. Oral Microb. Immunol. **8:** 89–93.
7. GU, M., G. HARAZTHY, A. COLLINS & E. BERGEY. 1994. Identification of salivary proteins inhibiting herpes simplex virus 1 replication. Oral Microb. Immunol. **10:** 54–59.
8. WEAVER, T., E. BERGEY, M. LEVINE & L. BOBEK. 1995. Effects of recombinant salivary cystatin on HSV-1 replication. J. Dent. Res. **74** (spec. iss.):84.
9. GAO, M., L. MATUSICK-KUMAR, W. HURLBURT, S. FEUER DITUSA, W. NEWCOMB, J. BROWN, P. MCCANN III, I. DECKMAN & R. COLONNO. 1994. The protease of herpes simplex virus type 1 is essential for functional capsid formation and viral growth. J. Virol. **68:** 3702–3712.
10. IRIE, K., H. HOSOYAMA, T. TAKEUCHI, K. IWABUCHI, H. WATANABE, M. ABE, K. ABE & S. ARAI. 1996. Transgenic rice established to express corn cystatin exhibits strong inhibitory activity against insect gut proteinases. Plant Mol. Biol. **30:** 149–57.
11. SILVER, P., L. KEEGAN & M. PTASHNE. 1984. Amino terminus of yeast GAL4 gene product is sufficient for nuclear localization. Proc. Natl. Acad. Sci. USA **81:** 5951–5955.
12. SUZUKI, K., T. SORIMACHI, T. YOSHIZAWA, K. KINBARA & S. ISHIMURA. 1995. Calpain:

Novel family members, activation, and physiological function. Biol. Chem. Hoppe-Seyler. **376:** 523–529.
13. HOSOYAMA, H., K. IRIE, K. ABE & S. ARAI. 1994. Oryzacystatin exogenously introduced into protoplasts and regeneration of transgenic rice. Biosc. Biotechnol. Biochem. **58:** 1500–1505.

Salivary Acidic Proline-rich Proteins in Rheumatoid Arthritis[a]

J.L. JENSEN[b]

Department of Oral Surgery and Oral Medicine, University of Oslo, Oslo, Norway

In an ongoing attempt to investigate qualitative salivary parameters in diseases affecting salivary glands, patients with rheumatoid arthritis (RA) were examined. Patients were selected from the Oslo RA register[1] for the present study if they fulfilled the following criteria: age 52–74 years, disease duration 10–20 years, and disability score as assessed by the Modified Health Assessment Questionnaire ≤ 2.5. From these 105 patients, two subgroups of patients were selected, one group with pronounced sicca symptoms from eyes and mouth, and one group without such symptoms. Sicca symptoms were assessed using a postal questionnaire with the questions on dry mouth and dry eyes of the European classification criteria for Sjögren's syndrome.[2] Patients were excluded from further examinations if they used medication that could cause dryness in eyes or mouth. Thus, nine patients remained in the sicca group (having four or more sicca symptoms), and ten matched RA patients were selected for the nonsicca group. A healthy sex- and age-matched control group (n=10) was also examined.

In a preliminary report we have shown that differences in flow rates between sicca and nonsicca RA patients were limited to lower values of unstimulated whole saliva.[3] To further evaluate salivary changes in RA, a disease frequently associated with secondary Sjögren's syndrome, we have studied qualitative salivary parameters in these patients, including secretory rates of proline-rich proteins (PRPs), statherins, and histatins.[4] In the present report, phenotypes of PRPs, the ratio of PRPs derived from the two loci (PRH1 and PRH2), and PRP concentration and output in parotid and submandibular saliva derived from the two loci are presented.

Parotid (PS) and submandibular saliva (SS) were collected from all individuals using 2% citric acid as a saliva stimulus. PRPs in PS and SS were identified using a SMART® microchromatographic system with a Mono Q® column and a Tris-HCl / NaCl gradient (method adapted from ref. 5). For PRPs, the primary polypeptide products are coded for on two loci (PRH1 and PRH2), which have three and two commonly occurring gene variants, respectively. On PRH1, the proteins PIF-s, Db-s, and Pa are coded for, whereas PRP-1 and PRP-2 are coded for on the PRH2 locus. As each protein variant has a postranscriptional cleavage product, individuals will exhibit four, six, or eight PRPs in their saliva, depending on whether they are homozygous at both, one, or neither of the two loci.[5] Accordingly, 18 possible phenotypes may exist, but as few as three phenotypes were found in 79% of the 127 healthy individuals examined by Hay et al.[5] The SMART system allows the determination of the different acidic PRPs present in saliva. Concentrations of the various phenotypes were calculated by peak integration versus pure PRP standards. Total PRP concentration derived from each locus was calculated as the sum of the concentrations of PRP variants from that locus.

---

[a] The work was supported by the Norwegian Research Council, Grant # 107574/320.

[b] Address for correspondence: Dr. Janicke Liaaen Jensen, Department of Oral Surgery and Oral Medicine, Faculty of Dentistry, University of Oslo, P.O. Box 1109 Blindern, 0317 Oslo, Norway. Tel: +47 22 85 22 05; fax: +47 22 85 23 41; e-mail: jljensen@odont.uio.no

TABLE 1. Concentrations of PRP Variants Derived from Locus PRH1 and Locus PRH2 in Parotid and Submandibular Saliva (μg/mL, medians and ranges) in Patients with RA with and without Sicca Symptoms and Healthy Controls

Parotid saliva	RA sicca (n=9)	RA nonsicca (n=10)	Controls (n=10)	p value Sicca/ nonsicca	p value Sicca/ control	p value Nonsicca /control
Locus PRH1	102.6 (36.6–134.7)	81.4 (59.7–156.0)	69.1 (28.1–128.9)	0.65	0.27	0.12
Locus PRH2	128.0 (47.7–188.4)	110.3 (69.2–334.1)	92.3 (56.1–148.1)	1.0	0.18	0.24
PRH2/ PRH1	1.30 (1.07–1.71)	1.31 (0.86–3.02)	1.59 (0.85–1.99)	0.84	0.54	0.73
Submandibular saliva						
Locus PRH1	19.4 (6.6–46.4)	40.8 (10.1–80.8)	32.1 (14.0–89.5)	0.14	0.15	0.96
Locus PRH2	31.1 (7.8–67.8)	61.6 (15.2–118.7)	51.0 (24.3–126.9)	0.11	0.15	0.54
PRH2/ PRH1	1.70 (0.70–2.65)	1.67 (1.03–2.51)	1.43 (1.00–2.34)	0.96	0.71	0.56

In the above-mentioned study,[5] the three phenotypes (PIF^{++}, Pr1^{++}), PIF$^+$, Pa$^+$, Pr1$^+$, Pr2$^+$), and (Db$^+$, PIF$^+$, and Pr1^{++}) accounted for 79% of the individuals. Phenotype distribution in the present study differed only slightly from those found previously: these phenotypes made up 63% and 70% in RA patients and controls, respectively. The phenotype (PIF^{++}, Pr1$^+$, Pr2$^+$) was found more often in RA patients (26% versus 10% in controls and 5% in ref. 4). In all groups, PRP production was higher on locus PRH2 than PRH1 and

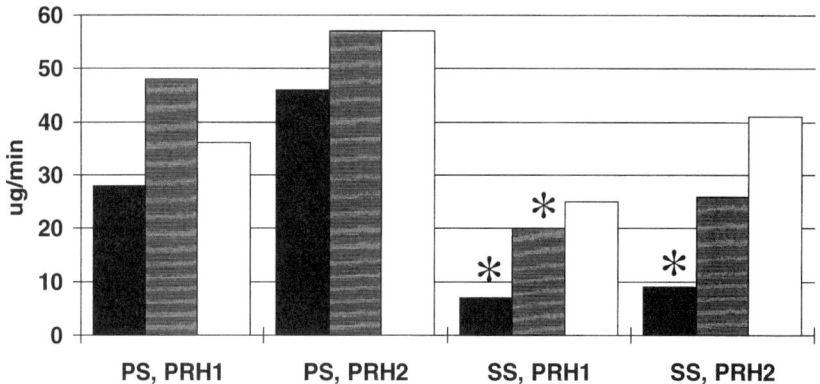

FIGURE 1. Output of PRP variants derived from locus PRH1 and locus PRH2 in parotid (PS) and submandibular (SS) saliva (μg/min, medians) in patients with RA with sicca symptoms (■, n=9), without such symptoms (▨, n=10), and healthy controls (☐, n=10).

higher in PS than SS (TABLE 1). However, the concentrations of PRPs derived from the two loci did not differ significantly between the RA and control groups (TABLE 1).

There were no significant differences in parotid salivary flow rates between groups, whereas submandibular flow rates were significantly lower in both RA groups than in controls. Consequently, when calculating the amount of protein secreted per time, that is, the output of proteins, the value for PRPs in SS was reduced by 75% in sicca RA patients versus controls (FIG.). This was valid for PRP output of variants derived from locus PRH1 as well as PRH2. By contrast, for nonsicca RA patients, output of PRPs derived from PRH1 in submandibular saliva was reduced by 20% only (FIG. 1). It can be concluded that in RA patients with sicca symptoms, both quantitative and qualitative salivary changes were seen related to the submandibular but not to the parotid gland.

ACKNOWLEDGMENTS

Dr. Frank Oppenheim at Boston University and Dr. Don Hay at Forsyth Dental Centre, Boston, MA are thanked for supplying PRPs.

REFERENCES

1. KVIEN, T.K., A. GLENNÅS, O.G. KNUDSRUD, L.M. SMEDSTAD & Ø. FØRRE. 1995. The prevalence and severity of RA: Results from a hospital based register and a population survey (20–79 years). Arthritis Rheum. **38:** 258.
2. VITALI, C., S. BOMBARDIERI, H.M. MOUTSOPOULOS et al. 1993. Preliminary criteria for the classification of Sjögren's syndrome. Results of a prospective concerted action supported by the European Community. Arthritis Rheum. **36:** 340–347.
3. JENSEN, J.L., T. UHLIG, T.K. KVIEN & T. AXÉLL. 1996. Salivary flow and oral health in rheumatoid arthritis (RA) patients. J. Dent. Res. **75:** 271.
4. JENSEN, J.L., T. UHLIG, T. K. KVIEN & T. AXÉLL. 1997. Characteristics of rheumatoid arthritis patients with self-reported sicca symptoms: Evaluation of medical, salivary and oral parameters. Oral Dis. **3:** 254–261.
5. HAY, D.I., J.M. AHERN, S.K. SCHLUCKEBIER & D.H. SCHLESINGER. 1994. Human salivary acidic proline rich protein polymorphism and biosynthesis studied by high-performance liquid chromatography. J. Dent. Res. **73:** 1717–1726.

Confocal Imaging of Gene Expression during Hamster Submandibular Gland Biogenesis

RUI FERNANDES,[a] MATTHEW FOX,[a] DOUGLAS COTANCHE,[b] KELLEY LENNON,[a] AND MARIA A. KUKURUZINSKA[a,c]

[a] *Division of Oral Biology, Boston University Goldman School of Dental Medicine, Center for Advanced Biomedical Research, 700 Albany Street, Boston, Massachusetts 02118, USA*

[b] *Department of Anatomy and Neurobiology, Boston University School of Medicine, 80 East Concord Street, Boston, Massachusetts 02118, USA*

INTRODUCTION

In the search for key players involved in salivary gland biogenesis, we have studied the evolutionarily conserved ALG7 gene, shown to be regulatory in yeast development.[1-4] ALG7 encodes the dolichol phosphate-dependent N-acetylglucosamine-1 phosphate transferase (GPT) and functions by initiating and regulating the dolichol pathway of protein N-glycosylation.[2,4,5] An essential housekeeping gene, ALG7 belongs to a class of highly regulated, early-growth response genes.[5] In yeast, adequate expression of this gene is required for the proper execution of such developmentally relevant genetic programs as proliferation, differentiation, and cell polarization.[1-3]

Our previous work with higher eukaryotes showed that downregulation of ALG7 expression on the level of transcript accumulation and the activity of its protein product, GPT, correlated with postnatal development of the hamster submandibular gland (SMG).[6] Inasmuch as perturbation of ALG7 activity is deleterious to developmentally relevant functions in diverse eukaryotic systems,[1-3,7] this progressive attenuation in ALG7 expression is likely to be critical for the normal development of SMGs. In the present study, we used immunohistochemical approaches, coupled with confocal microscopy, to further analyze this gene's expression at distinct stages of SMG cytomorphodifferentiation. We selected confocal microscopy for imaging ALG7 expression because it allows for the *in vivo* localization of gene products, while avoiding artifacts inherent to tissue sectioning. In addition, we confirmed these results with standard Western blot assays.

METHODS

Primary antibodies for the neonatal salivary protein marker protein C[8] were provided by Lily Mirels, University of California, Berkeley and used at a 1:2000 dilution for Western analyses and 1:200 for confocal staining. Rabbit polyclonal antibodies against the 11 C-terminal amino acids of hamster GPT were commercially prepared (BabCo) and used at a 1:5000 dilution for Western analyses and 1:100 for confocal staining. Secondary antibodies consisted of goat anti-rabbit IgG(Fc) derivatized with FITC (molecular probes) and used at a dilution of 1:1000 for Western analyses and 1:500 for confocal imaging. Timed-pregnant hamsters were purchased from Charles

---

[c] To whom correspondence should be addressed. Tel: (617) 638-4859; fax (617) 638-4924; e-mail: mkukuruz@bu.edu

River Labs; at 2, 5, 14, and 33 days postpartum, animals were sacrificed, and SMGs were isolated, as described previously.[6]

For confocal imaging, glands were fixed, stained, and analyzed using a Leitz confocal scanning microscope CLSM (with argon laser), essentially as described.[7] Typically, confocal images were set to represent scans through a plane of representative tissue sections 1 μm thick.

Western blot analyses of SMG homogenates were also carried out, as described.[7] Images were captured on Reflection autoradiography film (DuPont/NEN), and signal intensities were quantified using Kodak Digital Science 1D Software (Eastman Kodak), version 1.0.2. Amounts of samples and the exposure times were chosen to assure linearity of the signal.

RESULTS/CONCLUSIONS

In order to assess the relative levels of GPT during hamster SMG postnatal development, the following stages of cytomorphodifferentiation were examined: 2 days post-

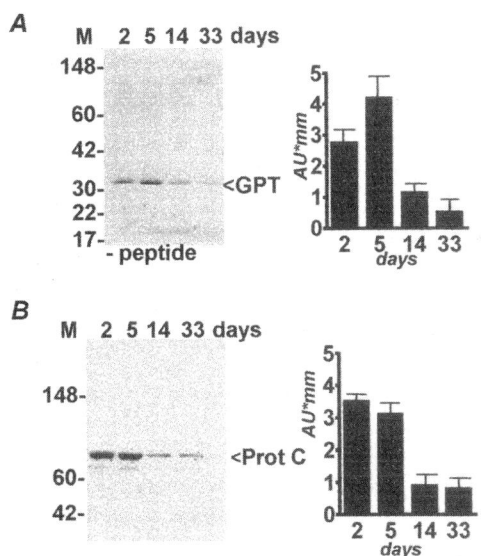

FIGURE 1. Western blot detection of GPT and protein C levels in tissue homogenates during postnatal development of hamster SMGs. Tissue homogenates (100 μg) from each developmental time point were subjected to electrophoresis on 12% polyacrylamide gels under reducing conditions and transferred to nitrocellulose using the Novex XCell II electrophoresis and blotting apparatus, as per manufacturer's instructions. Following transfer, blots were incubated consecutively with primary (anti-hamster GPT, 1:5000 in A; anti-rat protein C, 1:2000 in B) and secondary (horseradish peroxidase-conjugated anti-rabbit IgG, 1:1000) antibodies and developed with ECL detection reagents as per manufacturer's instructions (Amersham). Images were captured on Reflections film (NEN/DuPont), scanned into the computer using the HPScanJet 4C, and analyzed using Kodak Digital Science 1D software. The results are an average of four independent determinations; the standard error of the mean (SEM) is indicated. Au*mm, arbitrary absorbance units × height.

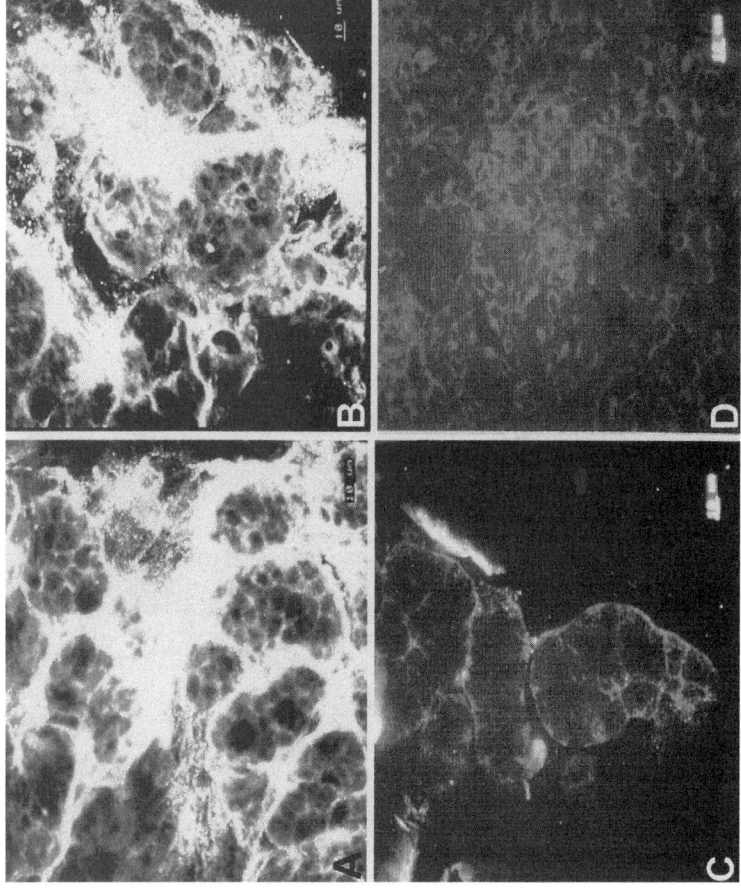

FIGURE 2. Confocal imaging of GPT expression in the postnatally developing hamster SMG: *in vivo* analyses of SMGs stained with polyclonal anti-hamster GPT (1:100) versus preimmune (1:100). The secondary antibody was goat anti-rabbit heavy and light chain IgG conjugated to FITC (1:500). **A:** Hamster SMG, day–2 postpartum; **B:** day 5; **C:** day 33; **D:** preimmune day 2. Bar, 10 µm.

partum, when cells begin to proliferate extensively; 5 days postpartum, reflecting a high mitotic index, and the transition from undifferentiated cells of the terminal tubules into terminal buds; 14 days after birth, when proliferation becomes abated and some acini acquire fully differentiated, functional phenotypes; and 33 days, reflecting functionally differentiated SMG, with acini completely replacing the terminal buds and cells filled with secretory granules.

Temporal Expression of GPT in the Postnatally Developing SMG: **In Vitro** *Analysis*

Tissue homogenates were prepared from distinct stages of SMG cytomorphodifferentiation and analyzed for reactivity with the anti-GPT antibody by Western blot procedure (Fig. 1A). The amount of GPT correlated with the proliferative activity of the gland, increasing from 2 to 5 days postpartum and then becoming progressively attenuated with diminished proliferation, reaching the lowest level in the functionally differentiated gland at day 33. These results support our previously reported RNA blotting and GPT activity studies,6 and they confirm the information from yeast about the growth-dependent nature of GPT expression.4,5 Furthermore, the modulated expression of GPT during postnatal development correlated with the previously reported transient production of the neonatal secretory protein, protein C8 (Fig. 1B), which was detected in the highest amounts at day 2 and declined more than 3-fold by 14 days postpartum.

Temporal Expression of GPT in the Developing SMG: **In Vivo** *Analysis*

The assessment of the expression of GPT in vivo using anti-GPT antisera and confocal imaging is shown in Figure 2. The highest level of staining was detected in the neonatal, 2- and 5-day-old glands (A and B), compared to later stages of postnatal development (C). No signal was detected when preimmune serum was used instead of primary antibody (D). Similar to GPT, positive staining was detected for 2- and 5-day SMGs with antisera raised against rat protein C, which were attenuated in the 14- and 33-day SMGs (data not shown). These results confirmed our immunoblotting analysis (Fig. 1), indicating that both GPT and protein C were present in the neonatal hamster tissues at much higher levels compared to the adult gland.

SUMMARY

The data presented here provide evidence that the abundance of the ALG7 protein product, GPT, correlates with high proliferative activity during the postnatal development of the hamster SMG development, and that it becomes downregulated with differentiation. Based on our previous studies with yeast,[1–3] changes in the levels of ALG7 expression may be necessary for the events directing salivary cell polarization, migration, differentiation, and apoptosis at distinct developmental stages.

REFERENCES

1. KUKURUZINSKA, M.A. & K. LENNON. 1995. Diminished activity of the first N-glycosylation enzyme, dolichol-P-dependent N-acetylglucosamine-1-P transferase (GPT), gives rise to mutant phenotypes in yeast. Biochim. Biophys. Acta **1247:** 51–59.
2. PRETEL, R., K. LENNON, A. BIRD & M.A. KUKURUZINSKA. 1995. Expression of the first N-

glycosylation gene in the dolichol pathway, ALG7, is regulated at two major control points in the G1 phase of the *Saccharomyces cerevisiae* cell cycle. Exp. Cell Res. **219:** 477–486.

3. LENNON, K., S. CERVANTES, A. BIRD, H. BATAL, J. KESSELHEIM & M.A. KUKURUZINSKA. 1998. Deregulated expression of the first *N*-glycosylation gene in the dolichol pathway, ALG7, results in developmental defects in the yeast *Saccharomyces cerevisiae*. Submitted.

4. LENNON, K.L., R. PRETEL, J. KESSELHEIM, S. TE HEESEN & M.A. KUKURUZINSKA. 1995. Proliferation-dependent differential regulation of the dolichol pathway genes in *Saccharomyces cerevisiae*. Glycobiology **5:** 633–642.

5. KUKURUZINSKA, M.A. & K. LENNON. 1994. Growth-related coordinate regulation of the early *N*-glycosylation genes in yeast. Glycobiology **4:** 437–443.

6. MOTA, O.M., G.T. HUANG & M.A. KUKURUZINSKA. 1994. Developmental regulation and tissue-specific expression of hamster dolichol-P-dependent *N*-acetylglucosamine-1-P transferase (GPT). Biochem. Biophys. Res. Commun. **204:** 284–291.

7. FERNANDES, R., M. FOX, D. COTANCHE, K. LENNON, & M.A. KUKURUZINSKA. 1998. Changes in the expression of the first dolichol pathway gene, ALG7, mark salivary cell differentiation. Submitted.

8. BALL, W.D., A.R. HAND & A.O. JOHNSON. 1988. Secretory proteins as markers for cellular phenotypes in rat salivary glands. Dev. Biol. **125:** 265–279.

Lacrimal Gland Functions Are Differentially Controlled by Protein Kinase C Isoforms

DRISS ZOUKHRI,[b] ROBIN R. HODGES, CHRISTIAN SERGHERAERT,[a]
AND DARLENE A. DARTT

Schepens Eye Research Institute and Department of Ophthalmology, Harvard Medical School, Boston, Massachusetts

[a] *Institut Pasteur de Lille, CNRS URA 1309, Lille, France*

INTRODUCTION

Lacrimal gland protein secretion is primarily under the control of cholinergic muscarinic and α_1-adrenergic receptors.[1] Cholinergic agonists are coupled to the activation of phospholipase C (PLC),[2] which leads to the production of two second messenger molecules: inositol 1,4,5-trisphosphate (IP_3) and diacylglycerol (DAG). IP_3 increases the cytoplasmic concentration of calcium ($[Ca^{2+}]_i$), and DAG activates protein kinase C (PKC), two events that are thought to trigger protein secretion.[1] Lacrimal gland α_1-adrenergic receptors are not coupled to the PLC pathway, although their activation leads to a slight increase in $[Ca^{2+}]_i$.[3] We have also shown that unlike the cholinergic receptors, α_1-adrenergic receptors are not linked to the activation of phospholipase D in lacrimal gland acini.[4] Thus the transduction pathway(s) used by the α_1-adrenergic receptors to trigger lacrimal gland protein secretion remains to be identified.

PKC was originally described as a Ca^{2+} and phospholipid-dependent protein kinase activated by DAG produced by the receptor-mediated breakdown of phosphoinositides. Molecular cloning and biochemical techniques have shown that PKC is a family of closely related enzymes consisting of at least eleven different isoforms that has been divided into three categories[5,6]: (1) conventional PKCs, including PKCα, -βI, -βII and -γ isoforms, have a Ca^{2+} and DAG-dependent kinase activity; (2) novel PKCs, including PKCε, -δ, -θ, -η, and -μ isoforms, are Ca^{2+}-independent and DAG-stimulated kinases; (3) atypical PKCs, including PKCζ, and -ι/λ isoforms, are Ca^{2+} and DAG-independent kinases. All PKC isoforms, except PKCμ, have a pseudosubstrate sequence in their N-terminal part that is thought to interact with the catalytic domain to keep the enzyme inactive in resting cells.[7]

In previous studies, we showed that lacrimal gland acini express three isoforms of PKC: PKCα, -δ, and -ε.[8] In the present study, we report the identification of two other PKC isoforms, namely PKCμ and -ι/λ. We show that these isoforms are differentially located and that they translocate differentially in response to phorbol esters and cholinergic agonists. We also show that PKC isoforms differentially control lacrimal gland protein secretion and cholinergic-induced Ca^{2+} elevation. Part of these results has been recently published.[9,10]

---

[b] Address for correspondence: Schepens Eye Research Institute, 20 Staniford Street, Boston, MA 02114, USA. Tel: (617) 912-7427; fax: (617) 912-0104; e-mail: zoukhri@vision.eri.harvard.edu

TABLE 1. Immunolocalization of PKC Isoforms in the Lacrimal Gland

PKC Isoforms	Immunolocalization
α	Basolateral and apical membranes of acinar cells and in membranes of the secretory granules.
δ	Cytosolic distribution in acinar cells and present in myoepithelial cells.
ε	Basolateral and apical membranes of acinar cells and present in myoepithelial cells.
μ	Basolateral and apical membranes of acinar cells and present in an intracellular filamentous network.
ι/λ	Cytosolic distribution in acinar cells near the Golgi area.

RESULTS AND DISCUSSION

The results summarized in TABLE 1 show that PKCα immunoreactivity was seen on the basolateral and apical membranes of all acini. Immunofluorescence was also detected near the apical membrane, suggesting that PKCα might be associated with the membranes of the secretory granules. PKCμ localization was similar to that of PKCα, in that immunofluorescence is clearly membranous, on the basolateral and apical membranes, outlining the individual acinar cells in an acinus, but was also found in an intracellular filamentous network. PKCε immunoreactivity was more cytoplasmic, though binding was also seen on the basolateral and apical membranes of acinar cells. PKCδ and PKCι/λ had a cytoplasmic distribution. PKCε and PKCδ immunoreactivity was occasionally associated with myoepithelial cells. These results show that five isoforms of PKC are present in the lacrimal gland, each with a different distribution.

Classical and novel, but not atypical, PKC isoforms translocate from the cytosol to the membrane in response to phorbol esters or other agonists.[5] As shown in FIGURE 1A, phorbol esters stimulated the translocation of PKCα, -δ, and -ε. Translocation occurred at 1 min and was still measurable at 10 min (not shown). By contrast, the cholinergic agonist, carbachol, stimulated the translocation of PKCδ and -ε, but surprisingly not -α. Similarly to PdBu, carbachol did not translocate the DAG-independent isoform, PKCι/λ (not shown). These results show that lacrimal gland PKC isoforms translocate differentially in response to phorbol esters and cholinergic agonists.

In order to study the role of PKC isoforms in agonist-induced lacrimal gland protein secretion, we have synthesized and N-myristoylated three peptides derived from the pseudosubstrate sequences of PKCα, -δ, and -ε. As shown in FIGURE 1B, preincubation of lacrimal gland acini for 1 h with the myristoylated peptides altered agonist-induced protein secretion. Myr-PKCα inhibited phorbol ester- and cholinergic agonist-induced protein secretion to a larger extent than did myr-PKCε, whereas myr-PKCδ had only a minor effect. By contrast, $α_1$-adrenergic-induced protein secretion was inhibited only by myr-PKCε, whereas myr-PKCα and myr-PKCδ had a stimulatory effect. The inhibitory effect of the peptides on cholinergic- and $α_1$-adrenergic-induced protein secretion was solely due to inhibition of PKC, as the peptides did not alter the changes in $[Ca^{2+}]_i$ induced by these agonists (data not shown).

It is well documented that cholinergic agonists stimulate the release of $[Ca^{2+}]_i$ and influx of Ca^{2+} in the lacrimal gland. Recent reports showed that preactivation of PKC results in negative feedback on cholinergic-induced Ca^{2+} release in the lacrimal gland, implicating PKC in the mechanism of desensitization of the cholinergic response. Our results show that when fura-2-loaded lacrimal gland acini are pretreated with the phorbol ester, PMA, carbachol-induced $[Ca^{2+}]_i$ elevation is inhibited by 50 percent. In order to determine which isoform of PKC is mediating the inhibitory effect of PMA, we used the myristoylated pseudosubstrate-derived peptides. Preincubation of lacrimal

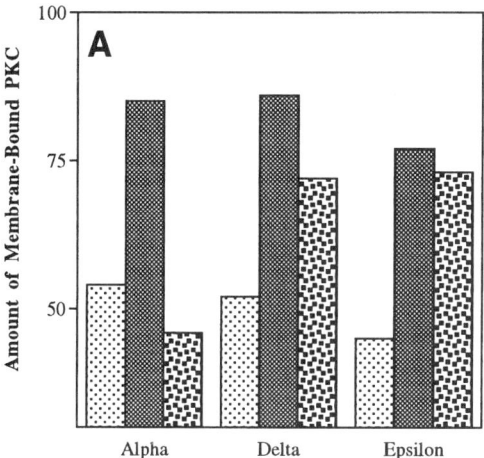
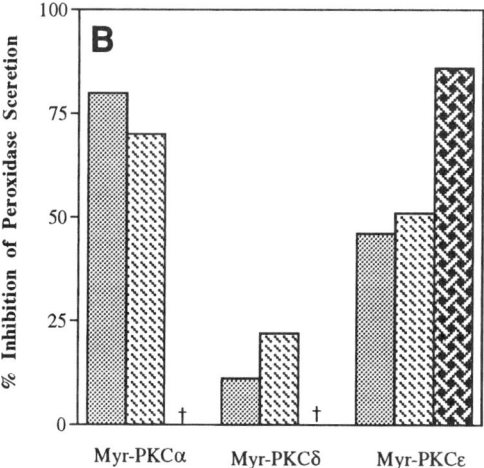

FIGURE 1. A: Effect of phorbol esters and a cholinergic agonist, carbachol, on the cellular distribution of lacrimal gland PKC isoforms. Lacrimal gland acini were incubated for 1 min in the presence or absence of phorbol 12,13-dibutyrate (PdBu, 10^{-6} M) or carbachol (10^{-3} M). Soluble and particulate fractions were prepared, and proteins from both fractions were separated by SDS-PAGE. The number of PKCα, -δ, and -ε isoforms were quantified by Western blotting. Data are an average from 2 to 3 experiments. ▨, control; ■, PdBu; ▦, carbachol. **B:** Effect of the myristoylated pseudosubstrate-derived peptides of PKCα, -δ, and -ε isoforms on agonist-induced lacrimal gland protein secretion. Lacrimal gland acini were incubated in the presence or absence of myr-PKCα, myr-PKCδ, or myr-PKCε (10^{-7} M) for 1 hour. The amount of peroxidase, a protein secreted by the lacrimal gland, was determined spectrophotometrically 20 min after addition of PdBu (10^{-6} M), carbachol (10^{-5} M), or the α_1-adrenergic agonist phenylephrine (10^{-4} M).† In fact, myr-PKCα and myr-PKCδ increased phenylephrine-induced protein secretion 1.9- and 2.5-fold, respectively. Data are an average from 5 to 6 experiments. ▨, PdBu; ▩, carbachol; ▩, phenylephrine.

gland acini with myr-PKCε or myr-PKCδ, but not myr-PKCα, prevented the inhibitory effect of PMA (PMA alone, 50% inhibition of carbachol-induced $[Ca^{2+}]_i$; PMA + myr-PKCε, 3%; PMA + myr-PKCδ, 17%, and PMA + myr-PKCα, 46%).

These results suggest that the Ca^{2+}-independent isoforms, PKCδ and -ε, negatively modulate cholinergic-induced $[Ca^{2+}]_i$ elevation in the lacrimal gland.

In conclusion, our studies show that lacrimal gland acini express five isoforms of PKC, each with a unique location, that these isoforms are differentially translocated by phorbol esters or cholinergic agonists, that they are differentially involved in agonist-induced protein secretion, and that they differentially control cholinergic-induced $[Ca^{2+}]_i$ elevation.

REFERENCES

1. DARTT, D. 1994. Regulation of inositol phosphates, calcium and protein kinase C in the lacrimal gland. Prog. Ret. and Eye Res. **13:** 443–478.
2. MAUDUIT, P., H. JAMMES & B. ROSSIGNOL. 1993. M_3 muscarinic acetylcholine receptor coupling to PLC in rat exorbital lacrimal acinar cells. Am. J. Physiol. **264:** C1550–C1560.
3. HODGES, R., D. DICKER, P. ROSE & D. DARTT. 1992. $α_1$-Adrenergic and cholinergic agonists use separate signal transduction pathways in lacrimal gland. Am. J. Physiol. **262:** G1087–G1096.
4. ZOUKHRI, D. & D. DARTT. 1995. Cholinergic activation of phospholipase D in lacrimal gland acini is independent of protein kinase C and calcium. Am. J. Physiol. **268:** C713–C720.
5. NEWTON, A.C. 1995. Protein kinase C: Structure, function, and regulation. J. Biol. Chem. **270:** 28495–28498.
6. NISHIZUKA, Y. 1995. Protein kinase C and lipid signaling for sustained responses. FASEB J. **9:** 484–496.
7. HOUSE, C. & B.E. KEMP. 1987. Protein kinase C contains a pseudosubstrate prototope in its regulatory domain. Science **238:** 1726–1728.
8. ZOUKHRI, D., R. HODGES, D. DICKER & D. DARTT. 1994. Role of protein kinase C in cholinergic stimulation of lacrimal gland protein secretion. FEBS Lett. **351:** 67–72.
9. ZOUKHRI, D., R. HODGES, C. SERGHERAERT & D. DARTT. 1997. Lacrimal gland PKC isoforms are differentially involved in agonist-induced protein secretion. Am. J. Physiol. **272:** C263–C269.
10. ZOUKHRI, D., R. HODGES, S. WILLERT & D. DARTT. 1997. Immunolocalization of lacrimal gland PKC isoforms. Effect of phorbol esters and cholinergic agonists on their cellular distribution. J. Membr. Biol. **157:** 169–175.

Autoantibodies in Salivary Hypofunction in the NOD Mouse[a]

THOMAS R. ESCH[b] AND MARTIN A. TAUBMAN

Department of Immunology, Forsyth Dental Center, 140 Fenway, Boston, Massachusetts 02115, USA

INTRODUCTION

The autoimmune condition known as Sjögren's syndrome (SS) is characterized primarily by dryness of the mouth and eyes, lymphocytic infiltration of the salivary and lacrimal glands, and circulating autoantibodies.[1,2] Although SS is presumed to be of autoimmune origin, investigation into the mechanism by which the immune system might induce loss of salivary and lacrimal function has been hampered by lack of a suitable and generally accepted animal model. Among the animal systems that have been proposed, the nonobese diabetic (NOD) mouse is unique in exhibiting all three of the above-mentioned characteristics of SS.[3–6] In addition, development of reduced salivary flow in this strain appears to require some contribution from lymphocytes, in that NOD mice carrying the *scid* mutation retain normal stimulated salivary flow rates.[7] Following the hypothesis that autoantibodies may be responsible for salivary hypofunction in these mice, we sought to answer three questions: (1) Is development of salivary hypofunction in the NOD mouse dependent upon massive infiltration of the salivary glands? (2) Do NOD mice exhibiting salivary hypofunction possess circulating autoantibodies to salivary tissues? and (3) Can salivary hypofunction be induced in healthy animals by transfer of serum from diseased mice? All of these question bear not only upon the utility of the NOD as a model for SS, but also upon its pathogenesis and upon mechanisms of interaction between the salivary and immune systems.

MATERIAL AND METHODS

NOD mice were bred in our animal facility from NOD/MrkTacfBR animals obtained from Taconic Farms and housed in specific pathogen-free conditions. C57B1/10 mice were purchased from the Jackson Laboratory. Serum was isolated from peripheral blood of animals bred in our facility or purchased directly from Taconic.

For immunoblotting experiments, fresh tissues were minced and solubilized in NP-40, followed by heating in SDS-PAGE sample buffer. Protein samples were separated on 10% SDS-PAGE gels under reducing conditions and transferred to nitrocellulose membranes. Blocked membranes were immobilized in a multislot immunoblotting apparatus and probed with diluted sera, followed by biotinylated secondary antibody and peroxidase-conjugated streptavidin, and developed with tetramethyl benzidine.

Stimulated salivary flow was measured by collecting total saliva onto preweighed cotton swabs following pilocarpine administration (0.5 µg pilocarpine per gram body

---

[a] This work was partially supported by PHS Grant DE-03420 from the National Institute of Dental Research.

[b] Corresponding author. Tel: (617) 262-5200; fax: (617) 262-4021; e-mail: tesch@forsyth.org

TABLE 1. Stimulated Salivary Flow Rates in NOD and C57Bl/10 Mice

Age and Strain	Stimulated Salivary Flow ± SD (mg/5 min)
6-week NOD	36.5 ± 15.5
6-month C57Bl/10	98.4 ± 52.3
6-month NOD	5.8 ± 6.6[a]

[a] Significantly less than both other groups ($p < 0.01$, Mann-Whitney test).

weight intraperitoneally). For histological analyses, submandibular salivary glands were removed postmortem and placed in formalin. Paraffin-embedded tissues were sectioned and individual sections selected at intervals throughout the gland for staining with hematoxylin and eosin. Infiltration was measured as the average number of small (< 50 mononuclear cells) and large (> 50 cells) foci per section.

RESULTS

To establish the degree of salivary hypofunction in our NOD colony, groups of female NOD mice either six weeks or six months of age were injected intraperi-

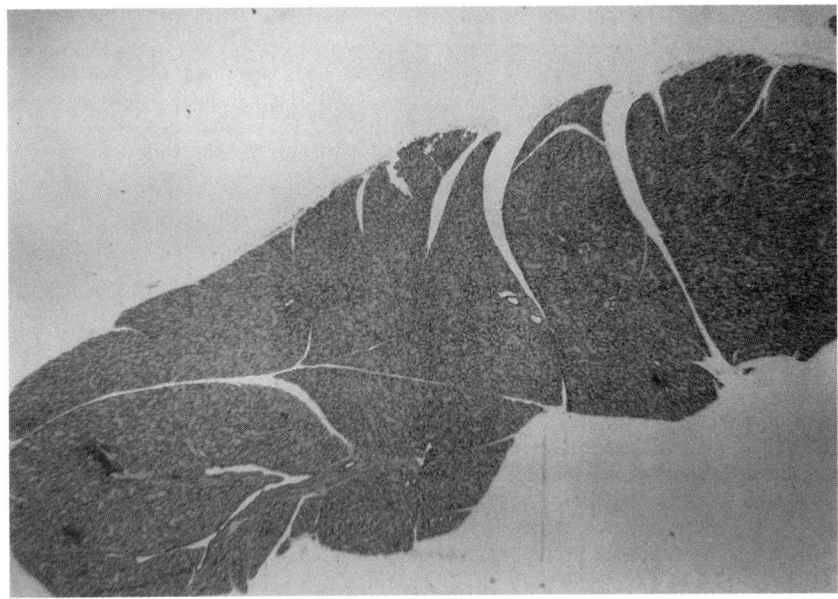

FIGURE 1. Minimal mononuclear cell infiltration in submandibular glands of NOD mice with salivary hypofunction. **A** (above): Six-month-old NOD mouse (40 ×, reduced here by 10%), showing >80% of the sectional area, with three foci (two large and one small). **B:** Six-month-old NOD mouse (100 ×, reduced here by 25%), showing approximately 20% of sectional area and both foci observed in that section. **C:** Six-month-old C57Bl/10 mouse (100 ×, reduced here by 10%).

toneally with pilocarpine, and stimulated salivary flow was evaluated by collecting saliva on a cotton swab inserted in the mouth. As a control, C57Bl/10 mice six months of age were similarly tested. TABLE 1 shows that stimulated salivary flow was significantly reduced in NOD mice six weeks of age as compared to both younger NOD mice and age-matched C57Bl/10 controls. None of the NOD mice in either group were diabetic at the time of evaluation, as determined by the absence of glycosuria.

To examine the relationship between salivary hypofunction and lymphocytic infiltration of the salivary glands, submandibular glands were taken from the mice used in the above experiment, sectioned, and stained for histological evaluation. One section from a six-month-old NOD mouse, encompassing most of the cross-sectional area of the gland, is shown in FIGURE 1A. Three foci (two large and one small) are seen, which is typical of the more severely inflamed glands seen in this set of profoundly hypofunctional mice. FIGURE 1B presents a higher magnification of a different section, showing approximately 20% of the section area and both of the foci observed, whereas FIGURE 1C shows a similar section from a six-month-old B10 mouse for comparison. The data from 21 randomly selected whole-gland sections from hypofunctional NOD mice are summarized in FIGURE 2. Each section was scored for the presence of small (< 50 cells) and large (> 50 cells) foci. In no case were more than three large or small foci observed in a single section, nor were any foci seen in sections from C57Bl/10 mice or younger (six weeks of age) NOD animals (data not shown).

The surprisingly sparse salivary gland infiltration observed in NOD mice with markedly reduced salivary function led us to hypothesize that a soluble factor or factors, possibly autoantibodies, were crucial to the mechanism that led to salivary hypofunction in the NOD mouse. To determine whether there animals possessed autoanti-

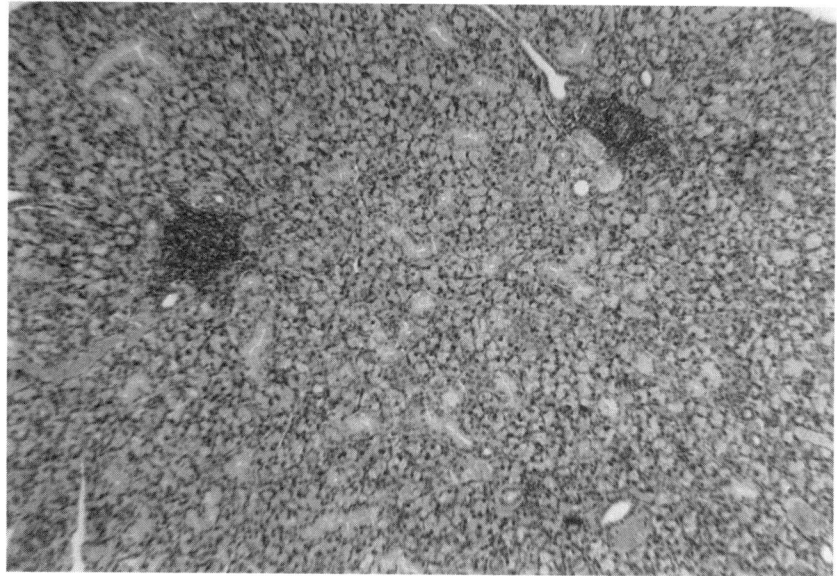

FIGURE 1B. See legend on page 222.

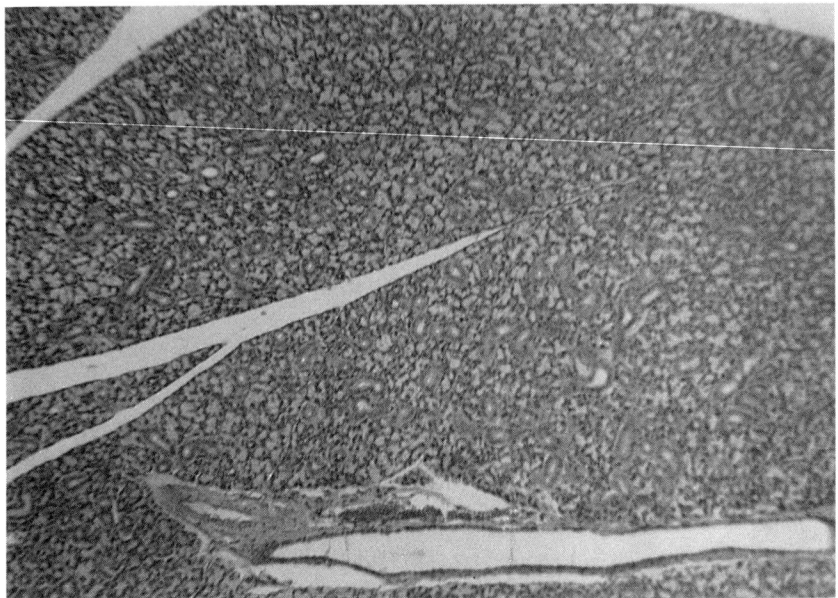

FIGURE 1C. See legend on page 222.

bodies specific for the putative target tissue, sera from young (six week) and old (six month) female NOD mice, as well as old B10 females, were used in Western blots to probe extracts of submandibular gland, brain (cerebellum), and liver. FIGURE 3 shows that sera from NOD mice with salivary hypofunction, but not from B10 controls or from NOD mice too young to have developed hypofunction, react specifically with proteins from both submandibular gland and brain, but not liver.

The persistent presence of relatively high titers of the autoantibodies demonstrated in FIGURE 3 suggested that this autoreactivity to potential target tissues might be manifested within the T-cell compartment as well. To test this point, splenocytes from NOD mice exhibiting salivary hypofunction were cultured in the presence of homogenates prepared from syngeneic submandibular gland, brain, and liver. FIGURE 4 illustrates that a proliferative response above background levels is seen when submandibular gland or brain serves as the stimulus, indicating the presence within the spleen of T cells reactive with these autoantigens.

If it is true that development of salivary hypofunction in the NOD mouse is mediated by autoantibody, then it should be possible to transfer the disease to healthy animals using serum from affected mice. To examine this possibility, serum was collected from female NOD mice with demonstrated loss of salivary flow and from female Swiss breeder mice. NOD mice of both sexes, six weeks of age, then received intraperitoneal injections (0.25 mL each on days 0, 3, 7, and 10) of one of these serum preparations. Pilocarpine-stimulated salivary flow was measured weekly beginning immediately before the first serum injections, and salivary flow measurements for each mouse were normalized to the baseline readings for comparison. TABLE 2 shows that transfer of serum from hypofunctional mice resulted in a transient decrease in stimulated salivary flow in the recipients as compared to animals receiving control serum.

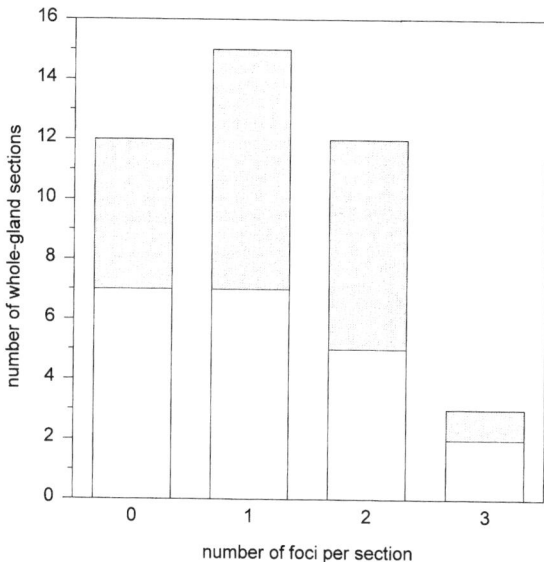

FIGURE 2. Distribution of mononuclear cell foci in submandibular gland sections from six-month-old NOD mice. Twenty-one randomly selected sections were scored for small (< 50 cells) and large (> 50 cells) foci; the resulting data were plotted as a frequency histogram. ☐, large foci; ☐, small foci.

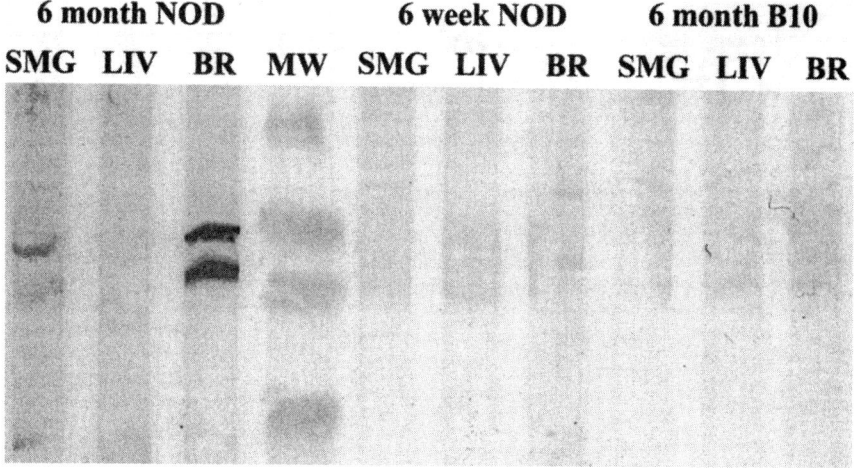

FIGURE 3. Autoreactivities to salivary and neural tissue in sera from hypofunctional NOD mice. Extracts of syngeneic submandibular gland (SMG), cerebellum (BR), and liver (LIV) were electrophoresed, transferred to nitrocellulose, and probed with sera from six-month-old, hypofunctional NOD mice, healthy six-week-old NOD mice, or six-month-old B10 mice. MW, molecular mass standards.

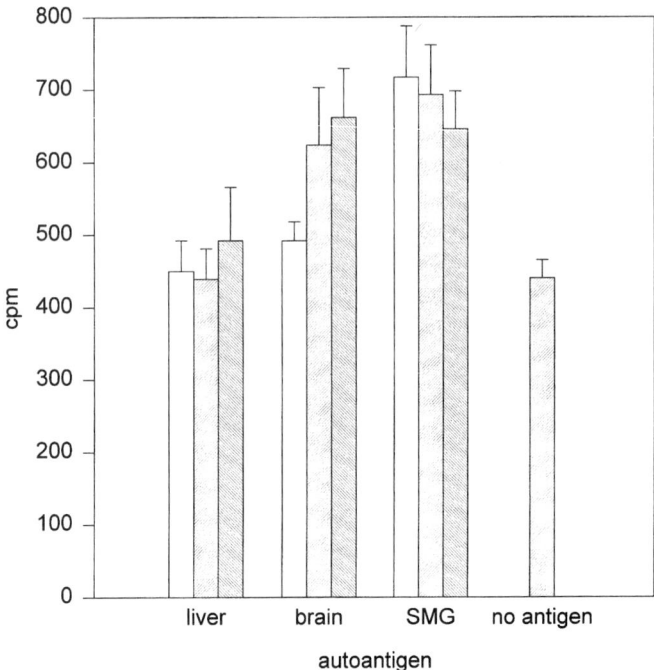

FIGURE 4. T-cell proliferative responses to salivary and neural autoantigens. Splenocytes from six-month-old, hypofunctional NOD mice were cultured with dilutions of homogenates prepared from syngeneic liver, brain, or submandibular gland (SMG). A proliferative response was measured at four days by incorporation of tritiated thymidine. Results shown are averages ± SEM of triplicate cultures in a representative experiment. ☐, 1:100; ☐, 1:300; ▨, 1:1000.

DISCUSSION

One of the more interesting findings of this study is that whereas NOD mice six months of age exhibit a dramatic loss of salivary function, the histopathology ob-

TABLE 2. Salivary Flow Rates in Young NOD Mice after Serum Transfers

	Relative stimulated salivary flow ± SE (mg/5 min)	
Days	NOD Serum	Swiss Serum
0	1.00	1.00
7	1.03 ± 0.15	1.32 ± 0.25
14	0.26 ± 0.05[a]	1.12 ± 0.37
21	0.84 ± 0.42	1.14 ± 0.42

[a] Significantly less than control group ($p < 0.03$, Mann-Whitney test).

served in the salivary glands seems disproportionately unimpressive. As shown in FIGURE 1, animals that produced less than 5 mg of whole saliva in five minutes following pilocarpine stimulation simultaneously exhibited an average of only two mononuclear cell foci (one large and one small) in the submandibular glands. Given that there appears to be no lymphocytic infiltration of the parotid glands in these mice,[7] the overall picture is one of drastic functional insufficiency in the absence of gross glandular destruction. Although it is possible that the degree of infiltration is further increased in still older NOD mice, it is clear that massive infiltration is not a prerequisite for hypofunction. The development of hypofunction also appears not to be linked to the occurrence of diabetes in this strain, as none of the NOD mice presented in TABLE 1 and FIGURE 1 tested positive for urinary glucose at any time.

The above results both confirm and extend the range of autoreactivities observed in the NOD mouse that may have relevance to salivary dysfunction. It has previously been shown that these mice have antibodies to salivary gland epithelium and β-adrenergic receptor.[8] We now demonstrate T-cell autoreactivity to both salivary and neural tissue, advancing the possibility of cognate help for continuous autoantibody production. Interestingly, the neural-specific reactivity that we have found may parallel the anti-Hu antibodies seen in a subset of SS patients with neurologic complications,[9] strengthening the similarity between the NOD mouse and SS.

The prominence of autoantibodies in SS and related disorders and previously shown in the NOD mouse made plausible the hypothesis that salivary hypofunction could be antibody mediated. As TABLE 2 shows, this is at least partially correct. It is interesting that the transferred hypofunction is neither permanent nor as profound as the naturally occurring disease (70–80% decrease in stimulated flow as compared to approximately 95% loss spontaneously). This first point indicates that the infused factor(s) have a limited half-life, as one would expect for antibody molecules,[10] and in combination with the second point suggests that the pathogenic mechanism may involve autoantibodies produced continuously with T-cell help.

The conclusion with perhaps the greatest practical relevance is that the NOD mouse may be an excellent model for study of immune-mediated salivary hypofunction, including SS. It would be unreasonable to expect salivary hypofunction in the NOD mouse to mimic faithfully all aspects of SS, but the NOD mouse clearly possesses analogues of the major clinical features of SS. More importantly, this condition in the NOD mouse appears to be mediated by immune factors, so that this model should serve to illuminate possible mechanisms of pathogenesis in salivary disorders. The fact that disease can be induced in healthy animals by passive transfer indicates that this model will be serviceable in experiments designed to identify various pathogenic immune factors (*e.g.*, autoantibodies, T-cell clones).

SUMMARY

The nonobese diabetic (NOD) mouse exhibits spontaneous salivary gland infiltration and loss of salivary function independent of its propensity to develop diabetes, and thus can serve as a model for salivary hypofunction in Sjögren's syndrome (SS). Studies by others have indicated that this pathology depends on lymphocytes and thus may be autoimmune mediated. We have found that NOD mice four months of age and older exhibit a 90–95% reduction in pilocarpine-stimulated salivary flow (5.8 ± 6.6 mg/5 min) as compared to age- and sex-matched C57Bl/10 controls (98.4 ± 52.3 mg/5 min). These mice simultaneously possess only sparse mononuclear cell infiltrates (averaging approximately one small and one large focus per whole-gland section) in the submandibular glands, suggesting that loss of salivary function does not require massive infiltration of the salivary glands. NOD serum autoantibodies to salivary gland proteins are demonstrable by Western blotting, and, as in a subset of SS patients, some NOD serum autoantibodies recognize neural antigens. Splenic T-cell reactivity to salivary and neural proteins can also be observed. Transfer experiments using NOD mouse serum suggest that loss of salivary function, evaluated as a decrease in pilocarpine-stimulated flow rate, can be transferred by humoral factors, possibly autoantibodies. These results suggest that autoimmune mechanisms dependent on both autoantibody and autoreactive T cells can mediate loss of salivary function, and that salivary and/or neural antigens may serve as a target for these autoimmune reactions.

ACKNOWLEDGMENTS

The authors wish to thank Justine Dobeck for histological preparations, Jo Buchanan for photograpic processing and advice, and Stephanie Baker and Subbiah Yoganathan for animal care.

REFERENCES

1. BLOCH, K. J., W. W. BUCHANAN, M. J. WOHL & J. J. BUNIM. 1965. Sjögren's syndrome: A clinical, pathological, and serological study of sixty-two cases. Medicine **44:** 187–231.
2. DANIELS, T. E. & P. C. FOX. 1992. Salivary and oral components of Sjögren's syndrome. Rheum. Dis. Clin. North. Am. **18:** 571–589.
3. MIYAGAWA, J.-I., T. HANAFUSA, A. MIYAZAKI, K. YAMADA, H. FUJINO-KURIHARA, H. NAKAJIMA, N. KONO, K. NONAKA, Y. TOCHINO & S. TARUI. 1986. Ultrastructural and immunocytochemical aspects of lymphocytic submandibulitis in the non-obese diabetic (NOD) mouse. Virchows Arch. B **51:** 215–225.
4. HU, Y., Y. NAKAGAWA, K. R. PURUSHOTHAM & M. G. HUMPHREYS-BEHER. 1992. Functional changes in salivary glands of autoimmune disease-prone NOD mice. Am. J. Physiol. **263:** E607-614.
5. HUMPHREYS-BEHER, M. G., L. BRINKLEY, K. R. PURUSHOTHAM, P.-L. WANG, Y. NAKAGAWA, D. DUSEK, M. KERR, N. CHEGINI & E. K. L. CHAN. 1993. Characterization of antinuclear autoantibodies present in the serum from nonobese diabetic (NOD) mice. Clin. Immunol. Immunopathol. **68:** 350–356.
6. HUMPHREYS-BEHER, M. G., Y. HU, Y. NAKAGAWA, P.-L. WANG & K. R. PURUSHOTHAM. 1994. Utilization of the non-obese diabetic (NOD) mouse as an animal model for the study of secondary Sjögren's syndrome. Adv. Exp. Med. Biol. **350:** 631–636.
7. ROBINSON, C. P., H. YAMAMOTO, A. B. PECK & M. G. HUMPHREYS-BEHER. 1996. Genetically programmed development of salivary gland abnormalities in the NOD and NOD-SCID mouse in the absence of detectable lymphocytic infiltration: A potential trigger for sialadenitis of NOD mice. Clin. Immunol. Immunopathol. **79:** 50–59.
8. HU, Y., K. R. PURUSHOTHAM, P. WANG, R. DAWSON, JR. & M. G. HUMPHREYS-BEHER. 1994. Downregulation of β-adrenergic receptors and signal transduction response in salivary glands of NOD mice. Am. J. Physiol. **266:** G433–443.
9. MOLL, J. W. B., H. M. MARKUSSE, J. J. J. M. PIJNENBURG, C. J. VECHT & S. C HENZEN-LONGMANS. 1993. Antineuronal antibodies in patients with neurologic complications of primary Sjögren's syndrome. Neurology **43:** 2574–2581.
10. GOMEZ, C. M. & D. P. RICHMAN. 1985. Monoclonal anti-acetylcholine receptor antibodies with differing capacities to induce experimental mayasthenia gravis. J. Immunol. **135:** 234–241.

Epilogue

The information presented at the meeting (of which this volume is a result) was discussed in a workshop session following the formal presentations. With the aid of facilitators Joram Piatigorsky, James Kennison, Malcolm Snead, and David Mooney, the participants identified the key themes from the conference and outlined strategies for the future. A synopsis of the conclusions and recommendations is presented below.

The key theme for the meeting was introduced by Mina Bissell during her opening address: "Do not ask what a cell can do, but ask what it does do." Thus, from the inception of the conference, the emphasis was on the importance of experimental models relevant to *in vivo* function. Furthermore, the meeting reiterated the much-accepted notion that the key regulators and basic mechanisms for proliferation, differentiation, and apoptosis are conserved in evolution. Great power lies in the use of such simple, genetically manipulatable organisms as yeast, flies, and worms for the assessment (or confirmation) of gene function and for the decipherment of genetic cascades and downstream targets. These can be used in conjunction with transgenic animals to further address more complex functional questions. The high cost of transgenic mice warrants reagents germane to rodent models and a national transgenic animal resource facility.

In all systems, cell shape and environment have great impact on cell function, and, according to Bissell, "form is the ultimate transcription factor." With regard to salivary cells, the roles of extracellular matrix, integrins, and macromolecular assemblies need to be defined in detail. Likewise, "gene sharing" is becoming recognized as common to diverse biological systems. It is increasingly clear that the same protein can perform distinct functions depending on the biological context: for example, different cell types, stages of development, and homeostasis. Although salivary cell–specific DNA sequences, with promoters and their cognate *trans*-factors, are being identified, more information is needed to understand the intricate interplay of salivary regulators and effectors. Indeed, regulation of salivary gland function has clinical connotations, as was emphasized by the understanding that "resting" salivary secretions do not imply "unregulated" secretions.

There was a consensus that future salivary therapeutics will be most expediently developed by using integrative approaches of molecular biology, genetics, biochemistry, and engineering. This has already been embraced by the new and rapidly growing discipline, biomimetics. Artificial tissues and organs are being developed from biocompatible materials capable of, in proper arrangements, orientation and combination, mimicking *in vivo* functions. This raises the possibility of designing and producing such artificial oral tissues as salivary glands, gingiva, and bone. The knowledge of molecular regulators may prove critical in tissue engineering, inasmuch as transcription factors may be the ultimate pharmaceuticals.

Maria A. Kukuruzinska
Lawrence A. Tabak

Index of Contributors

Allende, M. L., 49–54
Ambudkar, I., 171–180
Andrew, D. J., 55–69
Ann, D. K., 108–114

Bakkers, J., 49–54
Barkvoll, P., 156–162
Baserga, R., 76–81
Berninsone, P., 91–99
Bird, A., 195–198
Bissell, M. J., 1–6
Blitz, J., 16–27
Bobek, L. A., 204–208
Bouhadir, K. H., 188–194
Brizuela, B. J., 28–35

Camden, J. M., 70–75
Castle, J. D., 115–124
Cotanche, D., 212–216

Dartt, D. A., 217–220
DeLong, M. J., 82–90

Esch, T. R., 221–228

Faustman, D., 138–155
Fernandes, R., 212–216
Fox, M., 212–216
Fox, P. C., 132–137
Fu, Y., 138–155
Furth, P. A., 181–187

George-Weinstein, M., 16–27
Gerhart, J., 16–27
Grubman, S. A., 100–107

Hart, P. S., 125–131
Hennighausen, L., 181–187
Hirschberg, C. B., 91–99
Hodges, R. R., 217–220

Jefferson, D. M., 100–107
Jensen, J. L., 156–162, 209–211

Kennison, J. A., 28–35
Knudsen, K., 16–27
Kruse, D., 171–180
Kukuruzinska, M. A., ix, 195–198, 212–216, 229

Lafrenie, R. M., 42–48
Lennon, K., 195–198, 212–216
Li, D., 163–170
Li, M., 181–187
Lillibridge, C. D., 171–180
Lin, H. H., 108–114

Mattiacci-Paessler, M., 16–27
Menko, S., 36–41
Mooney, D. J., 188–194

O'Connell, B. C., 171–180
O'Malley Jr., B. W., 163–170

Park, M., 70–75
Philp, N., 36–41
Piatigorsky, J., 7–15

Reed, R., 16–27
Resnicoff, M., 76–81
Robbins, P. P., 49–54

Semino, C. E., 49–54
Sergheraert, C., 217–220
Shi, L., 138–155
Shida, T., 199–203
Simak, E., 16–27
Slavkin, H., xi
Soltoff, S. P., 100–107
Spaink, H. P., 49–54

Tabak, L. A., ix, 229
Takai, N., 199–203
Taubman, M. A., 221–228
Turner, J. T., 70–75

Uchihashi, K., 199–203
Ueda, Y., 199–203

Vázquez, M., 28–35
Veneziale, B., 36–41

Walker, J., 36–41
Weaver-Hiltke, T. R., 204–208
Weisman, G. A., 70–75

Yamada, K. M., 42–48
Yan, G., 138–155
Yoshida, Y., 199–203

Zoukhri, D., 217–220

OHIO UNIVERSITY LIBRARY
Please return this book as soon as you have